KHBl...

March 1927

DEPRESSION

Clinical, Biological and Psychological Perspectives

AMERICAN COLLEGE OF PSYCHIATRISTS

Depression

Clinical, Biological and
Psychological Perspectives

Edited by
GENE USDIN, M.D.

Clinical Professor of Psychiatry
and Behavioral Sciences,
Louisiana State University School of Medicine
(New Orleans)

BRUNNER/MAZEL, *Publishers* • New York

Library of Congress Cataloging in Publication Data
American College of Psychiatrists.
    Depression.
    Proceedings, plus three additional papers, presented at the annual
meeting of the American College of Psychiatrists held in Coronado,
Calif. 1976.
    Bibliographies.
    Includes index.
    1. Depression, Mental—Congresses.   2.   Manic-depressive psy-
choses—Congresses.   I. Usdin, Gene L.   II. Title.   [DNLM: 1.
Depression—Congresses.   WM170 A51d 1976]
RC537.A52   1977   616.89   76-49429
ISBN 0-87630-137-5

Contributors

NANCY ANDREASEN, Ph.D., M.D.
Assistant Professor of Psychiatry, University of Iowa College of Medicine

BRUCE H. BAILEY, M.D.
Chief Psychiatry Service, Veterans Administration Hospital, Phoenix, Arizona

JACK D. BARCHAS, M.D.
Professor of Psychiatry and Behavioral Sciences, Stanford University School of Medicine

PHILIP A. BERGER, M.D.
Assistant Professor, Department of Psychiatry and Behavioral Sciences, Stanford University School of Medicine

REMI J. CADORET, M.D.
Professor of Psychiatry, University of Iowa School of Medicine

WILLIAM A. CANTRELL, M.D.
Professor of Psychiatry, Baylor College of Medicine, Houston, Texas

HARRY K. DAVIS, M.D.
Clinical Associate Professor, Department of Psychiatry, and Clinical Associate Professor, Department of Family Medicine, University of Texas Medical Branch, Galveston.

JEAN ENDICOTT, Ph.D.
Assistant Professor of Clinical Psychology, Columbia University

v

JAMES R. GUIDY, Pharm.D.
Clinical Pharmacy Coordinator, Veterans Administration Hospital, Phoenix, Arizona

DAVID R. HAWKINS, M.D.
Professor and Chairman, Department of Psychiatry, University of Virginia School of Medicine

CHARLES K. HOFLING, M.D.
Professor of Psychiatry, School of Medicine, St. Louis University

KENNETH S. KENDLER, M.D.
Stanford University School of Medicine

HEINZ E. LEHMANN, M.D.
Professor of Psychiatry, McGill University and Douglas Hospital, Montreal

CARL P. MALMQUIST, M.D.
Professor of Law and Criminal Justice, University of Minnesota, Minneapolis

ROBERT L. PATRICK, Ph.D.
Research Associate, Department of Psychiatry and Behavioral Sciences, Stanford University School of Medicine

JOACHIM RAESE, M.D.
Research Associate, Department of Psychiatry and Behavioral Science, Stanford University School of Medicine

HERBERT S. RIPLEY, M.D.
Professor of Psychiatry and Behavioral Sciences, University of Washington School of Medicine, Seattle

ROBERT T. RUBIN, M.D.
Professor of Psychiatry, U.C.L.A. School of Medicine

JOSEPH J. SCHILDKRAUT, M.D.
Professor of Psychiatry, Harvard Medical School, Director,

Neuropsychopharmacology Laboratory, Massachusetts Mental Health Center

ROBERT L. SPITZER, M.D.
Professor of Clinical Psychiatry, Columbia University

EDWARD J. STAINBROOK, Ph.D., M.D.
Professor of Psychiatry, Department of Human Behavior, University of Southern California School of Medicine

VASANTKUMAR L. TANNA, M.D.
Assistant Professor of Psychiatry, University of Iowa School of Medicine

ROBERT B. WHITE, M.D.
Professor of Psychiatry, University of Texas Medical Branch, Galveston

ROBERT A. WOODRUFF, JR., M.D.
Professor of Psychiatry, Washington University School of Medicine

Contents

Introduction

This, the eighth publication of the American College of Psychiatrists, continues the pattern developed by the College in more recent years of bringing to readers provocative and topical presentations which can be useful in clinical practice. This volume, as all previous publications of the College, is a product of an annual meeting of the College. The meeting held in Coronado, California in early 1976 had depression as its theme. Credit for developing the program is due the Program Committee, whose chairman is Dr. Robert L. Williams.

This volume also brings an innovation to the College's publications. Because the scientific sessions are held in a three-day period and a significant portion of the meeting is devoted to small group discussions, some pertinent areas of the general topic were not formally presented by the speakers. Accordingly, this year the College invited three members, authorities in their particular areas, to prepare chapters supplementing the presentations at the meeting.

The goal of the College is to be a fountainhead of continuing education and self-development in the field of mental health. Its publications are an effort in this direction. The previous College publication concerned schizophrenia, providing an opportunity for a review of the role of drugs in the treatment and management of the first major psychiatric illness for which a newer breed, direct-acting psychotropic drug was used. It seems appropriate to follow a volume on schizophrenia with a study of another psychiatric disturbance for which there are an increasing number of effective psychotropic agents.

As with any collection of papers growing out of presentations at a scientific program (without prior awareness of other presentors' contributions), there are some repetition and overlap. However, readers should bear in mind that repetition often serves to underline and serve as a guideline as to what is significant.

Depression began to be used as a diagnostic label over 80 years ago. Lately, the condition has been considered under the term affective disorder, which some colleagues have questioned. Most recently, the phrase "mood disorder" appears to be gaining increasing acceptance. However, no term for this condition will be universally accepted, and the question of the viability of the term mood disorder must be recognized.

As several contributors to this volume point out, the introduction of the monoamine oxidase inhibitors, the tricyclic antidepressants, and lithium salts in the treatment of depression has had a major impact on clinical psychiatric practices and biological research in psychiatry. Study of the neuropharmacology of these drugs suggests that their effect on biogenic amine metabolism is a clue to their clinical effects. The early findings served to stimulate considerable interest and provided clues to the underlying pathophysiology of depressive and manic disorders. An intriguing possibility that subtypes of depression might be distinguished by differences in the metabolism of one or another biogenic amine is now supported by results of some recent studies. Biochemical measures related to biogenic amine metabolism may provide clinically useful criteria for classifying depressive disorders and, even more importantly, perhaps for predicting responses to individual treatment modalities. Although the choice of a particular drug is currently best determined by clinical appraisal, it soon may be influenced by biochemical determinations.

Many who vigorously advocate chemotherapy argue that it is more reasonable than psychoanalysis or psychotherapy in terms of cost to patients and in the number of patients who can be treated by the existing number of mental health personnel. Many psychotherapists counter that the impermanence of psychopharmacologic therapeutic cures is being overlooked. Accordingly, while the patient may be relieved of some of his depressive symptomatology, he still may not have the capacity of utilizing his skills for effective psychosocial functioning. Psychopharmacologists, on the other hand, point out that with diminution of symptoms, patients are better able to discuss their conflicts and work in therapy.

In the past few years, conflict between psychotherapists and psychopharmacologists has diminished. Both had felt the need for exclusiveness or priority of their treatment approaches and were reluctant to minimize the value of their own dedicated training and hard-earned expertise. There are still diehards in both camps who view methods other than their own as destructive to the patient. It is understandable that some who view depressive illness as essentially psychogenic in origin may minimize the usefulness of methods other than psychotherapy, and that those who view depression primarily as a genetically determined, biochemical abnormality may view psychotherapy as a secondary type of treatment modality.

Although such polar positions continue to be articulated, there is greater recognition of the need to consider multiple systems in understanding depression. Depression can be understood as *concurrently* a disorder of biogenic amine metabolism, a syndrome arising out of the intrapsychic consequences of object loss, a disturbance of family relationships, and a learned response pattern with adaptive utility. The systems viewpoint stresses the validity of each explanatory system as a way of understanding behavioral disturbance.

The question of whether depression is essentially psychogenic in origin or a genetically determined biochemical abnormality is clearly as complex as the disorder itself. Indeed, it is only when one's conceptual model excludes other approaches to understanding or minimizes their significance that progress in the field is halted. The task of the clinician is the development of a pluralistic orientation that enables him to appraise each relevant system and intervene with those treatment modalities which appear particularly suited for the individual patient.

If we accept the concept of multiple etiology for depressions and recognize that the quantitative proportions of genetic and psychogenic factors (including immediate stresses) vary in individuals, we are able to set more appropriate goals for therapy and eclectically utilize the best tools available. While psychotherapy is important in improving the depressed patient's capacity for interpersonal relationships and social adjustment, psychotropic drugs may more directly, or primarily, improve the symptom picture of the patient. Essentially, pharmacotherapy and psychotherapy affect different dimensions of the illness and, indeed, may have additive effects.

Some may consider this volume slanted toward the biological perspective. The predominance of material in this book lends some credence to that view. There is, however, a voluminous body of psychoanalytic and psychotherapeutic literature regarding depression, while the field of pharmacotherapy is a relatively new one in which dramatic strides presently are being made and an increased interest is being shown. At any rate, for the psychotherapist, much of the book's contents may be an intensive introduction to biogenic amine chemistry and psychopharmacology. For the psychopharmacologist, the book not only brings together the views of authorities regarding the current state of knowledge, but does so in the context of man's psychodynamic and social reality. Most of all, however, it is the hope of the College that this volume will prove useful to clinicians treating depressed patients.

GENE USDIN, M.D.

1

Depression and the Life Span – Epidemiology

Herbert S. Ripley, M.D.

In view of the many variables influencing the epidemiology of depression, comparisons between different groups of subjects are at best inexact even when the most carefully carried out studies are considered. The term depression itself has many meanings. It is used to designate reactions varying between an appropriate mood of depression through grief and the milder manifestations of illness to the severe forms of depressive psychosis. The criteria used in defining different types of depression show great variation.

Furthermore, there is lack of clarity in distinguishing depression from other psychiatric disorders such as schizophrenia. For example, the rates for these two diagnostic categories have shown much variation between New York and London. However, when a study of relative incidence was carried out (1) using clearly defined criteria, there was no significant difference between the two places. Rawnsley (2) has reported on the variation in use of diagnostic terms among psychiatrists in several countries. Summaries of 30 case histories not exceeding about 400 words were sent to psychiatrists in Denmark, Norway, Sweden, the United Kingdom, and the United States. In 22 of the 30 cases there was a substantial measure of agreement on diagnosis, but the amount of disagreement high-

1

lighted serious limitations in international comparisons of psychiatric morbidity statistics.

The affect of depression is a symptom in a wide variety of psychological problems and may be present in almost any clinical nosological entity. Furthermore, if a mood of depression does not occur when it is appropriate, such a lack of reaction in itself suggests psychopathology. Everyone is a reacting human being and has potential for developing depression either in response to such illnesses as brain tumor or kidney failure, or as part of the accompanying disordered brain function, or in response to interpersonal stress.

There has been much controversy about whether there are distinct types of depression or whether depression is a continuum with varying degrees of intensity. If a distinction is to be made between endogenous and exogenous depressions (and much evidence points to the validity of this distinction), it should be made not on the basis of the severity of the symptoms but rather on a qualitative evaluation. A severe psychoneurotic (exogenous or reactive) depression may be more disabling than a psychotic (endogenous) depression of mild or moderate degree. It has frequently been found that depressive neuroses are two to three times as common as depressive psychoses. Numerous recent physiological and biochemical investigations and studies now under way promise to help more clearly define the types of depressive reactions so that speculative controversies will be minimized.

Unfortunately, there has been a prevalent tendency to regard depression and suicide as due exclusively to either social, psychological or biological forces, and to base formulations on examination of a single system rather than the complexity of factors that require careful collection of data and perceptive evaluation.

When depression reaches a point dignified by the term illness, affective changes are the core manifestation accompanied by attitudes such as self-depreciation and hopelessness and by behavioral and physiological changes. As pointed out by many writers, such as Fabrega (3), there are two interrelated aspects of depression: (a) neurophysiologic changes underlying behavioral alteration that may show a measure of specificity, and (b) the culturally conceptualized expression of behavioral changes. The components of the disease mean different things to members of various social groups, creating special difficulties in making comparisons.

Although there is some disagreement in regard to the association between social class and the prevalence of depression, most commonly the rate has been considered greater for those in the higher socioeconomic groups. Variations in symptomatology from one cultural group to another have been noted. Feelings of alienation have been found to be characteristic of the middle and upper classes and feelings of futility, despair and hopelessness in the lower classes. Somatic symptoms have been considered especially prominent in minority groups who express relatively little self blame (4). However, this latter finding has not been confirmed by other investigators (5, 6).

Depression often reflects a response to loss, whether it be a loss of people, health, physical appearance, bodily function, money or status. The precipitating factors found to be most common are poor family or marital adjustment, financial problems, sexual maladjustment, poor health, inadequate work or school adjustment, death of relatives or friends, and painful symptoms (7). Especially prominent as a possible etiologic factor is concern about illness or disability, found to be present in 35 percent of a group of depressed patients (7), in 34.5 percent of those attempting suicide, and in 70 percent of those completing suicide (8).

Studies indicate that during a period before the onset of depression a variety of life events are more frequent in depressed patients than in matched controls. A quantitative measurement scale has been developed by Holmes and Rahe (9) which indicates that a high score in life changes is followed by various illnesses including depression. This finding has been corroborated by Paykel, Myers, Dienelt et al. (10) who found that events regarded as undesirable and those involving losses or exits from the social field particularly distinguished the depressed patients from the controls but that there was no excess of desirable events or entrances to the social field.

There is need to define more specifically the part that both remote and recent stressful situations may play in contributing to the etiology of different types of depressive illness. Among the variables to be considered are the influence of depression itself in reporting life events, fallaciously attributing to a situation a reaction which may have caused it, the relative impact of positive, neutral or negative changes, individual sensitivities to a given event, the role of chronically stressful situations which continue into the designated period preceding the illness, and the amount of readjustment required to cope with the specific stress.

THE EPIDEMIOLOGY OF INCIDENCE

Evaluation of the incidence of depression and suicide has been the concern of psychiatrists, sociologists and anthropologists for many years. As pointed out by Wittkower (11), Kraepelin, inspired by regional differences in behavior of the mentally ill which he observed in Germany and other European countries, studied cultural influences on the frequency and symptomatology of psychiatric disorders in Java. He noted that manic-depressive psychoses were relatively uncommon and that patients seldom had complaints of sinfulness. The focus of early investigations by psychiatrists and anthropologists was on the relationship between culture and personality. In recent years the emphasis has been on the frequency of such nosological entities as depression in contrasting cultures and subcultures and in the same culture with changes in the social milieu.

Depression is one of the commonest illnesses seen not only by the psychiatrist but in the office of the family doctor and on general hospital wards. Watts (12) found that about 1 in 10 patients in his rural practice in England had a depressive illness. They were equally divided between endogenous and exogenous types. In one evaluation of 536 patients seen by a psychiatrist on a medical inpatient service, Ripley (7) found that 150 (28 percent) had a pathological degree of depression.

Rawnsley (2) and Silverman (13) collected data on a number of epidemiological studies of depression. Both indicated that the great differences in criteria used by various investigators made it difficult to make comparisons. Silverman pointed out that distinction needs to be made between point prevalence, the frequency at a given time, usually a day, and period prevalence, the frequency during a period of time specified in weeks, months, years or a lifetime. However, considerations of four studies based on point prevalence in a rural county of Tennessee (14), a West Coast Swedish island (15), two rural parishes in Sweden (16), and a district of Prague, Czechoslovakia (17) found the range to be from 0.5 to 2.0 per 1,000 population. In six studies using period prevalence varying from six months to several years, of which two were in the Eastern Health District of Baltimore (18, 19) and one each in the North American Hutterite colonies in Manitoba and Alberta, Canada and in the Dakotas (20), in South Korea (21), in Formosa (22) and in Nova Scotia (23), the rates for depressive psychoses were slightly under 1 per 1,000 of population except in the Nova Scotia study where Leighton gave a rate of 3 per 1,000 based on current symptom patterns. Others have stated that the lifetime period rate of manic-depressive psychoses the world over is 3 to 4 per 1,000. Lehmann (24) considers that the lifetime expectancy of becoming depressed is approximately 10 percent. This is about 10 times higher than the risk for schizophrenia though, because of its chronic rather than episodic nature, schizophrenia is more common in psychiatric hospitals. He has estimated that 1 out of 5 of the patients who are depressed receives treatment by a doctor, 1 out of 50 is hospitalized, and about 1 in 200 commits suicide. Thus, many who could profit from treatment for active illness or from prophylaxis with lithium are not receiving it.

Standardization of diagnosis and other criteria will help to make epidemiological comparisons more accurate, but such factors as attitudes toward mental illness in the setting in which it develops will be important factors in its appraisal. In some cultures or subcultures, more people with identical symptoms will be seen as patients than in other situations. For example, many Japanese-Americans feel that the family should care for the mentally ill and medical attention is to be avoided.

The incidence of manic-depressive psychosis is said to be lower in Northern than Southern European countries. Highly contradictory reports are common. Many of the surveys, such as those making comparisons between different African regions, are based on superficial observations and are not valid. More careful studies are likely to indicate that care in collecting data, differences in the orientation of the investigators, and lack of evaluation of the role of the culture on the form of the illness would account for the marked range of incidence of depressive states varying between 1.1 in South Africa and 15 percent in Senegal in the reports collected by Collomb (25). Depression has been considered rare in Kenya and Ruanda Urundi and widespread in Ghana and Nigeria. I was told by psychiatrists at a Finnish hospital that all their psychotic patients had schizophrenia and that if I wished to see depression I should go to Italy!

Eaton and Weil (20) found a low incidence of psychosis in the Hutterites but that manic-depressive psychosis was four times as frequent as schizophrenia, a reversal of the usual predominance of schizophrenia. In this subculture dominated by religious restrictions on expression of emotions, similar to that of cultural patterns which have been considered conducive to the development of manic-depressive illness, the social pattern may be a predisposing factor. There is also the possibility that much inbreeding may contribute a strong hereditary factor, and that the older age of the group studied may have placed more subjects in the age period when depression is more prevalent than schizophrenia. Cohen (26) pointed out that possibly there has been a decline in incidence of manic-depressive psychosis in this century. For example, in 1900 17 percent of all admissions to the Boston State Hospital and 37 percent of the admissions to the McLean Hospital were so diagnosed. In 1950 the figures were 8 percent and 16 percent. In 1970 there were 69,339 admissions of manic-depressive patients to all U.S. inpatient and outpatient psychiatric services. They accounted for 3.5 percent of all admissions, a rate of 0.5 per 1,000 of population.

Mendels (27) suggested figures indicating a decrease in prevalence may represent a real reduction, but noted that it may be only apparent and the result of (a) changing criteria for diagnosis, (b) alterations in the clinical manifestations of the disorders leading to incorrect diagnoses, (c) modification of the course of the illness by more intensive therapeutic intervention, or (d) a retention of patients with milder forms of the disorder in the community. Recently, less mania has been seen except perhaps in primitive tribal societies in Africa and elsewhere either because of an overall decrease in manic-depressive illness or a relative increase in the purely depressive form of this condition.

Arieti (28) has related a decrease in manic-depressive illness in the United States to a decline in Puritan ethic with the decrease in influence of the doctrines of Luther and Calvin of "deeply felt concepts of responsibility, duty, guilt, and punishment" which colored every manifestation of life. Reisman, Glazer and Denney (29) have described an inner-directed personality with motivation derived from internal sources early in life which has gradually been replaced by the other-directed personality characterized by direction and motivation influenced chiefly by contemporaries. In the former there is a rigidity of personality similar to the life pattern of the manic-depressive.

Pederson, Barry and Babigian (30), using the Monroe County (New York) Cumulative Psychiatric Case Register, studied all patients who received a primary diagnosis of psychotic depression in the years 1961 and 1962. Of the 11,639 individuals reported to the register, 568 or 5 percent had a clear diagnosis of psychotic depression.

Lemkau, Tietze and Cooper (19) in a survey of 55,000 people in the Eastern Health District of Baltimore found a total of 48 adults (17 males and 31 females) to have psychotic depression for an overall incidence of 0.9/1,000/year. In a study of mental disorder on the island of Formosa, Lin (22) reported the incidence of manic-depressive psychosis to be 0.7/1,000. Yoo (21) in a comparison of the percentage of each type of mental disorder in various countries found that there was an unusually low percentage of manic-depressive psychosis in Japan, Formosa and South Korea in comparison with Bavaria, Denmark, Norway and Tennessee.

There have been relatively few efforts to relate the incidence of psychoses to race. The superficiality of classification by skin color, the mixture of racial groups, and the social and cultural differences of racial groups in various countries have made the differences noted of highly questionable validity. Rawnsley (2) cited a report by Foster on Maori patients in mental hospitals in New Zealand. Whereas the rate for schizophrenia was nearly 50 percent higher in Maoris than in Europeans, the rate of manic-depressive illness was over twice as high in Europeans; despite this predominance mania and circular types were more frequent among Maoris. In a study purportedly contrasting Jews and Gentiles racially, Grewel (31), who pointed out that several previous studies indicated that the frequency of mental disease in Jews was greater than in the host-populations, investigated the incidence of psychiatric illness among the Jews of Amsterdam. Although there has been considerable admixture between them, he made some distinctions between the Ashkenazic and the Sephardic Jews in regard to psychological characteristics and undertook a statistical study of both of these groups and of the Gentiles who were regarded as economically identical. In the Sephardim, who were of more schizothymic character, there was little difference between Jews and Gentiles. However, the most outstanding difference was the much higher percentage of manic-depressive psychoses in Ashkenazim than in Gentiles. He considers that his study shows the importance of race psychiatry, but he also points out that environmental factors, psychogenesis, and the cultural totality always have to be kept in view. Malzberg (32) found a significantly higher rate among Jews than Gentiles for admissions to New York hospitals with manic-depressive psychosis. However, Halpern (33) in Palestine and Hes (34) in Israel did not find an unusually high prevalence among Jews. Such conflicting reports and the difficulties in separating questionable racial identification from other complex variables point up that we have a paucity of substantial data relating psychopathology to race. It is to be noted that most studies in which different races are present have stressed other factors such as language and culture rather than race in making comparisons. There also has been a great divergence of findings in studies comparing different religious groups.

Comparative data on different cultures and races present still other difficulties. Even if the same investigator using identical criteria carries out the studies, cultural differences and the lack of vocabulary with identical meanings offer barriers to accurate comparisons. For example, in the study in Nigeria of the Yaruba by Leighton, Lambo, Hughes et al. (23), component symptoms of depression were elicited, but there was linguistic difficulty in describing the subjective feelings which had a distorting influence on the classification of patients. Therefore, comparisons by the same investigators between the Yaruba and the people of Nova Scotia were considered inaccurate.

A low incidence of depression and suicide has been reported by Prange, Wilson, Knox et al. (35) for African Americans in the southern United States, but not among Negroes in the North. Vitals (36) has postulated without supplying hard data that this finding may be ascribed to the southern Blacks having less to lose, being more limited in expectations and aspirations, and having more emotional security engendered by greater fundamentalist religious practice and family support. This apparent difference between Whites and Blacks in the South may be due to differences in diagnostic criteria and policies in regard to hospitalization. The study of McGough, Williams and Blackley (37) on the effects of racial integration in southern psychiatric hospitals suggests that the incidence of depressive psychoses is much higher than previously reported. Some observers have stated that mania is much less common among Blacks than Whites in the United States. If further careful observations confirm this finding, it may be that the manic form of manic-depressive illness is rarer among Blacks possibly due to genetic differences between the two racial groups.

Differences may be partly a function of the stereotypes investigators have of patients rather than their actual behavior. Another observer with a contrasting bias may report different findings. Prejudices can easily distort the interpretation of symptoms. For example, among Army personnel whom I saw during World War II, the incidence of psychiatric illness was higher among Negroes than Whites (38). Negroes considered hallucinations as representing severe psychopathology in other Negroes, whereas many physicians, especially southern White physicians, stated that hallucinations were normal for Negroes. The screening out by induction centers of those unfit for military service seems to have been less painstakingly performed for Negroes and influenced by applying different criteria so that the incidence was distorted.

Criteria other than findings based on subjective accounts, behavioral changes, and physiological determinations should be considered. Tests and scales such as the Rorschach, Thematic Apperception Test, Minnesota Multiphasic Personality Inventory, Beck Depression Inventory, Zung Self Rating Depression Scale, and Hamilton Depression Scale show a number of characteristic responses and have been used to identify depressive illness and to distinguish between neurotic and psychotic depression. The Depression Inventory devised by Beck (39) has been found to be highly effective in discriminating between depression and anxiety and to have consistently moderately high correlations with clinicians' rating. The MMPI frequently is useful in revealing hidden depression in subjects who have symptoms that have been considered to be depressive equivalents. However, in general, psychological tests appear to be of no greater validity in determining the overall amount of depressive illness and its distribution than statistical data based on clinical evaluations. Many variables complicate test assessments. For example, Harmatz and Shader (40) found that elderly subjects differ strikingly from young subjects in their responses to items in the MMPI self-ratings of depression. Though the preponderant evidence is to the contrary, Zung (41) found no significant differences in incidence with age among a group of 261 normal subjects as measured by the Self Rating Depression Scale.

A number of symposia and surveys of depression have served as a means of presenting data and stimulating contact between investigators. Frequently, reports and discussions are of an impressionistic nature which may obfuscate rather than clarify. Criticisms of a report by such highly regarded investigators as Murphy, Wittkower and Chance (42), who surveyed by questionnaire the impressions of voluntary collaborators in many countries about primary symptoms of depression, point out some of the problems of such broad approaches. Carstairs commented that "instant research" of this type can only give rise to speculative hypotheses and ephemeral conclusions, but Kiev stated that such attempts are laudable and add to communication but that the results are questionable. Murphy (43) has defended this type of general survey and stated that it has provided pointers to the potentialities and problems likely to be uncovered if the work were done more systematically.

INCIDENCE BY SEX AND AGE

In Western countries many more females than males have been found to have depressive illnesses. However, in other cultures the sex ratio is the reverse. In India, Rao (44) in a study of endogenous depression in 62 patients found that 64 percent were males and 36 percent females. He states that others have found a male predominance and that the rate for depression is low in South India compared to North India. Differences in sexual prevalence dependent on the socioeconomic class have been found in the United States. For example, Schwab, Bialow, Holzer et al. (45) report that males are more likely to suffer depression in the lowest socioeconomic class. In New Zealand (2) there is a preponderance of manic-depressive illness in women among Europeans but an equal incidence in men and women among the Maoris.

Depression and suicide are particularly prone to occur at certain critical age periods. Statistical analyses by various investigators of age and sex distribution show minor variations in the decade of life when the frequency is greatest. Social changes may predispose to shifts in prevalence. For example, in the United States many children and adolescents are in greater conflict about their roles in society. On the one hand, they are permitted to be more assertive and to assume more responsibility for such things as choosing their own books, clothing, food and leisure time activities. With more mothers working they are forced to be more independent. On the other hand, they are under pressure to achieve and are expected to conform in a changing world to rigid patterns set by their parents. With the increase in years of education far beyond childhood, immaturity into adulthood is fostered.

There is evidence that depression in adolescents is increasing. Instead of the former pattern where depression increased with age, there are peak periods in the ages 17 to 22 and after 45. Much of the drug use among youth is based upon the need for relief from depression. The rise in suicide among youth has been especially high among Black and American Indian males. For example, Hendin, using vital statistics and an in-depth study of 25 Black men and women who attempted suicide (46), discussed the finding that in New York City the suicide rate for Black American men aged 20 to 35 is twice as high as among White men in the same age group. He pointed out, "A sense of despair, a feeling that life will never be satisfying, confronts many Blacks at a far younger age than it does most Whites. For most discontented White people the young adult years contain the hope of significant changes for the better. The marked rise in White suicide after 45 reflects, among other things, the decline in such hope that is bound to accompany age. The Blacks who survive past the dangerous years between 20 and 35 have made some accommodation with life—a compromise that has usually had to include a scaling down of their aspirations." He further stated that failure to find pleasure in sex, friendship, work or even drugs is at least partially a reflection of the repressed anger and blunted emotional life that characterize the depressed patient. In many individuals an overt expression of the anger is evidenced by the fact that Black homicide reaches its peak at the same age period as Black suicide. Incidentally, Hendin makes some interesting comparisons of depression and suicide between the Negroes in New York City and the Scandinavians on whom he carried out a previous psychodynamic survey (47). In contrast to the Blacks, in Sweden suicide was related to rigid concern about achievement that characterizes the culture, while in Norway suicide reflected a concern with sin and punishment.

In some mothers who must cope with caring for a baby who

seems fragile and vulnerable to sudden illness or death, some degree of depression from a mild mood of depression to a severe postpartum depression may occur. In other parents, difficulty in coping has led to an increase in child abandonment and the battered child syndrome. The change in sexual mores may create as many problems as it solves. The cultural changes foster feelings of insecurity. The high rate of marital maladjustment and divorce may partially account for the large numbers of depressed young adults seen in physicians' offices, community mental health centers, and emergency rooms of general hospitals.

Middle age is another period of vulnerability. In men there is frustration over failure to achieve occupational goals, over unemployment or the pressures of being promoted. Advancement may cause either a reaction to unanticipated stress with the development of the so-called "promotion depression," or give the feeling that there is nothing left to strive for. Those who feel they do not have anything to look forward to may try to establish a new life style. Divorce is one attempted solution. In women there may be a feeling of emptiness created by alienation of husband and of children who are becoming independent and leaving home.

The elderly feel social isolation since in many places society puts a premium on youth. Retirement is often conducive to people's feeling useless. There is a loss of vigor. Illnesses are more frequent, multiple, chronic, and life threatening.

For endogenous depression Watts (12) reported peak incidence for women is between 45 and 50 and for men after 60. Between 55 and 60 there was an equal incidence in men and women.

Schwab, Holzer and Warheit (48) investigated a sample of 1,645 people of a county population in Florida using an interview schedule including 15 questions about commonly studied symptoms of depression. The respondents were classified by seven age groups. The mean depression scores were highest in youngest (16-19) and oldest (70+). Those 20-29 and 30-39 had the lowest and the mean scores rose in almost linear fashion for those above the age of 40. They raised questions such as, "Is our society geared in such a way that its values are acceptable and its rewards available only to those in the prime of life?" and "Does this mean that both today's youth and the elderly are dispensable?" In the study by Pederson et al. (30), the prevalence and incidence rates for a Monroe County (New York) population 15 years of age and older were computed. The overall age-adjusted yearly prevalence of psychotic depression was 0.7/1,000/year. This rate for men was 0.53/1,000/year and for women 0.87/1,000/year. The rate considering only those with the first diagnosis made during the two-year study period was 0.33/1,000/year. For men the rate was 0.27/1,000/year and for women 0.37/1,000/year. Thirty-five percent were men and 65 percent were women. Sixty-six percent were married and 18 percent widowed. The proportion from the different socioeconomic levels closely reflected the distribution in the county at large. In terms of age, 63 percent were between 50 and 70 and less than 5 percent were younger than 40 years of age.

Several Scandinavian investigations have conducted detailed comprehensive surveys and analyses of the prevalence of depression in limited areas of their countries. Sjögren (15) carefully evaluated the occurrence of psychoses on two islands of the West Coast of Sweden and found 17 male and 33 female patients with manic-depressive psychosis, which represented 9.0 and 12.0 per 1,000 births. Essen-Möller (16) in a study of the entire population of two parishes in Southern Sweden reported the prevalence to be 17 per 1,000 for males and 28 per 1,000 for females. Similar rates of 18.0 for males and 24.6 for females were recorded by Helgason (49) in Iceland. In contrast, Böök (50) found manic-depressive psychoses to be rare in a North Swedish population and a large majority of the psychoses to be schizophrenia.

In a survey of 4,399 people on the Danish island of Samso by Sorenson and Strömgren (51), on a given day 3.9 percent of the population over the age of 20 were suffering from a depressive disease (1.7 percent of the men and 6.1 percent of the women). The highest incidence for women was in the 30-39 and the 40-49 groups (8.4 percent each) and for men in the 50-59 age group (2.7 percent). Diagnostically, 77 percent were considered to have a depressive neurosis and 23 percent a psychosis.

In the previously referred to evaluation of general hospital patients by Ripley (7), 41 percent of them were males and 59 percent females. They ranged in age from 15 to 69. Similarly, Schwab, Brown and Holzer (52) in an evaluation of medical inpatients found that 16 percent of the males and 25 percent of the females aged 15 to 90 were depressed. The incidence by age tended to be younger in the latter study.

DEPRESSION AND SUICIDE

In view of the inadequacy of the statistics on depression, some investigators have considered that since more adequate data are available on completed suicide and there is a relatively high correlation between suicide and depression, suicide is the single best measure of depressive illness. However, statistics on suicide are also notoriously unreliable. It has been estimated that one-half to three-quarters of suicides go unreported due to attitudes which are disposed to hide suicide more in some cultures than in others. If it is true as generally considered that in the United States there is a greater incidence of depression in women than in men, the higher completed suicide rate in men would indicate a lack of reliability of suicide as a measure of depression. In this instance, attempted suicide which is higher among women than men might be a better indicator. Perhaps the very lethal method, shooting, the most common method used by men, decreases the accuracy of suicide as a gauge in the United States. In some other places where the methods used by both sexes are similar, the suicide rate is higher in women or close to the same rate in men and women. For example, in the Netherlands and Scotland where there is less discrepancy between the rates in the sexes, suicide may more accurately represent the incidence of depression.

In a study comparing suicide in Seattle and Edinburgh, Ripley (53) found that in Edinburgh in recent years an increasingly higher proportion of women have been committing suicide so that distribution between sexes is almost equal, whereas in Seattle there has been a constant ratio of twice as many men as women for a number of years.

Kato (54) has noted that in Japan there has been a great decline in the suicide rate among youth of both sexes, particularly those from 15 to 24, since World War II, coinciding with the greater Westernization of the country. There has been a corresponding increase in homicide and other crimes among the youth. He hypothecated that there has been a change from being passively dependent with loyalty to one's lord and fidelity to one's parents to being individually independent and rebellious to society and parents. Among young women the rate has gone down in almost direct proportion to their increased personal freedom. In other words, they show more extrapunitive and aggressive behavior in contrast to their former intropunitive suppression or repression of aggression which is conducive to the development of depression. There has been no appreciable change in suicide rate in older men and women or the ratio of higher incidence in men than women.

Sainsbury (55) who studied suicide in London found that 27 percent, an unusually low rate, suffered from a depressive psychosis. In reviewing the literature he noted that various factors such as differences in definition of mental disorder, the type of selection of patients, and the adequacy of the data are among the causes of wide disagreement. Both suicide and mental disorder had a higher incidence in the more mobile and socially disorganized districts. He concluded that the complexity of the relationship of suicide to mental disorder is due to the fact that both are determined by the same order of social, psychological, and biological causes compounded in one individual to dispose to suicide, in another to mental illness, and in a third to both.

Robins, Murphy, Wilkerson et al. (56), based on interviews with key people, found that 94 percent of their patients in St. Louis who were successful suicides were mentally ill and 55 percent had a manic-depressive psychosis. In a follow-up study of the Monroe County (New York) Survey (30), after three or four years 14 percent of those with psychotic depression had committed suicide.

In a study of suicide in Seattle by Dorpat and Ripley (57), data obtained from those who were acquainted with the subjects indicated that nearly all had depression but some could not be classified as having an affective illness per se. Depression was often associated with other types of psychiatric illness, notably personality disorders (9.3 percent), alcoholism (26.9 percent), and schizophrenia (12.0 percent). Gardner, Bahn and Mack (58) noted that suicide rates for neurotic or personality disorders, as well as for affective psychoses, were more than twice as high after age 55 as before that age.

Silverman (13) in her review of the work of others reported that the percentage of suicides with mental disorder ranged from 47 to 90 and the percentage of depressive illness in all those with mental illness from 27 to 74. There was no diagnostic category which approached the order of magnitude of the contribution of depression to suicide. In citing data obtained in New York State hospitals by Malzberg, she noted that the average annual suicide rates for manic-depressive psychoses were 87.4 per 100,000 resident patients and for involutional melancholia were 80.4; these rates were far above those for the next two diagnostic categories, cerebral arteriosclerosis (31.9 percent) and dementia praecox (30.1 percent). Silverman concluded that whatever the combination of psychological, biological, and socio-cultural forces which make up the illness of depression, it can become lethal in certain situations and that suicide is the mortality of depressive illness.

Symptoms by Age

There has been much disagreement about the age at which depression begins (59). Until recently, many considered that the individual had not developed psychologically to the point where depression could be experienced until reaching puberty. There is still a lack of agreement concerning the existence of depression as a clinical entity before adolescence, especially in regard to manic-depressive psychosis which many consider has yet to be demonstrated in prepubertal children. At present, depression may be more common in children than is generally recognized because the presenting symptoms may be deceptive. For many years a few writers have considered depression to be present at all ages. Abraham (60) in 1924 described "primal parathymia" as the infantile prototype of a later depressive psychosis. Spitz (61) was the first to describe anaclitic depression which he related to maternal deprivation. It is characterized initially by crying and struggling, later by despair and withdrawal, and finally, in some subjects, by failure to eat, wasting away, and death. In those who survive there is likely to be permanent personality damage. He considered severe narcissistic trauma in early childhood because of disappointments in early relationships as primary in severe depressive states throughout life.

Many investigators—Zilboorg (62), Batchelor and Napier (63), Brown (64), Beck et al. (65), Gregory (66), Bowlby (67) and Dorpat, Jackson and Ripley (68)—have noted a significantly higher rate in childhood of bereavement or broken homes among adult depressive patients who reactivate early experiences of helplessness. Whiting and Child (69) have related weaning and toilet training to the development of depression, and Goldman-Eisler (70) found that early weaning was a significant factor in the etiology of oral pessimism and probably depression. Comparison of different cultural groups or changes in practices within the same cultural group in regard to such variables as discipline and weaning would be of great interest.

Freud (71) in 1917, influenced by the earlier work of Abraham in 1916, had emphasized that there are ambivalent feelings toward a lost loved one who is incorporated into the self and that the socially unacceptable hostility toward that person can be directed toward the self. When the need for melancholia is ended, the energy incorporated in the self becomes free and makes mania possible. Psychodynamic understanding of depression is largely based on these early psychoanalytic formulations and later modifications by such leading theorists as Bibring (72), Jacobson (73) and Rado (74). However, often the particular depressive syndrome on which the theory is based has not been clearly defined and in spite of Freud's reference to constitutional predisposition and his warning never to try to analyze depressed patients, hereditary, somatic, and cultural factors have been largely ignored by other psychoanalysts. Many investigators such as Kraines (75), who postulated that depressive psychoses are due to hereditary susceptibility and physiologic factors, vigorously protest the psychoanalytic theories of etiology and consider that psychic manifestations are secondary.

Sandler and Joffe (76), in a careful examination of the material of 100 cases of children of all age groups at the Hampstead Child-Therapy Clinic, found that a number of them showed what could be termed depressive reactions of great variation in intensity and duration with a wide range of internal and external precipitating circumstances. Although the authors make a psychodynamic formulation of depression, they state that a constitutional predisposition also must be important. They postulate that the influence of the parents through the maturation period is progressively replaced by the superego. Guilt occurs as a consequence of the ego's perception that the actual self cannot live up to one's ideals. In those who cannot tolerate this disparity the response to the mental pain is depression. They emphasized that repression of aggression and displacement of anger from a frustrating individual to the self may occur in vulnerable children. In some there may be a reversal of affect. Then depression becomes complicated and obscured by either excitement and clowning or by psychophysiologic reactions in an attempt to deny or prevent the experiencing of helplessness in the face of frustration or disappointment. These clinical manifestations, although they have their own child-related qualities and vary with age, are to be found in similar form in adults. They further stated that depression in children derives from the same factors as in adults. Their conception of the basic depressive reaction in children is similar to that of Bibring (72) except that they stress the basic biological nature related to pain rather than the concepts of undermining or diminution of self-esteem and attribute greater importance to the role of aggression. Their diagnosis is based on the following criteria: looking sad or unhappy, withdrawal, little capacity for pleasure, feelings of rejection, difficulty in accepting help, passivity, insomnia, and autoerotic or other repetitive activities. Special emphasis was placed on both feelings of helplessness and passive resignation.

Further evidence that depressive illness in children is similar to that in adults is given by the results in several drug studies. Frommer (77) pointed out that the diagnosis of childhood depression is often missed. She investigated 32 children after months or years of illness in a double-blind cross-over trial comparing a combination of phenelzine, a monoamine oxidase inhibitor, and chlordiazepoxide with phenobarbitone and an inert capsule and found that 28 improved on antidepressants and only one on phenobarbitone. Three were withdrawn from the trial because of hysterical behavior.

Weinberg, Rutman, Sullivan et al. (78) in an evaluation of 72 children found that 45 had symptoms permitting a clinical diagnosis of depression. The most common manifestations were agitated behavior, crying, moodiness, sleep disturbances, and somatic complaints—symptoms common in adult depression. Severe psychomotor retardation was not noted but rather a gradual loss of interest, social withdrawal, feelings of sadness, and irritability. Fifteen expressed a serious desire to die and three had attempted suicide. Developmental symptoms such as hyperactivity, school phobia, enuresis, temper tantrums, poor social judgment, and destructive behavior were common and hindered recognition of depression. They hypothecated that hyperactivity as a change in behavior may correspond to manic behavior in adults. It was thought likely that with the lessening of these symptoms in adolescence, depressive illness becomes more easily recognized. After three to seven months, those treated with tricyclic antidepressive drugs, amitriptyline, or imipramine, demonstrated significant improvement in symptoms of depressive illness.

Cytryn and McKnew (79) pointed out that in infancy there is a limited repertoire of defense mechanisms available. Fantasy life is primitive and does not always allow for containment or discharge of depressive affect. Verbalization is unavailable for either abreaction or depression or seeking solutions to depression-inducing situations. Thus, the infant is vulnerable to flooding by depressive affect and grossly depressed mood and behavior. Substituting others for a lost or unsatisfactory mother figure can counteract depression so that it may be short-lived. In early childhood, verbalization increases, although, because it remains relatively rudimentary, affect is translated into action or fantasy. With increasing age the depression breaks through into overt mood and behavior. With greater development of conscience, guilt feelings and low self-esteem ensue. In those with more mature defenses, the ability to verbalize feelings and solve problems develops. Where more primitive defenses such as denial prevail, there is poor reality testing and development of depressive equivalents.

Toolan (80) also described an evolution of symptoms of depression with age. In infants, depression is often evidenced by eating and sleeping disturbances, colic, crying, and head-banging. At a somewhat later stage of infancy, withdrawal, apathy, and regression are evidences of the same difficulty. Severe emotional deprivation may lead to permanent emotional and intellectual impairment and even death. In childhood, depressive feelings are displaced by behavioral problems, tantrums, disobedience, truancy, running away from home, accident proneness, getting beaten up by peers, self-destructive behavior, and inferiority feelings. In adolescence, boredom, difficulty in concentration, restlessness, fatigue, hypochondriasis, and insomnia are common symptoms. Adolescents use denial as a main method of handling conflicts. Rarely do they discuss significant problems. When concerned with philosophical problems, it is usually a cover for matters of more personal concern.

I am reminded of a patient who came to me for psychoanalysis at the age of 23. He reported that when he had had analytic treatment from the ages of 14 to 16 he had talked a great deal but said nothing. He now felt he had matured to the point where he wanted to discuss his conflicts freely.

In youth, dreams and fantasies help in the recognition of depression. Fantasies of being unloved are frequent. They may daydream of their death and of others being sorry for mistreating them. Dreams may reveal a preoccupation with dead people, of being attacked or injured, or of the dead beckoning them to join them. Dreams also often relate to dissolution or loss of body parts.

In contrast to the findings in children and adolescents, in adults the most prominent symptoms are those associated with changes in affect, especially sadness or apathy, self-depreciation, lack of interest, helplessness, crying, unrealistic distortions, decreased libido, poor concentration, withdrawal, suicidal preoccupation, and hypochondriasis, and with physical manifestations such as insomnia or hypersomnia, anorexia, weight changes, constipation, psychomotor retardation or agitation, fatigue, impotence or vaginismus, and lowered bodily metabolism.

More people are living longer and are in the age groups most prone to depressive illness. As in the children the recognition may be difficult since not infrequently a depressive illness may be mistaken for a senile or arteriosclerotic brain syndrome or may be complicated by structural cerebral changes. Grief and depression in older people show a wide range of differences. In some, there may be an intensification of depressive reactions. In others, emotions are less strongly expressed than at younger age periods either due to an emotional blunting associated with the aging process or as a defense against powerful feelings.

COMMENT

Since there is a lack of agreement in regard to diagnostic criteria for depressive illnesses and especially the failure to apply with exactness those we now have, epidemiological surveys and comparisons lack a solid data base. Even under the best of circumstances the complexity of biological, psychological, and cultural variables makes it difficult to identify the significance of any one factor or to clarify the importance of a constellation of factors influencing depressive reactions. However, many studies have given valuable information and as pioneer efforts can stimulate investigations aimed at more accurate estimates of the prevalence and factors influencing the incidence and course in various places under varying conditions throughout the human life span.

In view of the complexities, especially in making transcultural and subcultural comparisons, collaborative studies between psychiatrists and experts in other disciplines need to be carried out with scrupulous attention to clear definition of terms, careful collection of data, perceptive evaluations and attention to reliability. Some helpful suggestions about methodology of epidemiology in psychiatry are offered by Cooper and Morgan (81). The application of specific universal criteria in making comparative studies in the same culture and between cultures will help to give more accurate epidemiological knowledge so as to illuminate the factors causing depression and augment improved approaches to its prevention and treatment.

REFERENCES

1. COOPER, J. E., KENDALL, R. E., GURLAND, B. J., SHARPE, L., COPE-
   LAND, J. R. M. and SIMON, R.: *Psychiatric Diagnosis in New
   York and London.* London: Oxford University Press, 1972.
2. RAWNSLEY, K.: Epidemiology of affective disorders. *In* Recent
   Developments in Affective Disorders. *Brit. J. Psychiat. Spec.
   Pub.*, 2:27-36, 1968.
3. FABREGA, H.: Problems implicit in the cultural and social study
   of depression. *Psychosom. Med.*, 36:377-398, 1974.
4. FRANK, J.: Adjustment problems of selected Negro soldiers. *J.
   Nerv. Ment. Dis.*, 105:647-660, 1947.
5. TONKS, C. M., PAYKEL, E. S. and KLERMAN, J. L.: Clinical depression among Negroes. *Am. J. Psychiat.*, 127(3):329-335,
   1970.
6. WAGNER, P.: A comparative study of Negro and White admissions to the psychiatric pavilion of the Cincinnati General Hospital. *Am. J. Psychiat.*, 95:167-183, 1938.
7. RIPLEY, H. S.: Depressive reactions in a general hospital. *J.
   Nerv. Ment. Dis.*, 105:607-615, 1947.
8. DORPAT, T. L., ANDERSON, W. F. and RIPLEY, H. S.: The relationship of physical illness to suicide. *In* Resnik, H. L. P. (Ed.),
   Suicidal Behaviors: Diagnosis and Management. Boston: Little,
   Brown & Co., 1968.
9. HOLMES, T. H. and RAHE, R. H.: The social readjustment rating
   scale. *J. Psychosom. Res.*, 11:213-218, 1967.
10. PAYKEL, E. S., MYERS, J. K., DIENELT, M., KLERMAN, G., LIN-
    DENTHAL, J. and PEPPER, M.: Life events and depression. *Arch.
    Gen. Psychiat.*, 21:753-760, 1969.
11. WITTKOWER,, E. and RIN, H.: Recent developments in transcultural
    psychiatry. *In* De Reuck, A. and Porter, R. (Eds.), *Trans-
    cultural Psychiatry.* Boston: Little, Brown & Co., 1965, pp. 4-16.
12. WATTS, C. A.: *Depressive Disorders in the Community.* Bristol,
    England: John Wright & Sons, Ltd., 1966.
13. SILVERMAN, C.: The epidemiology of depression: A review. *Am. J.
    Psychiat.*, 124(7):883-891, 1968.
14. ROTH, W. F. and LUTON, F. H.: Mental health program in Ten-
    nessee. *Am. J. Psychiat.*, 99:662-675, 1943.
15. SJOGREN, T.: Genetic-statistical and psychiatric investigations of a
    West Swedish population. *Acta Psychiat. Neurol. Suppl.*, 52:
    1-102, 1948.
16. ESSEN-MOLLER, E.: Individual traits and morbidity in a Swedish

population. *Acta Psychiat. Neurol. Scand.* Suppl., 100:1-160, 1956.
17. IVANYS, E., DRDKOVA, S. and VANA, J.: Prevalence of psychoses recorded among psychiatric patients in a part of the urban population. *Cesk Psychiat.*, 60:152-163, 1964.
18. COHEN, B. and FAIRBANK, R.: Statistical contributions from the mental hygiene study of the Eastern Health District of Baltimore. *Am. J. Psychiat.*, 94:1377-1395, 1938.
19. LEMKAU, P. V., TIETZE, C. and COOPER, M.: Mental hygiene problems in an urban district: II. The psychotics and the neurotics. *Ment. Hyg.*, 26:100-119, 1942.
20. EATON, J. W. and WEIL, R. J.: *Culture and Mental Disorders: A Comparative Study of the Hutterites and Other Populations.* New York: Free Press, 1955.
21. YOO, P. S.: Mental illness in Korean rural communities. *Proceedings of the Third World Congress of Psychiatry*, Montreal, Canada, June 1961 (pp. 1305-1309).
22. LIN, T.: A study of the incidence of mental disorders in Chinese and other cultures. *Psychiat.*, 16:313-336, 1953.
23. LEIGHTON, A. H., LAMBO, T. A., HUGHES, C. C., LEIGHTON, D. C., MURPHY, J. M. and MACKLIN, D. B.: *Psychiatric Disorder Among the Yaruba.* Ithaca, New York: Cornell University Press, 1963.
24. LEHMANN, H. E.: Epidemiology of depressive disorders. *In* Fieve, R. R. (Ed.), *Excerpta Medica*, 1971, *Depression in the 70's* (pp. 21-30).
25. COLLOMB, H.: Methodological problems in cross-cultural research. *Int. J. Psychiat.*, 3:17-19, 1967.
26. COHEN, R. A.: Manic-depressive illness. *In* Freedman, A. M., Kaplan, H. I. and Sadock, B. J. (Eds.), *Comprehensive Textbook of Psychiatry, II.* Baltimore: Williams & Wilkins Co., 1975, pp. 1012-1024.
27. MENDELS, J.: *Concepts of Depression.* New York: John Wiley & Sons, 1970.
28. ARIETI, S.: Manic-depressive psychosis. *In* Arieti, S. (Ed.), *American Handbook of Psychiatry.* New York: Basic Books, 1959.
29. REISMAN, D., GLAZER, N. and DENNEY, R.: *The Lonely Crowd.* New York: Doubleday Anchor Books, 1953.
30. PEDERSON, A. M., BARRY, D. J. and BABIGIAN, H. M.: Epidemiological considerations of psychotic depression. *Arch. Gen. Psychiat.*, 27:193-197, 1972.
31. GREWEL, F.: Psychiatric differences in Ashkenazim and Sephardim. *Psychiatria, Neurologea, Neurochirurgia*, 70:330-347, 1967.
32. MALZBERG, B.: The distribution of mental disease according to religious affiliation in New York State, 1949-51. *Ment. Hyg.*, 46:510-522, 1962.

33. HALPERN, L.: Some data of the psychic morbidity of Jews and Arabs in Palestine. *Am. J. Psychiat.*, 94:1215-1222, 1938.
34. HES, J.: Manic-depressive illness in Israel. *Am. J. Psychiat.*, 116: 1082-1086, 1960.
35. PRANGE, A. J., WILSON, F. C., KNOX, A., MCCLANE, T. and LIPTON, M. A.: Enhancement of imipramine by thyroid stimulating hormone: Clinical and theoretical implications. *Am. J. Psychiat.*, 127(2):191-199, 1970.
36. VITALS, M. and PRANGE, A.: Cultural aspects of the relatively low incidence of depression in Southern Negroes. *Int. J. Soc. Psychiat.*, 8:104-112, 1962.
37. MCGOUGH, W., WILLIAMS, E. and BLACKLEY, J.: Changing patterns of psychiatric illness among Negroes of the Southeastern United States. *Proceedings of the IVth World Congress of Psychiatry*, Excerpta International Congress Series No. 150. Amsterdam: Excerpta Medica Foundation, 1966.
38. RIPLEY, H. and WOLF, S.: Mental illness among Negro troops overseas. *Am. J. Psychiat.*, 103(4):499-512, 1947.
39. BECK, A. T.: *Depression: Clinical, Experimental and Theoretical Aspects.* New York: Harper & Row, 1967.
40. HARMATZ, J. S. and SHADER, R. I.: Psychopharmacologic investigations in healthy elderly volunteers: MMPI Depression Scale. *J. Am. Geriat. Soc.*, 23(8):350-354, 1975.
41. ZUNG, W.: Depression in the normal adult population. *Psychosomatics*, 12(3):164, 1971.
42. MURPHY, H., WITTKOWER, E. and CHANCE, N.: Crosscultural inquiry into the symptomatology of depression: A preliminary report. *Int. J. Psychiat.*, 3:6-22, 1967.
43. MURPHY, H.: The epidemiological approach to transcultural psychiatric research. *In* DeReuck, A. and Porter, R. (Eds.), *Ciba Foundation Symposium: Transcultural Psychiatry.* Boston: Little, Brown & Co., 1965, pp. 303-323.
44. RAO, A. V.: A study of depression as prevalent in South India. *Transcult. Psychiat. Res. Rev.*, 7:166-167, 1970.
45. SCHWAB, J. J., BIALOW, M., HOLZER, C. E., BROWN, J. M. and STEVENSON, B. E.: Sociocultural aspects of depression in medical inpatients. *Arch. Gen. Psychiat.*, 17:533, 1967.
46. HENDIN, H.: *Black Suicide.* New York: Basic Books, Inc., 1969.
47. HENDIN, H.: *Suicide and Scandinavia.* New York: Grune and Stratton, 1964.
48. SCHWAB, J., HOLZER, C. and WARHEIT, G.: Depression symptomatology and age. *Psychosomatics*, 14(3):135-141, 1973.
49. HELGASON, T.: Epidemiology of mental disorders in Iceland. *Acta Psychiat. Scand.* Suppl., 40:173, 1964.
50. BOOK, J. A.: A genetic and neuropsychiatric investigation of a North Swedish population with special regard to schizophrenia

and mental deficiency. *Acta Genet. et Stat. Medica,* 4:1-100, 1953.

51. SORENSEN, A. and STROMGREN, E.: Frequency of depressive states within the geographically delimited population groups: 2. Prevalence (The Samso Investigation). *Acta Psychiat. Scand.,* 37 (Suppl.), 162:62-68, 1961.

52. SCHWAB, J., BROWN, J. and HOLZER, C.: Sex and age differences in depression in medical inpatients. *Ment. Hyg.,* 52(4):627-630, 1968.

53. RIPLEY, H.: Suicidal behavior in Edinburgh and Seattle. *Am. J. Psychiat.,* 130(9):995-1001, 1973.

54. KATO, M.: Self destruction in Japan: A crosscultural, epidemiological analysis of suicide. *Fol. Psychiat. et Neur. Japonica,* 23(4):291-307, 1969.

55. SAINSBURY, P.: *Suicide in London: An Ecological Study.* London: Chapman & Hall, 1955.

56. ROBINS, E., MURPHY, G. E., WILKINSON, R. H., GLASSNER, S. and KAYES, J.: Some clinical considerations in the prevention of suicide based on a study of 134 successful suicides. *Am. J. Pub. Health,* 49:888-898, 1959.

57. DORPAT, T. L. and RIPLEY, H. S.: A study of suicide in the Seattle area. *Comprehens. Psychiat.,* 1(6):349-359, 1960.

58. GARDNER, E. A., BAHN, A. K. and MACK, M.: Suicide and psychiatric care in the aging. *Arch. Gen. Psychiat.,* 10:547-553, 1964.

59. GARFINKEL, B. D. and GOLOMBEK, H.: Suicide and depression in childhood and adolescence. *Can. Med. Assoc. J.,* 110:1278-1281, 1974.

60. ABRAHAM, K.: A short study of the development of the libido, viewed in the light of mental disorders. *In: Selected Papers on Psychoanalysis.* London: Hogarth Press, 1927.

61. SPITZ, R.: Anaclitic depression. *In: The Psychoanalytic Study of the Child.* New York: International Universities Press, 1946.

62. ZILBOORG, G.: Suicide among primitive and civilized races. *Am. J. Psychiat.,* 92:1346-1369, 1936.

63. BATCHELOR, I. R. C. and NAPIER, M. B.: Broken homes and attempted suicide. *Brit. J. Delinquency,* 4:1-10, 1953.

64. BROWN, F.: Depression and childhood bereavement. *J. Ment. Sci.,* 107:754-777, 1961.

65. BECK, A. T., SETHI, B. B. and TUTHILL, R. W.: Childhood bereavement and adult depression. *Arch. Gen. Psychiat.,* 9:295-302, 1963.

66. GREGORY, I.: Studies of parental deprivation in psychiatric patients. *Am. J. Psychiat.,* 115:432-442, 1958.

67. BOWLBY, J.: Childhood mourning and its implication for psychiatry. *Am. J. Psychiat.,* 118:481-498, 1961.

68. DORPAT, T. L., JACKSON, J. K. and RIPLEY, H. S.: Broken homes and attempted and completed suicide. *Arch. Gen. Psychiat.,* 12:213-216, 1965.

69. WHITING, J. and CHILD, I.: *Child Training and Personality*: A *Cross-Cultural Study*. New Haven: Yale University Press, 1953.
70. GOLDMAN-EISLER, F. Breast feeding and character formation. *In* Kluckhohn, C. and Murray, H. (Eds.), *Nature, Society and Culture*. New York: Knopf, 1953, pp. 146-184.
71. FREUD, S.: Mourning and melancholia. *In: Collected Papers, Volume IV*. London: Hogarth Press, 1946.
72. BIBRING, E.: The mechanisms of depression. *In* Greenacre, P. (Ed.), *Affective Disorders*. New York: International Universities Press, 1953, pp. 13-48.
73. JACOBSON, E.: Contributions to the meta-psychology of cyclothymic depression. *In* Greenacre, P. (Ed.), *Affective Disorders*. New York: International Universities Press, 1953, pp. 49-83.
74. RADO, S.: Hedonic control, action-self, and the depressive spell. *In* Hoch, P. H. and Zubin, J. (Eds.), *Depression*. New York: Grune & Stratton, 1954, pp. 153-182.
75. KRAINES, S. M.: *Mental Depressions and Their Treatment*. New York: The Macmillan Co., 1957.
76. SANDLER, J. and JOFFE, W. G.: Notes on childhood depression. *Int. J. Psychoanal.*, 46:88-96, 1965.
77. FROMMER, E. A.: Treatment of childhood depression with antidepressant drugs. *Brit. Med. J.*, 1:729-732, 1967.
78. WEINBERG, W. A., RUTMAN, J., SULLIVAN, L., PENICK, E. C. and DEITZ, S. G.: Depression in children referred to an educational diagnostic center: Diagnosis and treatment. *J. Peds.*, 83(6): 1065-1072, 1973.
79. CYTRYN, L. and McKNEW, D. H.: Factors influencing the changing clinical expression of the depressive process in children. *Am. J. Psychiat.*, 131(8):879-881, 1974.
80. TOOLAN, J.: Depression in children and adolescents. *Am. J. Orthopsychiat.*, 32:404, 1962.
81. COOPER, B. and MORGAN, H. G.: *Epidemiological Psychiatry*. Springfield, Illinois: Charles C Thomas, 1973.

2

Depression: The Psychosocial Context

Edward J. Stainbrook, Ph.D., M.D.

In one of those historically rare forecasts of a great unifying principle which can come only from the inspiration of a genial and creative thinker, the British neurophysiologist, Sir Charles Sherrington, suggested during the first years of this century: "Mind and energy—perhaps we are the tie that binds them" (1).

At the time Sherrington wrote that statement, psychoanalysis had barely begun its cultural ascendancy, the academic takeoff in American psychology of the various learning theories of behavior had yet to occur by two score of years, and the present revolution in behavioral biology and in the psychobiology of cognition and of information-processing was a full half century away. Yet, now, we who are thinking of an integrative conceptual model of human behavior based on the rapidly accumulating knowledge and the associated explanatory power of contemporary behavioral science can apply Sherrington's principle more resourcefully and effectively than was ever possible in the context of its origin.

Particularly since the creation over 20 years ago of the Watson-Crick model of genetic structure and the subsequent developments in working out the details of the control by genetic information of biologic form and process, it is now possible to reformulate the

28

Sherrington assumption in contemporary terms. Indeed, soon after the demonstration that DNA was the source of genetic specificity, theoretical biologists were describing the organism as the seat of a triple flux of matter, energy and information.

For the purposes of providing a basic thesis for the understanding of how psychosocial information and meaning evoke and maintain the complicated and varying psychobiologic processes and behavior which we call depression, we can make a similar reductionistic definition of the person. A person is an intricate organization of interrelating biologic systems composed of structures and processes in which energy transformations, manifested covertly or overtly as behavior, are constantly going on under the direction of information. Some of this information directing and controlling biologic action comes from genetic sources. Some comes from the here-and-now appraisals of present self and situation. And because man is the animal who not only remembers his past but by conceptual foresight can also remember his future, some of the information influencing biologic processes of brain and body comes from the scan and anticipated consequences of the future.

Hence, not only a general theory of human nature and behavior but a more specific theory of disease can be based on the principle of the control of biologic processes by information, or by misinformation, which evokes and maintains both adaptive and maladaptive responses. This information or misinformation ultimately consists of neuroelectric, neuroendocrine, or other biochemical or physiologic signals.

In human life-settings and cultures, psychosocial information is called meaning. This meaning is transduced into neurophysiologic phenomena both as signal process and as altered structure in the nervous system and into neuroendocrine patterns of secretory activity for further communication to cells and organs. The cells may then respond by altering physiologic structures or functions.

When in the study of biologic responses to psychosocial happenings we monitor physiologic processes or titer biochemical activity, we are studying the signals and the signaled effects of the transduced psychocultural meaning, not the meaning itself. The specific psychosocial meaning can be restored to the signals only by collating them with the evoking or maintaining psychosocial events, that is to say by decoding them back into the meaning. Hence, he who studies only the transduced biologic signals and evoked processes of psychosocial events will not know what they mean.

Perhaps no more urgent reason exists for our continuing devotion of time, energy and increasing resourcefulness to the study of individual subjectivity than to increase the certainty of our knowledge about the interrelationships between the physiologic patterns of process created by the biologic transduction of psychologic meaning and that same meaning and behavior described both subjectively and objectively in psychosocial language and thought.

Serious explorations in the recording of authentic self-expressed subjectivity correlated with monitored physiologic processes do not characterize very much of the contemporary research in either laboratory or clinical psychobiology. Even during the course of a clinically designated depressive reaction the subjective self-report of the prevailing character of the frequently shifting balance of anxiety, anger, loss-distress, shame and guilt is often ignored.

Essentially, then, in the formulation of a psychobiologic conception of depressive behavior, the biologic mediators of behavior perform a double role as both dependent and independent variables. Neurophysiologic and endocrine processes, particularly, are obviously dependent variables in their responses to psychosocial information of the past, present and future. These are the pathways by which present self-environmental transactions, person-environment interactions remote in time and space, and environmental experiences anticipated in the future all influence biologic processes and bring emotional and other behavior into being and sustain it.

Just as demonstrably, biologic processes also function as independent variables which may evoke, modify and maintain behavior.

To reinforce the conception of psychobiologic integration as insistently as possible, therefore, we must not, in a discussion of the psychosocial determinants of depression, conceptualize individuals as disembodied selves even though some current theories of depression seem to be referring to depersonalized bodies. The self is a socialized body and the mind is the socialized and experientially organized brain—a brain which genetically may also be considered to have inherited a mind of its own. The older mind-body problems disappear, therefore, except as very inept ways of talking about the character and the sources of the information that direct the energy transformations constituting the biologic processes of behavior. Information and energy, to rephrase Sherrington—we are the tie that binds them.

Over the last 20 years, research in general and in evolutionary behavioral biology—in animal behavior, in experimental psychology, in the social sciences, and in clinical psychiatry and medicine— has provided us with several currently plausible assumptions about the determinants and characteristics of depressive behavior.

Initially, the considerable study being devoted to the elucidation of innately specific neurobiologic organizations of emotional behavior has led to several different models for parsing out separately distinct emotions. J. P. Scott (2) suggests a classification of basic adaptive behavioral systems and their associated emotional behavior such as, for example, the association of allelomimetic behavior (doing the same thing as others) with loneliness and fear. This is similar to Plutchik's categories (3) which include an innate programming of sadness and grief in association with experiences of losing contact. David Hamburg (4) and others use the naturalistic observations of primate behavior to demonstrate genetically distinct emotional action.

With Sylvan Tomkins (5), and most recently Carroll Izard (6), we may assume that innate and distinct emotions would satisfy the following criteria:

1. A specific regional and integrative neurophysiology and the associated neutral circuitry should be demonstrable.

2. Specific expressive, postural and behavioral movement should be associated with the emotional process.

3. In man, a subjective feeling quality should be distinctive enough to be correctly and differentially self-interpreted.

Identifying basic innately organized emotional systems enables us to recognize the possible meaningful components of what we now too glibly, both in the folk-speech and in the nosology of psychiatry, are calling anxiety and depression. It is not necessary to agree completely with Izard's list of the basic emotions to appreciate the pragmatic diagnostic value inherent in his analysis of the emotional pattern called depression. The pattern of depression can be described as a frequently changing combination of distress, anger, anxiety, guilt, shame, contempt, and various degrees of loss of interest. These emotions comprise the psychobiologic arousal modulating the seeking of information, the attaining of goals, the approach to or avoidance of sources of possible positive and negative reinforcement, and the appraisal of the feedback from the consequences of action.

More narrowly, the current knowledge from evolutionary psychobiology, from the animal laboratory, and from the observations on the development of the human infant now seems to make quite clear what Freud had been confused about in his early discussions of anxiety. Freud had defined basic anxiety as the loss of maternal love and care. Implicitly, anxiety was the fear of being abandoned and, therefore, of being helpless. The concept of anxiety was thus used to refer to both the distress-loss reaction and the inferred anxiety of helplessness in relation to the consequences of loss.

If we assume that anxiety is a fear-related emotion whose emergence both phylogenetically and ontogenetically is dependent upon human cognitive development involving particularly the ability to anticipate (7), then before sufficient cognitive ability develops, distress and fear rather than anxiety would seem to be the appropriate interpretations of the infantile responses to separation and loss. Anxiety is a cognitively modified fear response emerging with sociocultural development which functions to signal uncertainties about whether loss will occur, or, if it has already occurred, whether it can be repaired. Because of cognitive capacity, threats of distress occurring as an anticipation of consequences about impending or actual loss and of the probabilities of restoration arise from the broadest range of human experience. These threats include those of person loss, social role loss, social and physical space loss, loss of possessions and the threatened or actual loss of conceptions of the psychologic self and of the meaning of existence.

At the level of primate behavior, Charles Kaufman (8) has been able to demonstrate that brief separations of the infant monkey from maternal nurturance and protection evoke fear-distress reactions; however, as the loss becomes seemingly irreparable, depressive behavior occurs. Moreover, the developmental age at which separation or loss occurs and the possible availability of substitute mothering are important variables. These observations associate readily with the conception of learned helplessness, advanced by Seligman (9) and others, as a factor in understanding depressive behavior.

In view of all these considerations, it is tempting to revise "mourning becomes melancholia" to "separation-anxiety becomes depression." For the human situation, however, this is much too simple a statement.

At least two simplifying questions are at the basis of an adequate evaluation of the psychosocial situations which may evoke, maintain or change depressive behavior. The cognitive appraisal induced by the first question: "What is the danger of my losing something?" results primarily in the feeling of anxiety. Such anxiety functions both as signal-awareness of impending psychologic threat as well as motivational modulation to reduce uncertainty and to increase the effectiveness of coping. Worry, whether constructive, ineffective or destructive, about impending loss begins.

Anticipatory distress as a distinctive depressive feeling is also a resultant of the cognitive analysis of the threat of loss. How frequently, how intensely, and for what duration anticipatory loss-distress will be subjectively manifest will depend largely on the effectiveness of both defensive and coping worry and worry-related action in relation to the reality of the situation. The loss may be forestalled or prevented or, if the loss actually occurs, confidence in some degree about restoration or replacement may be achieved.

In general, in uncertain states of impending loss, anxiety is in the foreground and loss-distress emotion is in the background. However, if worry is ineffective or is heavily invested with a sense of helplessness or is motivated significantly by self-destructive and self-punitive needs, the anticipatory loss-distress may be experienced as significant depression even before the loss actually occurs. It is at least of incidental value to consider here the possible implications of anticipatory loss-distress behavior for the concept of endogenous depression. As with all contrasting polarities, no one is ever happy with the exclusive extremes. It seems acceptable to assume, therefore, that in an individual with a biologic vulnerability of the neurophysiologic and endocrine processes underlying distress behavior, clinically visible depressive behavior could occur as a response to only subjectively anticipated loss. A clinical exploration and assessment of the psychosocial surroundings for significant life-stress might not disclose acceptable evidence supporting any reactive contribution to what might then be diagnosed as an endogenous disorder.

The extensive experimental use of the life-events rating scale, originally developed by Holmes and Rahe (10), Paykel (11), and others provides considerable evidence that the accumulation of the stress of minor life-events, some of which by themselves might not seem significant either to the depressed patient or to the evaluating physician, may summate through time to the equivalent of major stress. Paykel's specific study of the relationship of stressful life-events to the onset of depression demonstrates the considerable time-span over which stressful happenings may precede the ultimate emergence of depressive behavior. His studies also suggest that after the depressive process is in being, additional stress-events may be more closely related to suicidal responses.

When disengagement and loss actually do occur, a second question comes to dominate the control of emotional processes: What are the consequences of this loss going to be for me? What will happen to me if I cannot or if I will not recommit myself or re-relate to other persons, social roles, values, objects, or places? In this assessment the behavior of helplessness, pessimism, estrangement, alienation, and disengagement may be admixed with hopefulness, some degree of optimism, and a consideration of other gratifications which modulate the feeling of acute and pervasive loss-distress.

With actual loss-occurrence, anxiety, conditioned by past experiences relating to confidence or helplessness about loss-mastery and by cognitive appraisals and reappraisals of present and future, becomes a significant component of the depressive pattern of behavior. The thought, feeling and conduct of disengagement and recommitment, succeeding or failing, constitute the course of the depression (12). The behavioral importance of the emotional components of the depressive process, particularly of distress and anxiety, is related to the vicissitudes of the experience of detaching and disengaging and of relating and recommitting.

A similar analysis of the emotional components of depression comes from the germinal work of George Engel (13), Arthur Schmale (14), and their colleagues. For some time they have been describing the possible psychosomatic implications of the precarious balancing of anxious anticipation and depression. Anxiety and the implied presence of hope motivate and sustain behavior designed to reduce uncertainty and helplessness while maintaining the person's interest in living. If an individual gives up anxious hope, distress-depression urges psychobiologic withdrawal and conservation as the ultimate defense against wept-out exhaustion and hopelessness.

The two components of anxiety and distress are usually the dominant concerns of psychiatric diagnosis and treatment. However, anger, shame and guilt are also highly significant determinants of the total depressive behavior.

The adaptive value of anger is to intensify and prolong the assertive or aggressive determination to take a stand and do something to achieve goal outcomes or conflict resolution. What is done by any one individual may be destructive to self or to others, may be constructively effective, or may be ineffective or impairing. Guilt and shame may similarly modulate adaptive behavior and effective problem-solving or be associated with impairment, incompetence and ineffectiveness.

As Karl Pribram (15) observed some time ago, the general objective in dealing with affective behavior is to transform it into effective behavior. Recently, Arnold Mandell (16) has also suggested that more attention must be given to the feeling signals and processes of dysphoric emotions as sources of motivation for problem-seeing and problem-solving. Between physician and patient, especially, emotions are information to be collaboratively and effectively used as well as sufferings to be unilaterally treated.

One dimension of the psychosocial context of behavior has been insufficiently endowed with research attention by both clinical and preventive psychiatry. This is the study of the relationship between the values, knowledge and practices directing the current socialization of children and the adaptive worth of such values, beliefs and information in the development of behavior which will be effective and resourceful for a future changing society. Most estimates of the cultural changes of the future suggest a significant increase in frequency during an individual's lifetime of disengagement-recommitment behavior in relation to more rapidly changing personal relationships, social spaces, occupational and other social roles, ideologies, knowledge, values, and life-meaning.

The present life time of an ideology (witness the private enterprise psychotherapies), is about three to five years. In the child-rearing socialization of future adults for the effective mastery of the anticipated frequency of these various commitment-disengagement experiences, have we been paying too little attention to the management of the tender loving care of separation in contrast to our concerns with the tender loving enhancement of attachment?

The present increased study of attachment behavior now being reported from child development research is due largely to the well-known writing of John Bowlby (17), behind whom stand the ethologists, Lorenz, Tingbergen, Eibes-Eibelfeldt and others who made the imprinting of attachment so dramatically visible. The biobehavioral anlage of loss-distress can be considered as the internal biologic system of negative reinforcement activated when the survival behavior of keeping attached to and in contact with parental and other sources of protection, nurturance and adaptive learning is threatened. The tremendous importance for depressive behavior later in life of the experiences of helplessness or of confidence in restoring loss or in renewing contact seems obvious. So much of the existing clinical studies on the relation of parental death during childhood and subsequent depressive vulnerability suggests an as yet to be proven relationship between parental death-loss with its high likelihood of realistic associated helplessness and the anticipated effectiveness of being able to master the losses, symbolic and actual, of later life.

Even in the primate research laboratory we have been so busy observing the vicissitudes of the attachment behavior of monkeys that only recently have we begun to notice how the monkey mother at an appropriate time trains her offspring to confidently separate and disengage from attachment. To paraphrase Ecclesiastes, there is a time for attachment and a time for separation.

A salutary trend in the sociology of preventive medicine is being proposed by Cassell (18) who advises a shift of emphasis from attending only to the sociologic sanitation of psychosocial stress-reduction to concern about the strategies for developing increased psychobiologic and sociocultural supports and resources for more gratifying, adaptive and effective living. So, similarly, enhanced psychologic and social resources for successful separation and disengagement and for loss-restoration, renewal and recommitment must engage our preventive efforts. Among other consultation tasks to the general society, behavioral scientists must be prepared to advise parents on the child-rearing behavior best adapted to the probable social and cultural characteristics of the adult life ahead.

We have been attempting to bring together conceptually some of the major aspects of the psychobiology of depressive behavior. This has been done in order to emphasize in contemporary terms the possible interrelationships between biologic processes described in the language of biology and these same processes when they have, in the meaning of Piaget, assimilated and accommodated to their experiences in living, when they have been informed, organized and reorganized by learning, and are then described in the language of psychology and the social sciences.

One additional significant consideration, however, is particularly relevant in evaluating correlations between described psychosocial context and behavior and concomitant physiologic and biochemical events. This has to do with further reflection on the various possible genetic influences on the depressive emotional process. A considerable amount of individual biologic variability of the structure and function of the nervous and endocrine systems is genetically determined. Such genetic influence may affect variably the transduction of neuroelectric signals into hormonal outputs, the intensity and duration of neural reverberatory activity and feedback, particularly in the limbic and associated systems, and the sensitivity and action of the neural and neurohumoral "switch-on" and "switch-off" mechanisms involved in emotional processes, to mention only a few.

Some recent research relevant to these considerations suggests, for example, that the elevated corticosteroids associated with depressive behavior do not co-vary consistently with the observed or experienced psychosocial stress of the individual but are, instead, correlated with the existence of the depressive process itself. If this is true, it is tempting to think of this as due to the modulation of depressive behavior by internal neuro-endocrine systems with possible feedback or "switch-off" defects.

It is of at least incidental interest to consider the adaptive value of the quick "switch-on" reactions of the innate emotional responses of fear, anger, distress and the feelings of pain, appetite and thirst and the relatively slow "switch-off" of these same responses. Under many civilized conditions, pain is an unnecessarily prolonged and redundant psychobiologic signal even though under other conditions it assures an enduring and adaptive protective attention to injury. Similarly, a much quicker cut-off of the neurobiologic conditions sustaining eating behavior in the food-affluent environment prevailing for many people today would be more adaptive than the slow fade-out of appetite which facilitates eating as much as possible at every opportunity in a food-scarce society. In general, it appears that a slow "switch-off" of emotional and other biologic need-arousal has been basically adaptive. In many contemporary social situations, however, it has become maladaptive. Indeed, just as so much of psychosocial stress, monitored in individuals as emotional behavior, becomes significant because it evokes too intense, too frequent, or too long enduring emotion, so one can say that much of our emotional behavior evoked as adaptation to the past is now too intense, too frequently evoked, and too long maintained to be desirably adapted to our present psychosocial environment.

We have also just begun to parse out the possible various genotypes which may condition depressive behavior. There is accumulating evidence pointing to psychophysiologic and personality differences between the bipolar and the unipolar cluster of depressive symptoms. The success with lithium in treating some depressive individuals and its failure with others suggest possible genotypic differences. Yet, as with the schizophrenic syndromes, the clinician deals with phenotypes and cannot yet sufficiently distinguish the genotypic variations in what to him is a diagnostic grouping of similar phenotypes.

As has already been indicated, the assumption of genetic susceptibility as a determinant of the frequency, intensity or duration of a depressive emotional process may not be an absolute differential distinguishing the endogenous from the reactive depressive disorder. I would rather insist that the introduction of biologic vulnerability, genetically or otherwise determined, allows a diminished but not extinguished role as independent variable to the existing evoking and maintaining psychosocial conditions. There is always some of the exogenous influence in the endogenous depression and there may be some of the endogenous process in the reactive depression. People who are depressed sufficiently to encounter psychiatric diagnosis are likely to represent many combinations of high and low stress and high and low biologic vulnerability.

Indeed, in terms of intensity and duration of impairment, individuals with significant biologic vulnerability might be those most benefited by psychobiologic and sociocultural attempts to minimize loss-distress and to aid re-engagement and recommitment when loss and disengagement do occur.

In order to relate person-environment transactions to the onset and course of depressive behavior with some hope of specificity, it may be helpful to consider some of the current conceptions about emotional behavior in general. This is particularly relevant, of course, when the term depression is used as the name for the emotional process of anticipatory or actual loss-distress which is a potential response of everyone to certain appraisals of the personal impact of various life-events. In this sense depression is an ubiquitously occurring normal emotion with adaptive significance.

The attribution to any individual of a medical diagnosis of an affective or emotional disorder results from additional biologic, psychologic and sociocultural variables combining in various patterns. Quantitative increases in the intensity, frequency or duration of the emotional process or qualitative changes in the character of one or more of the influencing variables are the most likely factors determining the perception of the depressive behavior as an illness.

Obviously, one of the reasons why studies of the interrelations between depressive illness and sociocultural context are contradictory and inconclusive lies in the difficulty of analyzing and controlling the large number of variables involved in determining what transforms an individually occurring depressive emotional process into a socially visible illness.

As an illustration of this, one of the more consistent findings of several studies on the relationship of depressive illness to social class and occupation suggests that depressive behavior is more frequent in persons with relatively high socioeconomic status. Schwab (19) and his colleagues have shown, however, that the method of assessment may be a significant variable. The finding appeared true when the assessment of behavior was made by medical diagnostic interview. If the behavior was assessed by a protocol rating from case histories and records, no social class differences seemed demonstrable. And when objective rating scales of behavior were used as a basis for evaluation, depression appeared to be most frequent in the lower socioeconomic representatives.

So, similarly, the reported positive correlation between high occupational status and depression must certainly be conditioned across the occupational range of skills and degree of responsibility by the differential challenge to competence and effectiveness posed by depressive impairment. Other obvious variables are also operative.

In spite of the uncertainty about the relationship of the normal depressive process to the diagnosed affective disorders, an understanding of the normal emotional process is essential.

When behavioral intrapersonal or interpersonal variables are considered to be independent, an emotional process may be described as being evoked and maintained by the existing psychosocial behavior and as varying with that behavior. From this point of view, the emotional process is a result of behavior. The behavior is frequently a direct or indirect response to the presenting social surround, involving cognitive appraisals and reappraisals of the meaning and of the action resources of the situation and of the meaning and competence of the self in the situation. Decisions about action or inaction are made and executed and the consequent feedback information is utilized in interpreting and influencing the ongoing behavioral process. If the behavioral action is effectively adaptive, the emotional process drops out of being as an attention-demanding aspect of consciousness. When the behavior is ineffectively adaptive, the emotional process may remain in being. In the language of the street, it is "hung-up."

At this point the emotional process is then described frequently as an independent variable influencing or motivating behavior. Many of the individual's behavioral concerns are now directed to the management of emotion. Anxiety or loss-distress, for example, must be diminished or controlled. Behavior motivated by the immediate short-term goal of distress-reduction is then observed. This behavior is frequently defined medically as symptoms and may be composed of developmentally early-learned and culturally influenced responses with a history of previous high reinforcement. Frequently this behavior of attempted emotional control, such as avoidance, withdrawal and the reactivation in the present of earlier learned defensive responses, may interfere strongly with other intrapersonal and interpersonal behavior. Pharmacologic and other interventions designed to alter the neurobiology of the emotional process are an attempt to control this emotion-motivated behavior and so to reduce both dysphoric feeling and the interference of defensive and symptomatic behavior with effective and adaptive psychosocial problem-seeing and problem-solving.

When the evocation and maintenance of an emotional process are dependent upon psychosocial behavior, then an understanding of both the individual and of his sociocultural surround is necessary.

Until an adequate theoretical integration is achieved, the analysis of the self-environment transactions identified as depressive behavior must be based upon the descriptive and explanatory resources of at least three current psychologic theories of behavior: the psychoanalytic, the cognitive and the behavioristic. Each of these theories emphasizes, conceptually explores, and attempts to validate scientifically a significant aspect of the total psychosocial behavior.

Since any emotional process, including the depressive, is an evaluative modulation of the existing information processing of the person, much of the character of the depressive emotion will depend upon the individual's interpretation of the meaning and probable consequences of the situational events in which he is participating. These events also have a social and cultural reality of their own which conditions the individual's appraisal of them and which determines the realistic amount of control, threat, deprivation or gratification which may actually exist in relation to the individual.

We all cognitively construct ourselves and our investing world out of past, present and anticipated future information, using our learned characteristic ways of thinking. Decisions then ensue to activate or inactivate certain responses from our individually and characteristically organized repertory of behavior.

To make this concretely relevant to depressive emotion, consider Aaron Beck's (20) well-known conception of the cognitive triad assumed to be basic to depressive behavior. These three cognitive constructions refer to: 1) a negative, self-deprecatory conception of the self, 2) an aversive, pessimistic interpretation of the world, and 3) an assumption of negative reinforcement or of non-reinforcement for the behaving self continuing into the foreseeable future.

The negative conception of the self which induces and maintains the depressive process and which may augment it through interpersonal feedback as well as by self-fulfilling assumptions is usually defined by adjectives such as unworthy, unesteemed, unloved, unlovable, ineffective, inadequate, incompetent, shameful, guilty, or sinful.

Even from a common-sense point of view, these adjectives suggest that since the individual is a highly socially and culturally shaped being, the psychosocial context of child-rearing, of general developmental learning, and of the contemporary social and cultural here-and-now must significantly determine such conceptions of the self. Moreover, the variable occurrence and importance of these adjectives in depressive self-conception suggest their relationship, both across cultures and in the same culture through historical change, to a range of varying values, beliefs and knowledge and to different or changing social and economic organization.

Clinical psychoanalytic investigation has demonstrated the influence of early socialization and social learning on preconditioning the intensity and frequency of subsequent depressive reactions.

Some of these predisposing conditions and experiences which have been delineated by psychoanalytic study are: 1) the failure to learn the effective mastery of being independent and of being a confident, separate self without severe distress, 2) the amount of ambivalence toward parental and other persons who give security and affirmation but who also demand socialized compliance and commitment, 3) the conflicts induced by cultural values relating to need-gratifications, achievement, competition and personal responsibility, and 4) the level of expected performance being taught and learned in any family or social context as necessary to elicit the approval and acceptance of others.

Both the socializing family and the embedding culture are significant determinants of the learned outcome of this socialization process. Insofar as primary prevention is a serious concern of medicine in general and of psychiatry in particular, the social institutions of family, school and church need to be insistently informed about the contemporary behavioral knowledge relevant to the socialization experience.

The self-reproaching behavior of the depressed self, therefore, is dependent significantly on past socialization experience. As child-rearing attitudes, values and transactions change, the content of negative, depression-evoking self-conception changes. There are strong suggestions from cross-cultural research that self-deprecation and guilt do not occur as frequent depressive behavior in non-Western societies, particularly the African. Moreover, in the African cultures the extent to which the society inculcates a sense of self-accountability seems to determine the amount of self-reproach occurring in depressive reactions (21).

The psychosocial context of psychiatric treatment may exacerbate as well as diminish the self-reproach, shame or guilt of the depressed person. Even the pursuit of the desirable value of self-reflection and of collaborative therapeutic self-study may increase self-reproach and self-rejection and so cognitively intensify the depressive emotion.

In relation to the currently increased behavioristic emphasis on how behavior is evoked, maintained and altered by environmental stimuli and response-consequences, it is of more than incidental importance for therapists to analyze as clearly as possible the environmental resources available to the depressed person for adaptive, rewarding behavior and to understand thoroughly their own behavior as social reinforcers. The transformation of a transference analyst into a social reinforcer does not release the psychotherapist or his treatment associates from the burden or the opportunities of self-knowledge.

The predisposing self-conceptions to depressive behavior constructed out of the experiences of the past are constantly reinforced and transformed by the experiences of the here-and-now and the associated anticipations of the future. Both common-sense knowledge and clinical observation indicate that personal relationship losses and social role losses are major precipitants of depressive emotion.

The loss or anticipated loss of a significant other person may occur by death, by physical absence with or without psychologic withdrawal of interest, or by withdrawal of psychologic interest alone. The situation of loss may be permanent or temporary, and either threaten or occasion partial need-deprivation or what may seem subjectively to be total deprivation.

Withdrawal or diminution of psychologic interest and gratification is a highly transactional process. Anticipated loss or withdrawal of another significant person will evoke behavior designed to prevent disengagement. Resentment and increased aggressive demandingness may escalate the withdrawal or need-refusal of the other. The feedback into the negative self-concept of the distressed person intensifies the depressive process by the feeling that one has become blamefully unlovable and destructive.

If the present instance is a repetition of similar past interpersonal experiences, feelings of helplessness and possibly of hopelessness about the successful mastery of intimate interpersonal relationships may become part of one's conception of oneself. The maintenance of resentful or self-demeaning loss of interest may generalize to much of the person's world and prevent any attempts at re-engagement. The future is conceived as the enduring unchanging present, and hope, the other side of despair and the forward look of desire and confidence, is given up.

Since the interpersonal behavior of the depressed person is composed not only of the predispositional and current cognitive constructions of self and investing world but also of actual social behavior, social learning theorists and behavioristic psychologists can suggest very cogently that both the depressive-ready and the depressed person might be taught the social skills and behavior which elicits interested, responsive and gratifying responses from others and be given opportunity to unlearn that behavior which evokes non-interest or negative reinforcement.

It is, incidentally, an interesting commentary on this society with its great fund of information about behavior that there exists almost nowhere in our educational systems, general or professional, any formal curriculum devoted to the teaching and learning of effective and gratifying interpersonal behavior. Perhaps, as we can accept that such opportunities for the study and practice of selves-behaving-with-others need not be conducted as psychotherapy or even specifically as the prevention of psychologic illness, then we may begin the teaching and learning of resourceful human behavior simply as basic education in how to be effectively human.

One of the most helpful conceptions from sociology in the understanding of depressive behavior is the idea of social role. Human experience is organized largely into social role behavior. Conceptions of the self can, to a considerable extent, be viewed as determined by the experiences arising out of past and present social role enactment. Depressive behavior may come into being as the result of the loss of a significant social role as well as because of happenings within a maintained role enactment which diminish or end valued reinforcements or which engender aversive consequences.

The significances of role loss may be obscured frequently when the most visible loss or separation is that of role-validating other persons such as spouse or children. Prolonged grief and mourning are frequently a depressive response to the loss of social role gratifications and meaning. Object-loss mourning may be kept in the foreground as an unwitting defense against the anxiety of seeking a new social role commitment.

If any single social epidemiologic fact can be relied on in the assessment of a risk population for depressive behavior, it is the finding that depressive disorders are much more frequent in women than in men, both in younger women and in the middle age ranges. There are many variables to be considered in explaining this difference but obviously the differential relationships of men and women to the variety and accessibility of available social roles, to the number of social roles in being at any one time for any individual, and to the character of the gratifications and rewards arising out of social role enactment are highly relevant.

Confident and unconfident self-conceptions and the dependency-independency balance of individuals have, of course, much to do with the depressive potential of social role change and of social role loss. The depressive aspects of the retirement crisis are the more apparent in persons whose worth, significance and competence largely depend on occupational role enactment. However, a unique characteristic of retirement role-loss, perhaps also occurring in pre-retirement chronic illness, is that it is usually seen as an absolute ending of occupational role-enactment. A sense of irreplaceable loss is thus frequently engendered. Psychologically this means the loss of a significant positive conception of the self.

The conception that aging persons tend to disengage from various social role participations and commitments with a resultant vulnerability to loss-distress and depression merits considerable analysis. For biologic, psychodynamic and cultural reasons, self-conceptions of esteem, competency and effectiveness may be threatened by the increasing stresses of role performance and by diminishing psychologic rewards for behavior, whether actually existing or self-provoked. Disengagement may thus be both protective against stress as well as the expression of loss of interest.

A possible relationship of depressive behavior to economic stress and particularly to unemployment is strongly suggested by considerations of temporary role loss and the resultant reinforcement failure for security, significance and self-esteem.

The variable pattern of existing total social role involvement at any one time is an important determinant of how intensely loss of roles or of change within role may evoke depressive behavior. Gratifying and affirming experiences in other concomitantly enacted roles may offset even rather significant self-concept loss in one role. To the extent that an individual is restricted to a very narrow range of social participation, distress as a reaction to role loss is apt to be severe. This is relevant for both men and women in the retirement transition and for women in role loss experience at any time in adulthood.

In his recent study on feelings of loneliness in suburban housewives, Robert Weiss (22) has suggested emotional isolation and social isolation as two distinguishable components. He points out that a happily married couple can nevertheless be lonely because of their lack of social interaction. Social isolation, however, may occur because of the unavailability in the environment of meaningful social roles and of other social and cultural resources, or such isolation may be the result of social and cultural alienation. Alienation can be defined as the consequence of the individual's inability or unwillingness to engage with existing social roles and resources.

In an analysis of the psychosocial factors which may be influential in either the amelioration or the prevention of the depressive spectrum of behavior, as it has been called by Schuyler (23) and others, some applications of behavioristic psychology may be pertinent. If we are not unwittingly conditioned by the original image of the experimenter controlling the subject, the image suggested by the phrase behavioral control, we can find use for the concepts of the experimental analysis of behavior as conceptual methods for the analysis and design of resourceful social and cultural environments dedicated to the effective and rewarding self-control of behavior.

The social and cultural provision of available and accessible social roles and institutional and cultural resources is the obvious way to enhance and maintain a health-inviting environment. When such environments are in being, individual help in managing disengagement, alienation and other precursors or expressions of depressive behavior is likely to succeed. This is so because when the psychobiologic emotional process of interest is restored by whatever means, there is a surrounding world which is structured to respond to that interest and to maintain it.

In this respect the future fate of preventive medicine needs serious and innovative consideration. It is becoming increasingly apparent that precursor conditions to subsequent symptomatic expressions of disease can be specifically identified. Quite beyond the implications of responding amelioratively to the precursors of depressive disorder and of suicide, it is apparent that even for the diseases of cancer, hypertension, diabetes and many others, corrective intervention at the precursor stage is not biomedical but largely psychosocial. Modification of learned behavior, attitudes, values, lifestyles, and environmentally engendered psychosocial stress is becoming increasingly the real province of preventive medicine.

Yet only three years ago the president of the American Medical Association said the care of the acutely ill is the primary task of the physician and anyone who thinks the physician is going to be concerned about the prevention of illness just doesn't understand the situation.

Recently, however, the medical economists are suggesting that the greatest future returns in the conquest of disease morbidity and mortality may very well lie in the liveware of the behavioral sciences rather than in the hardware of biomedical technology.

Two trends, both of which are vitally connected with psychiatric theory and practice, have emerged. The prepaid premium health maintenance organization concept is a trend which will probably not by the very nature of its economics, based on minimizing costs and maximizing savings, provide for the psychosocial management of the behavioral precursors of disease. The second trend is the incursion of private nonmedical enterprise into the preventive field, for example, in the areas of control of eating and smoking. A whole gamut of social organizations for the support and repair of interpersonal relations and the changing of life-styles has come into being outside of medicine and under the auspices of a wide range of ideologies and objectives.

If, indeed, it is close to the truth that a very large number of severely depressed persons do not engage themselves in any kind of psychiatric transaction, then we are obviously reaching even a lesser proportion of persons for whom the successful modification of a precursor might prevent a later symptom of severe impairment or distress.

Finally, since a pessimistic, negative conception of the world as no longer meaningful or no longer interesting is a cognitive component of depressive behavior, a consideration of the contribution of the prevailing cultural reality as a context of depression should be briefly mentioned. There is no concise way to relate changes in cultural values or the changing knowledge and assumptions about the nature of man and of the universe to behavior included within the depressive spectrum. The Age of Depression is as interesting and inconclusive a journalistic phrase as was the psychoanalytically inspired Age of Anxiety.

Yet we have become a secular society. For many, the absolutes of religion have gone, although I suppose it is still possible to say that God is not dead; he is alive and well in DNA. Values, which are the directives for decisions about behavior, are rapidly changing. The meaning of life and hence of personal significance and meaning changes with the discovery and validation of knowledge. Hence values and ontologic meaning can be lost and evoke pervasive depressive feeling and anxiety. Thus, in relationship to the abstract and symbolic, the emotional and behavioral processes of disengagement and recommitment must repeatedly occur. Certainly, W. B. Yeats' oft-quoted sentence, "things fall apart; the centre cannot hold," is an implicitly depressive declaration.

Perhaps, however, it is not outlandishly speculative to suggest that the ecological sciences and the biobehavioral sciences, particularly, are heralding the advent of a new center of stability and significance for us. The ecologic repossession of ourselves as being *in* nature and the biobehavioral repossession of ourselves *as* nature may enable Western man to rejoin the natural reality from which historically he has alienated himself. His meaning and his definition of himself will not then depend so precariously on the immediate social and cultural situation in which he finds himself, but will be sustained by his knowledge that nature is forever renewing its self-consciousness in him.

REFERENCES

1. COHEN, H. C.: *Sherrington: Physiologist, Philosopher and Poet.* Liverpool: Liverpool University Press, 1958.
2. SCOTT, J. P. and SENAY, E. C. (Eds.): *Separation and Depression: Clinical and Research Aspects.* Washington: American Association for Advancement of Science, Publication #94, 1973.
3. PLUTCHIK, R.: Emotions, evolution and adaptive process. *In* M. B. Arnold (Ed.), *Feelings and Emotions.* New York: Academic Press, 1970.
4. HAMBURG, D. A.: Emotions in the perspective of human evolution. *In* P. H. Knapp (Ed.), *Expression of Emotion in Man.* New York: International Universities Press, 1963.
5. TOMKINS, S. S.: *Affect, Cognition and Personality.* New York: Springer, 1965.
6. IZARD, C.: *Patterns of Emotions.* New York: Academic Press, 1972.
7. LZARUS, P. S. and AVERILL, J. R.: Emotion and cognition with special reference to anxiety. *In* C. D. Spielberger, *Anxiety: Current Trends in Theory and Research.* Vol. II. New York: Academic Press, 1973.
8. KAUFMAN, I. C.: On animal models. *In* R. J. Friedman and M. M. Katz (Eds.), *The Psychology of Depression: Contemporary Research and Theory.* New York: John Wiley & Sons, 1974, p. 251.

9. SELIGMAN, M. E. P.: Depression and learned helplessness. *In* R. J. Friedman and M. M. Katz (Eds.), *The Psychology of Depression: Contemporary Research and Theory.* New York: John Wiley & Sons, 1974, p. 983.
10. HOLMES, T. H. and RAHE, R. H.: The social readjustment scale. *J. Psychosom. Res.*, 11:213, 1967.
11. PAYKEL, E. S., et al.: Life events and depression: A controlled study. *Arch. Gen. Psychiat.*, 21:753, 1969.
12. KLINGER, E.: Consequences of commitment to and disengagement from incentives. *Psychol. Rev.*, 82:1, 1975.
13. ENGEL, G. L.: A life-setting conducive to illness: The giving-up-given-up complex. *Bull. Menninger Clin.*, 32:355, 1968.
14. SCHMALE, A., JR.: On development and the conversation-withdrawal reaction. *In* R. J. Friedman and M. M. Katz (Eds.), *The Psychology of Depression: Contemporary Research and Theory.* New York: John Wiley & Sons, 1974.
15. PRIBRAM, K. H.: Feelings as monitors. *In* M. B. Arnold (Ed.), *Feelings and Emotions.* New York: Academic Press, 1970.
16. MANDELL, A.: Neurobiologic barriers to euphoria. *Am. Science*, 61:565, 1973.
17. BOWLBY, J.: *Attachment and Loss.* New York: Basic Books, 1969.
18. CASSEL, J.: Psychosocial processes and stress. *Int. J. Health Services*, Summer, 1974.
19. SCHWAB, J. J. and SCHWAB, R.: The epidemiology of mental illness. *In* G. Usdin (Ed.), *Psychiatry: Education and Image.* New York: Brunner/Mazel, 1973.
20. BECK, A. T.: The development of depression: A cognitive model. *In* R. J. Friedman and M. M. Katz (Eds.), *The Psychology of Depression: Contemporary Research and Theory.* New York: John Wiley & Sons, 1974.
21. MURPHY, H. B. M., WITTKOWER, E. D. and CHANCE, N.: A cross-cultural inquiry into the symptomatology of depression. *Int. J. Psychiatry*, 3:6, 1967.
22. WEISS, R. S.: *Loneliness: The Experience of Emotional and Social Isolation.* Cambridge, Mass.: MIT Press, 1973.
23. SCHUYLER, D.: *The Depressive Spectrum.* New York: Aronson, 1974.

3

The Treatment of Depression: A Selective Historical Review

Charles K. Hofling, M.D.

This is not a comprehensive survey of the history of concepts of depression and its treatment, but an impressionistic overview. It focuses on certain highlights in this long development which appear to have the most to say to twentieth century investigators and practitioners.

In considering even briefly the history of concepts of depression, one can scarcely help noticing that some of the basic issues have been with us for a very long time, such as the relative importance of intrinsic and situational factors. Among the former, there are questions about the relative importance of purely psychological factors and of physicochemical factors; the nature of the relationship between depression and grief (is it, for example, meaningful to speak of a "normal depression"?); variability in the natural history of the disorder; the nature of the optimal therapeutic measures. All of these issues have arisen and have been struggled with over long periods.

Although incomplete and intellectually tantalizing in many ways, the Old Testament story of King Saul's madness is one of the best ancient accounts of what appears to have been a psychotic depression, and as such, it deserves careful consideration. The story appears as part of the running account of the later years of Saul's reign given in *I Samuel*, chapters 15-31. Samuel tells Saul that God has commanded him to destroy utterly the Amelekites: the king, all of the people, and all of their herd animals. Saul wins the victory but spares the king and the livestock. God is represented as angered by Saul's exercise of his own judgment, and Samuel reproaches Saul, saying:

> . . . Rebellion is the sin of witchcraft. . . . Because thou hast rejected the word of the Lord . . . the Lord hath rent the kingdom of Israel from thee this day, and hath given it to a neighbor of thine, that is better than thou. . . .
>
> Then Saul said, I have sinned: yet honour me now, I pray thee, before . . . Israel, and turn again with me, that I may worship the Lord thy God. So Samuel turned again after Saul; and Saul worshipped the Lord.

After this public face-saving, Samuel personally kills Agag, the king of the Amelekites and then leaves the court unmollified.

> And Samuel came no more to see Saul until the day of his death; for Samuel mourned for Saul: and the Lord repented that he had made Saul king over Israel. . . .
>
> Then Samuel took the horn of oil, and anointed him David in the midst of his brethren: and the spirit of the Lord came mightily upon David from that day forward. . . .
>
> Now the spirit of the Lord had departed from Saul, and an evil spirit from the Lord troubled him. And Saul's servants said unto him . . . Let our Lord now command thy servants to seek out a man who is a cunning player upon the harp: and it shall come to pass, when the evil spirit from God is upon thee, that he shall play with his hand, and thou shalt be well. . . .
>
> And David came to Saul, and stood before him: and he loved him greatly. . . . And it came to pass, when the evil spirit from God was upon Saul, that David took the harp and played with his hand: so Saul was refreshed, and was well, and the evil spirit departed from him. . . .
>
> And David went out withersoever Saul sent him, and behaved himself wisely: and Saul set him over the men of war. . . .
>
> And it came to pass as they came, when David returned

from the slaughter of the Philistine, that the women came out
of all the cities of Israel, singing and dancing . . . and said,

Saul hath slain his thousands,
And David his ten thousands.

. . . And Saul was very wroth, and this saying displeased him
. . . and Saul eyed David from that day and forward.

And it came to pass on the morrow, that an evil spirit from
God came mightily upon Saul, and he prophesied [spoke
wildly] in the midst of his house: and David played with his
hand, as he did day by day: and Saul had his spear in his hand.
And Saul cast the spear; for he said, I will smite David even
unto the wall. And David avoided out of his presence twice.
And Saul was afraid of David, because the Lord was with him,
and was departed from Saul. . . .

And Saul spake to Jonathan his son, and to all his servants,
that they should slay David. But Jonathan . . . delighted much
in David. . . . And Jonathan spake good of David unto Saul
his father. . . . And Saul hearkened unto the voice of Jonathan:
and Saul sware, As the Lord liveth, he shall not be put to
death. . . .

[But later] Saul and his men went to seek him . . . and
pursued after David in the wilderness of Macon. . . . And he
came . . . where there was a cave; and Saul went in alone to
cover his feet [to sleep]. Now David and his men were abiding
in the innermost parts of the cave. . . . Then David arose, and
cut off the skirt of Saul's robe privily. . . .

And Saul rose up out of the cave, and went on his way.
David . . . cried after Saul, saying, My lord the king. And
when Saul looked behind him, David . . . did obeisance. And
David said to Saul . . . the Lord had delivered thee today into
my hand in the cave: but mine eye spared thee: and I said I
will not put forth mine hand against the Lord's anointed. Moreover, my father, see . . . the skirt of thy robe in my hand:
for in that I cut off the skirt of thy robe, and killed thee not,
know thou and see that there is neither evil nor transgression
in my hand. . . .

And Saul . . . wept. And he said unto David, Thou are more
righteous than I: for thou hast rendered unto me good, whereas
I have rendered unto thee evil. . . . And now, behold, I know
that thou shalt surely be king, and that the kingdom of Israel
shall be established in thine hand. . . .

> Now the Philistines fought against Israel: and the men of Israel fled before the Philistines. . . . And the Philistines followed hard upon Saul and his sons; and the Philistines slew . . . the sons of Saul. And the battle went sore against Saul, and the Philistine archers overtook him. . . . Then Saul said to his armourbearer, Draw thy sword, and thrust me through herewith; lest these uncircumcised come and thrust me through and abuse me. But his armourbearer would not; for he was sore afraid. Therefore Saul took his own sword, and fell upon it. . . .

Making due allowances for the fact that this account was put into its present form centuries after the events described and by priests wishing to portray Samuel as the righteous instrument of God and not as a political intriguer, this is a remarkable narrative. Although Saul's mental affliction is said to have come from the Lord, the condition is well described, and many clues to the psychological forces at work are given. The depression is portrayed as coming on in middle age to a man of strong and conflicted passions. There is the background of ambivalence toward Samuel, the demanding father-figure, who turns against Saul, allegedly for the king's disobedience to the Lord but actually for his having behaved in a wiser and more humane way than that ordered by the old prophet. Against the background of his own angry, anxious, and guilty feelings, Saul becomes depressed, and he is then introduced to young David (whom, one has every reason to suppose, he knew or suspected to be Samuel's candidate for the succession).

Saul comes to love David, and the young man's kindness, loyalty, and strength as well as his soothing music exert a therapeutic effect upon the king. It is not until Saul experiences the narcissistic injury of hearing himself surpassed in public esteem by David (with all that that implies) that his aggression mounts and cannot be expressed or contained merely in the depressive symptoms. Saul resorts to episodic violence against the young man, but even here, the other side of Saul's ambivalence (reinforced by superego factors) is clearly indicated by the circumstance that this superb old warrior never hits David with his thrown spear.

The story is markedly condensed in the *I Samuel* account, but it is clear that Saul has periods of lucidity and effectiveness until the end of his life. At such times—as in the cave episode—he perceives David's kindness and good-will and is responsive to them, although perhaps made inwardly even guiltier thereby.

The picture is, of course, incomplete, but the main features of a serious depression (perhaps involutional, with some paranoid features) are clearly sketched. The idea of a complex etiology is present, with psychological factors, possibly physiological factors, and still other factors (the "evil spirit from the Lord") being indicated. The relationship of the psychological state to guilt-feelings, to narcissistic injury, and to loss (of Samuel's approval and thus of the Lord's) is indicated, and the therapeutic effects of music and of a calm, strong figure in attendance are suggested.

It is worthy of note that the term *melancholy,* although perfectly current in the vocabulary of the Jacobean (English) translators of the Bible, is never used by them, either in the Old or the New Testament. *Sorrow, sorrowful, sad,* and *sadness* are, of course, used some hundreds of times and in varying senses, as witness the following, more-or-less random quotations.

> Gen. 3:17. And unto Adam he said, because thou hast hearkened unto the voice of thy wife, and has eaten of the tree, of which I commanded thee, saying, thou shalt not eat of it: Cursed is the ground for thy sake; in sorrow shalt thou eat of it all the days of thy life.

> Deut. 28:65. And among those nations shalt thou find no ease, neither shall the sole of thy foot have rest: but the Lord shall give thee there a trembling heart, and failing of the eyes, and sorrow of mind.

> Nem. 2:2. Wherefore the king said unto me, Why is thy countenance sad, seeing thou are not sick? This is nothing else but sorrow of heart. Then I was very sore afraid. . . .

> Isa. 53:34. He is despised and rejected of men; a man of sorrows, and acquainted with grief: and we hid as it were our faces from him; he was despised and we esteemed him not.

Eccl. 7:3, 4. Sorrow is better than laughter: for by the sadness of the countenance the heart is made better. The heart of the wise is in the house of mourning; but the heart of fools is in the house of mirth.

Two important points can be gleaned from these quotations: 1) no semantic distinction is made between low spirits appropriate to circumstances and those inappropriate, and 2) no semantic distinction is made between low spirits due to divine action and those having mundane etiology. One notes also—in the last two quotations—that, in this Semitic literature (as in other material to be mentioned later), there is already the notion that melancholy is somehow related to wisdom and virtue.

In all biblical references to depression the cure is considered to lie in a reconciliation with God. It seems to be recognized that a drastic lowering of the self-esteem may derive from more than one etiological factor, but the remedy is perceived as a sense of reinstatement in the love of God. Of course, due recognition is given to the complexity of the latter factor, so the solution is not necessarily so simple as may appear at first glance.

A brief survey of the contributions of the Greeks and Romans to the thinking about depression can be conveniently focused upon three principal figures: Hippocrates, Aristotle, and Galen.

The Hippocratic school held that the body was essentially composed of four "humours" (liquids): blood, phlegm, black bile (melancholy), and yellow bile (choler). Excess or defect of one or more humours gave rise to disease. A predominance of black bile was held responsible for melancholia (among other ills). Mania was also recognized—although not very clearly defined—but it was not related to melancholia. In fact, neither condition was defined very sharply. Hippocrates recognized that the brain was somehow involved, but he placed his emphasis upon physiology, not psychology.

Aristotle, synthesizing the work of more ancient writers, considered that there were four primary and opposite fundamental qualities—in the material world and represented in the human body: the hot, the cold, the wet, and the dry. The four "elements" were compounded out of these qualities in specific ways: thus earth was hot and wet; fire, hot and dry; water, cold and wet; and air, cold and dry. (Later writers combined the Hippocratic and Aristotelian views, relating the humours to the elements.) Aristotle was typically more interested in theory than in practice, but the writings of subsequent Greek physicians indicate that occupational therapy and music therapy were utilized in the treatment of the mentally disturbed, including melancholics.

Galen achieved the final medical synthesis of classical antiquity and provided most of the scientific medical knowledge of Europe for the next twelve or thirteen centuries. His physiology supposed the existence of three types of "spirits," each associated with a characteristic type of activity of living beings. The "natural spirits" were formed in the liver and distributed by the veins; the "vital spirits" were formed in the heart and distributed by the arteries; and the "animal spirits" were formed in the brain and distributed by the nerves. Mania and melancholia were associated with brain malfunction. Galen noted, however, that symptoms were not invariably an expression of primary disease in the bodily organs producing them.

Leaving aside the not unimportant, but, for the writer, rather vague and confused period of the Middle Ages, we may turn with profit to the great Renaissance English compendium, Robert Burton's *The Anatomy of Melancholy* (1621). This work was a great and immediate success, going through five editions in its author's lifetime.

Burton, himself a victim of what we would now call a mild, chronic neurotic depression with features of neurasthenia, had, however, such an encyclopedic knowledge of ideas then current in Europe about melancholia—ideas of which samples are to be found in Marlowe, Shakespeare, Donne, and other Elizabethans and Jacobeans—that his work is more than merely a summary of the ancients and serves as a helpful background to the discoveries of the nineteenth and early twentieth centuries.

Burton classifies melancholy as a "disease of the head or mind," of which he recognizes the following varieties: "dotage, phrenzy, madness, extasy, lycanthropia, chorus sancti viti [epilepsy], hydrophobia, possession of devils, and melancholy." Of the last-mentioned he writes: "Melancholy is either in disposition or habit. In disposition, is that transitory melancholy which goes and comes upon every small occasion of sorrow, need, sickness, trouble, fear, grief, passion, or perturbation of mind, any manner of care, discontent, or thought, which causeth anguish, dulness, heaviness and vexation of spirit. . . . and from these melancholy dispositions no man living is free . . . none so wise, none so happy, so well-composed, but more or less, some time or other, he feels the smart of it. Melancholy in this sense is the character of morality" (1).

Burton subscribes, at times, to the humoural theory, and he gives considerable weight to theories of divine displeasure, but he is preeminently an eclectic. He thus writes: "The name is imposed from the matter, and disease denominated from the material cause. . . . Melancholia, a sort of melania (black) chole (choler), from black Choler. And whether it be a cause or an effect, a disease or a symptom . . . I will not contend about it. . . . Fear and Sorrow are the true characters and inseparable companions of most melancholy, not all . . . for to some it is most pleasant, as to such as laugh most part; some are bold again, and free from all manner of fear and grief . . ." (1).

Thus Burton lists as causes of melancholy: God, witches, stars, old age, heredity, bad diet, [morbid] bowel function, bad air, immoderate exercise, sleep patterns, and psychological causes. He is, however, clearly more interested in psychological causes, and he lists these essentially as follows:

[Excessive] imagination
Sorrow
Fear
Shame and Disgrace
Envy, Malice, Hatred
[Excessive] Emulation
Anger
Cares, Miseries, Discontents
Concupiscible Appetite, as Desires, Ambition
Covetousness

> Self-love, Vain-glory, Pride
> Love of Gaming and Pleasures immoderate
> [Excessive] love of Learning or over-much Study

To this list Burton adds certain "outward, adventitious, or accidental causes." These are really an extension of the psychological causes, differentiated on the basis of their not being the responsibility of the subject.

> From the Nurse
> [Faulty] Education
> Terrors and Affrights
> Scoffs, Calumnies, bitter Jests
> Loss of Liberty, Servitude, Imprisonment
> Accidents: Death of Friends, Losses, etc.

Burton clearly recognizes the existence of a continuum both between psychological and non-psychological factors and, among the former, between what we would now call predisposing factors and precipitating factors.

Burton discusses "cures" of melancholy at great length, beginning with the following hopeful and not unwise passage.

> Inveterate melancholy, howsoever it may seem to be a continuate, inexorable disease, hard to be cured, yet many times it may be helped, even that which is most violent, or at least it may be mitigated and much eased. Never despair. It may be hard to cure, but not impossible for him that is most grievously afflicted, if he but be willing to be helped.

Burton rejects as "unlawful" cures accomplished through appeal to witches and (good Protestant that he was) to saints. He approves appeals to God through the clergy and prayer, but suggests that this be combined with medical measures.

> It is lawful to appeal to God's immediate ministers to whom in our infirmities we are to seek help. Yet not so that we rely too much, or wholly upon them . . . we must first begin with prayer, and then use physic; not one without the other, but both together.

For the sufferer himself Burton has a great deal of advice, some of it quaint-sounding and fanciful, little of it harmful, and much of it quite sound. He recommends matters of good general hygiene, a reasonable amount of exercise (even if the patient is not so inclined), wholesale diversions, confession of shortcomings to one's friends, the company of cheerful companions, soothing music, and a serious attempt to alter the course of one's life, "removing obstacles and all manner of discontents."

Burton gives a large and delightful section of his book to a consideration of "Heroical or Love Melancholy." He clearly recognizes the part played in the disorder by a narcissistic disturbance, citing examples reminiscent of Romeo in the first act of Shakespeare's *Romeo and Juliet*. He also recognizes that the melancholic can be at times capable (as was Shakespeare's Jaques in *As You Like It*) of a biting wit. The significance of jealousy as a precipitating cause is discussed, and the possibility of a paranoid tinge in the melancholic's productions is noted.

Burton also realizes that, in mild degrees, melancholy may even be related to a kind of creativity; artistically valuable sonnets may, for example, be written by a melancholic. (This idea is, of course, carried even further by Milton in *Il Penseroso:* "Hail, divinest Melancholy!") It looks to us now as if a somewhat coincidental feature were being confused with a typical feature. One can, after all, react to certain kinds of frustration or loss by *both* a moderate lowering of spirits and a partially effective sublimatory effort.

All of this reminds one of the outstanding literary portrayal of melancholia, Hamlet. Although less formal and systematic than Burton's, Shakespeare's knowledge was by far the more profound. Hamlet's melancholy is exquisitely revealed, as in the great soliloquy on suicide.

> O that this too too solid flesh would melt,
> Thaw and resolve itself into a dew!
> Or that the Everlasting had not fix'd
> His canon 'gainst self-slaughter! O God! God!
> How weary, stale, flat, and unprofitable
> Seem to me all the uses of this world. . . .
>
> (I, ii, 129ff.)

The dynamic factors involved in the depression are rather fully indicated and have been discussed in a scholarly fashion, originally and incompletely by Jones (2) and more penetratingly by Eissler (3) and Lidz (4). It now seems reasonably clear that Hamlet's devastating loss of self-esteem, which Shakespeare indicates as the chief factor in his melancholia, is to be considered as primarily resulting from what he considered to be an unforgivable betrayal by his mother; this is shown to be coupled with the blocking of his murderous rage at her (4).

Portrayals such as that of Hamlet or those of some of Burton's more complex examples cannot really have been accounted for (in their authors' views) by a humoral theory of behavior. But then, as Barroll has pointed out, the humoral theory was no longer, by the seventeenth century, taken as a comprehensive psychological statement (5).

When the question of "Elizabethan psychology" is taken in hand, we find that the answers have not only tended to be traditional but various. We hear much of the "humors," for instance, and it is true that sixteenth- and seventeenth-century physicians might indeed have spoken in terms of "black bile" . . . or "sanguine" propensities. That a writer might have shaped character in such terms, however, offers us not simplification but aesthetic and ideological complexities. For to depict according to the humors would lead to results equivalent to those produced by allegory. . . . Ultimately, the theory of "complexions," when not used strictly for medical purposes, was perhaps only the Renaissance shrug of the shoulder at the basic differences among men. Why does one man seek riches, another, power, and a third, love? Humor theory could in part account for such inclinations. . . .

Burton could write an *Anatomy of Melancholy*, but it is not by mere coincidence that such a work ultimately had to become a compendium of all that was thought not only about "complexions" but about the whole matter of psychology, considerations moving far beyond questions that had to do with the purely physical basis of emotion. . . .

Humor theory, in the end, was not useful in the kind of tragedy which sought to analyze the deviations of an imagined character from some ethical norm since, by definition, there was no "cause" for humors and since "innate" bases for more complex activity were not definitive of anything but themselves. . . .

The great work of classification of mental disorders, including affective disorders, so urgently needed despite the wealth of knowledge of human nature shown by the late Renaissance and early modern writers, was undertaken in the eighteenth and nineteenth centuries. Pinel (1745-1826) separated psychotic illnesses into melancholias, manias without delirium, manias with delirium, and "dementia" (intellectual deterioration on whatever basis and idiocy). He believed that severe psychiatric illness might be due to a central nervous system lesion or lesions, but he was convinced that such illness was not something mysteriously superimposed upon the patient, but a result of heredity and life experiences, both of which, in theory at least, were capable of being specified. His treatment measures were a humane and scientific turning away from the purging, blistering, bloodletting and induced vomiting of his predecessors (e.g., Cullen: 1712-1790) and involved a rudimentary kind of milieu therapy and occupational therapy.

Benjamin Rush (1745-1813) discussed melancholia in his *Medical Inquiries and Observations upon the Diseases of the Mind,* the first American textbook of psychiatry. He objected to the term, *melancholia,* however; nor did he like *hypochondriasis* (a frequent synonym) much better. Rush's preferred term was the highly descriptive *tristimania.* He noted that the condition was often not induced by mere external causes but could be causally related to the patient's "person . . . or condition in life." The symptom-picture Rush described was still a confused one; yet he at times grasped the essence of severe depression, noting that somatic delusions, delusions of guilt, disturbed bowel function, and "durable distress of mind" are frequent findings.

Rush's prescriptions for *tristimania* were both physical and psychological. Under the former heading he places bloodletting, purging, emetics, dietary modifications, baths both hot and cold, exercise including hard physical labor, and, perhaps most interestingly, the production of pain. Aside from advocating blistering of the skin through various applications, Rush is not specific as to the means of producing pain, nor does he seem to have grasped the nature of the psychological connection between imposed suffering and relief of depression. He is, however, quite definite as to the existence of such a connection in some cases, and he gives the following illustrative anecdote.

> I once attended a gentleman from Barbadoes who suffered great distress of mind from a hypochondriac gout which floated in his nerves and brain; but no sooner did the gout fix, and excite pain in his hands and feet, than he recovered his spirits, and became pleasant and agreeable to all around him (6).

Those of Rush's remedies which he considered psychological are similar to those given by Burton (whom he quotes several times) and include activity therapies of various sorts, guided conversation, bibliotherapy, and music therapy.

Griesinger (1817-1868) believed that mental illness, including severe depression, were basically due to brain malfunction, but he also gave weight to psychological factors as precipitants. He went so far as to say that "cerebral activity may be modified quite effectually, directly, and immediately by the evocation of frames of mind, emotions and thoughts," adding that "almost no recovery can be perfected without psychical remedies (which may only consist of work, discipline, et cetera)." He regularly recommended work and occupational therapies along with somatic measures of dubious validity.

Kahlbaum (1828-1899), believing that all psychiatric symptoms could be organized into syndromes having at least heuristic value, introduced the term *cyclothymia* in very much its current sense.

Kraepelin (1856-1926) was, of course, the great classifier. Building upon the work of Griesinger, Kahlbaum, and the latter's student, Hecker (1843-1909), he delineated the syndromes of dementia praecox (catatonic, hebephrenic, and paranoid types) and of manic-depressive psychosis.

All of the work touched on above, while leading directly to the great advances of the twentieth century, was not immediately productive of much in the way of therapeutic advances beyond those utilized by the more discerning physicians of the early nineteenth century. Nor did it quickly lead to any meaningful ideas regarding etiology. In the author's collection is the first American edition of Krafft-Ebing's *Lehrbuch der Psychiatrie*. Of the etiology of melancholia—the term depression as a diagnosis did not come into general use until the 1920's—Krafft-Ebing writes the following account (7), quaint-sounding but not without pertinence.

> The fundamental phenomenon in melancholia consists of the painful emotional depression, which has no external, or an insufficient external, cause, and general inhibition of the mental activities, which may be entirely arrested.
> Concerning the inner basis and relation of these two fundamental anomalies of the psychic mechanism in melancholics we have only hypotheses.
> While some regard the painful depression as the expression of a disturbance of nutrition in the psychic organ (psychic neuralgia) from which, as a result, arises the inhibition of the mental activities, a more recent theory regards the inhibition as primary, and the psychic pain as a secondary manifestation due to consciousness of the mental inhibition. Both these theories are at best one-sided. The hypothesis that makes psychic pain secondary does not accord with experience. It could be only so regarded if the intensity of the psychic pain stood in proportional relation to the degree of inhibition, which, however, is not the case, and if the inhibition preceded the psychic pain in time; but even this hypothesis finds no support. The first manifestation is psychic pain; then inhibition follows, which, of course, becomes a new source of psychic pain. The facts force us to conclude that psychic pain and inhibition are co-ordinated phenomena, between which, of course, a mutual reaction is not excluded. At the same time a common fundamental cause may be thought of: a disturbance of cerebral nutrition (anemia?), which leads to lessened production of vital force.

Krafft-Ebing offers the following "general principles for the treatment of melancholia":

1. Give the patient complete physical and mental rest. . . .
2. Surveillance of the patient to protect him from himself and others from him. . . .
3. Care of the general condition and of the amount of food taken.
4. Treatment . . . of sleeplessness, which is very exhausting and favors the development of delusions and hallucinations. Morphine is of little service; chloral hydrate is more valuable, though it cannot be used freely for a long time. Opium is better, as are also sulphonal and trional. Assistance is given by lukewarm baths, especially when prolonged: mustard-baths and Preissnitz packs. In anemic patients, alcoholic stimulants, especially strong beer, have a good effect. . . .
5. Use of symptomatic remedies approved by experience. [In effect, merely a restatement of 1-4.]

The therapy of mania is given as follows:

The most important means of treatment is isolation adapted to the degree of the exaltation, and the prevention of all abnormal irritation, especially excesses. For many cases hospital treatment is sufficient, where an isolated room may be temporarily necessary. To overcome sleeplessness and restlessness at night, chloral hydrate, sulphonal, and trional are useful. Narcotics, especially opium and morphine, so frequently useful in periodic cases, are here disadvantageous, and often have the effect to increase the excitement.

On the other hand, it is rare for lukewarm baths, especially when prolonged, to fail to produce a quieting effect on the central nervous system; but this effect lasts usually only a few hours.

Where states of excitation have their origin in the sexual system, it is well to administer bromides. At the same time, under such circumstances, the patient must be carefully watched on account of the tendency to onanism.

Perhaps, on the whole, one would have preferred to have Burton as a consultant. He would have approved of the baths and the beer, but he would have added "exercise . . . wholesome diversions . . . and an alteration of his course of life."

A more modern-sounding presentation is to be found in textbooks of the 1920's and 1930's. The following excerpts are taken from Sadler's *Theory and Practice of Psychiatry* (published in 1936 but bearing the stamp of the preceding decade) (8).

For more than a quarter of a century I have felt that these disturbances [the affective psychoses] are basically rooted in the endocrine system. While I still hold to this theory, I must confess that no amount of endocrine therapy has been at all helpful. One thing is certain: They are not a simple psychologic defense mechanism, a release technic, or anything of that kind. . . .
As to the far-flung etiology, it most *certainly is constitutional.* There is a *large element of heredity* in this type of disorder. . . . It usually appears by the twenty-fifth year, and the first attack is often the climax of an accumulation of emotional tension. I believe, especially in the milder or prepsychotic types, that there is a very definite subconscious motive of *escape from difficulties.* . . .
I believe there are two types: One, *the constitutional,* in which heredity plays the dominant role, the attacks being severe and almost wholly due to this supposed endocrine disturbance. The second is *the reactive type,* in which patients with the constitutional predisposition to these upheavals, utilize this tendency as a means of fleeing from reality, escaping difficulties, and securing unearned recognition, and otherwise carrying on much as does one indulging in a neurotic defense reaction. Many geniuses are found in the families afflicted with this disorder.

With respect to treatment, Sadler writes:

The backbone of my treatment [presumably in both depression and mania] is isolation and rest. I keep the patients in bed during the early stages and treat them with massage and hydrotherapy. Insomnia is controlled by the judicious use of sodium amytal. As a rule, I give bromides only in the agitated types of depression.
It is my practice, except in stupors, to keep the family away from the patient for a considerable period. He does not have access to either newspapers or telephones. In the milder cases during convalescence, occupational therapy is very helpful.

Very much depends upon the attitude of the medical attendants. Wise discipline proves helpful, but there is no use, in the midst of depression, in trying to "cheer up" the patient. All efforts at real reconstruction and improvement of insight must be carried out between attacks.

One of the reasons for isolating the more serious types is to prevent sexual and alcoholic excesses and waste of money during exaltation as well as to guard against suicide during depression. . . .

The reason for my having chosen Sadler's book in this highly selective survey is, of course, that it represents the very latest date at which a textbook of psychiatry could have been conscientiously written without reference to (a) the highly sophisticated efforts, at Simmel's hospital in Berlin and at the Menninger Clinic, to apply psychoanalytic theory to the all-out, scientific development of milieu (including attitude and occupational) therapy, and (b) the development of shock therapy (insulin, camphor, metrazol, electric), plus the often successful efforts to treat neurotic depressions by classical psychoanalytic techniques. With these advances, the therapy of the affective disorders in the acute stage began to come of age. (Sadler did, of course, refer to "efforts at real reconstruction and improvement of insight," by which he seems to have meant primarily psychoanalytically derived efforts to help the patient mature psychologically to a point at which his vulnerability to subsequent psychotic episodes would be diminished.)

Freud (1856-1939) was, from a very early stage of his researches, interested in depressive phenomena. He at first thought of episodic depression as a form of the neurasthenic reactions, along with neurasthenia proper and anxiety neurosis, being quite aware that a lowering of self-confidence is regularly present (9). His great work *Mourning and Melancholia* (10) traced clearly the course of hostility turned against the self. Abraham (1877-1925), following intimations offered by Freud, was the first to publish on the profound connection between depression and orality (11). As a result of these and other contributions, the psychoanalytic treatment of depressions of less than psychotic intensity became an often effective method. With respect to affective disorders of a graver nature, a development of greater therapeutic significance was that of the hospital based upon psychoanalytic principles. It was in 1926 that Simmel (1882-1947) in Berlin opened *Tegelsee*, the first such hospital in Europe and one which Freud visited on several occasions. It is a matter of pride for American psychiatrists, however, that, in the development of the modern, psychoanalytically-oriented psychiatric hospital, the priority goes to the Menningers. Inspired by the leadership of Karl Menninger (1893-   ), what is now the C. F. Menninger Memorial Hospital in Topeka had its modest beginning when, in September, 1925, the first six psychiatric patients were moved into a remodeled farmhouse on the outskirts of the city (12). The classic paper of William C. Menninger (1899-1966), "Psychoanalytic principles applied to the treatment of hospitalized patients," appeared in 1937 (13). In this article was stated the principle of bringing the entire hospital effort in any given case together under one guiding theme. Thus, the theme in many instances of severe depression was "Encouraging the relief from a sense of guilt for introjected hostility." Occupational therapy, work therapy, and the attitudes of all personnel would be coordinated to implement such a theme.

During the 1930's also were developed the shock therapies for depression. This line of development took place almost entirely in Europe, and it stemmed, in the first instance, from the widely-held (although not entirely correct) notion of a biological incompatibility between epilepsy and schizophrenia. In 1935 von Meduna (1896-1964) reported the induction of convulsions in schizophrenics by the injection of camphor-in-oil (14). This procedure was soon supplanted by the use of pentylenetetrazole (Metrazole, Cardiazole). In 1933 Cerletti (1877-1963) and Bini (1908-1964) had already begun using the administration of an alternating electric current to produce convulsions for therapeutic effect (15), and this method began, by the late 1930's and early 1940's, largely to supplant chemically-induced convulsions, by reasons both of its relative simplicity and precision and its avoidance of the needless moment of terror produced in patients by the chemical methods. Simultaneously with the purely technical developments of the shock therapies occurred the growing realization that they were far more effective in severe depressions than in the schizophrenias.

The development for therapeutic purposes of prefrontal lobotomy by Moniz (1874-1955) after his period of study in Fulton's laboratory was also a product of the 1930's (16). Subsequent technical modifications by Freeman (1895-1972) and others vastly increased the popularity of the procedure for a time, but it is now used only very seldom for affective disorders (17).

The modern era in the treatment of depression, particularly in serious form, may be considered to have begun in the 1950's. The year 1951 marked the first use of isoniazid and iproniazid in the treatment of tuberculosis, and it was quickly noted that both compounds, but particularly iproniazid, exerted mood-elevating effects upon the tuberculous patients. By the following year Delay began studying the effects of iproniazid upon depressed patients (18). Although iminodibenzyl was synthesized in the last century, the synthesis of its derivative, imipramine, was not performed until 1948 (Häfliger), and the discovery of the usefulness of the latter compound was made by Kuhn in 1958 (19). From the work of Delay and Kuhn to the present, the line of development is unbroken.

Several impressions emerge from this brief and somewhat arbitrary glance at the long developmental history of ideas about depression and its treatment. There is, on the one hand, the recognition that the concept of a continuum among conditions marked by low spirits and an aversion to activity has been traditionally noted by the more thoughtful observers. On the other hand, it is equally clear that only through persistent efforts at classification within this large area have modern advances become possible. Perhaps most important of all are the interrelated ideas of a multifactorial etiology and a multiple approach to therapy, with due consideration being given both to those factors best comprehended in somatic terms and those best comprehended in psychological terms.

REFERENCES

1. BURTON, R.: *The Anatomy of Melancholy.* Oxford, 1621. Reprinted, with translation of French and Latin passages, F. Dell and P. Jordan-Smith (Eds.). New York: Tudor Publishing Co., 1941.
2. JONES, E.: *Hamlet and Oedipus.* New York: W. W. Norton, 1949.
3. EISSLER, K.: *Discourse on Hamlet and Hamlet.* New York: International Universities Press, 1971.
4. LIDZ, T. *Hamlet's Enemy: Madness and Myth in Hamlet.* New York: Basic Books, 1975.
5. BARROLL, J. L.: *Artificial Persons.* Columbia, S. C.: University of South Carolina Press, 1974.
6. RUSH, B.: *Medical Inquiries and Observations Upon the Diseases of the Mind* (1812). Reissued, New York: Hafner Publishing Co., 1962.
7. KRAFFT-EBING, R. VON: *Textbook of Insanity* (Chaddock, C. G., tr.). Philadelphia: F. A. Davis, 1904.
8. SADLER, W. S.: *Theory and Practice of Psychiatry.* St. Louis: Mosby, 1936.
9. FREUD, S.: The aetiology of the neuroses (1893). *In The Standard Edition of the Complete Psychological Works of Sigmund Freud,* Vol. 1. London: Hogarth Press, 1950.
10. FREUD, S.: Mourning and melancholia (1917), *Standard Edition,* Vol. 14. London: Hogarth Press, 1957.
11. ABRAHAM, K.: The first pregenital stage of the libido (1916). *In: Selected Papers on Psychoanalysis.* London: Hogarth Press, 1948.
12. WINSLOW, W.: *The Menninger Story.* Garden City, N. Y.: Doubleday, 1956.
13. MENNINGER, W. C.: Psychoanalytic principles applied to the treatment of hospitalized patients. *Bull. Menn. Clinic,* 1:35, 1936-1937.
14. MEDUNA, L. J. and FRIEDMAN, E.: The convulsive-irritative therapy of the psychoses. *J.A.M.A.,* 112:6, 1939.
15. CERLETTI, U. and BINI, L.: L'Elettroshock. *Arch. Gen. Neurol. Psichiat. Psicoanal.,* 19:266, 1938.
16. MONIZ, E.: *Tentatives Opératoires dans le Traitement de Certaines Psychoses.* Paris: Masson, 1936.
17. GREENBLATT, M.: Psychosurgery. *In* A. M. Freedman and H. Kaplan (Eds.), *Comprehensive Textbook of Psychiatry.* Baltimore: Williams & Wilkins, 1967.
18. GOODMAN, L. S. and GILMAN, A.: *The Pharmacological Basis of Therapeutics,* 3rd ed. New York: Macmillan, 1965.
19. KUHN, R.: The treatment of depressive states with G22355 (imipramine hydrochloride). *Am. J. Psychiat.,* 115:459, 1958.

GENERAL BIBLIOGRAPHY

ADAMS, F.: *The Genuine Works of Hippocrates*. New York: Wood, 1886.

ALEXANDER, F. and SELESNICK, S. T.: *The History of Psychiatry*. New York: Harper & Row, 1966.

ANTHONY, E. J. and BENEDEK, T.: *Depression and Human Existence*, Boston: Little, Brown, 1975.

BELLAK, L., PASQUARELLI, B., PARKES, E., BELLAK, S. S. and BRAVER-MAN, S.: *Manic-Depressive Psychosis and Allied Conditions*. New York: Grune & Stratton, 1952.

The Bible, King James Version.

The Encyclopaedia Britannica, 14th Ed. New York: Encyclopaedia Britannica, Inc., 1929.

GOSHEN, C. E.: *Documentary History of Psychiatry*. New York: Philosophical Library, 1967.

HINSIE, L. E. and CAMPBELL, R. J.: *Psychiatric Dictionary*, 3rd Ed. New York: Oxford University Press, 1960.

HUNTER, R. and MACALPINE, I.: *Three Hundred Years of Psychiatry: 1535-1860*. London: Oxford University Press, 1963.

PINEL, P.: *A Treatise on Insanity* (David, D. D., tr.). London: Cadell and Davies, 1906.

RAYMOND, A.: *Sciences in Greek and Roman Antiquity*. London: Methuen & Co., 1927.

SCHNECK, J. M.: *A History of Psychiatry*. Springfield, Ill.: Thomas, 1960.

SHAKESPEARE: *Hamlet*. The Yale Shakespeare. New Haven, Conn.: Yale University Press, 1947.

ZILBOORG, G.: *A History of Medical Psychology*. New York: Norton, 1941.

4

Classification of Mood Disorders

*Robert L. Spitzer, M.D., Jean Endicott, Ph.D.,
Robert A. Woodruff, Jr., M.D. and
Nancy Andreasen, Ph.D., M.D.*

Mood disorders are perhaps the oldest of the recognized psychiatric disorders. Saul's melancholic state, described in I Samuel, portrays the syndrome clearly, even as to its episodic nature. Our problem is not in recognizing the severe form of the disorder, such as that manifested by Saul, but rather in understanding its limits and the most satisfactory scheme for subclassifying its many forms. This paper will describe a classification system being considered by the Task Force on Nomenclature and Statistics of the American

All authors are members of the American Psychiatric Association Task Force on Nomenclature and Statistics.

Following the presentation of this paper at the 1976 American College of Psychiatrists annual meeting, discussion with members of the College indicated the need for further revisions in the classification, particularly with regard to the major-minor distinction. The current approach towards the classification eliminates the minor categories and subdivides the major depressive disorders into levels of severity. Finally, a residual group of other mood disorders allows the classification of individuals with a disturbance of mood who are not classifiable in any of the previous categories.

Psychiatric Association for inclusion in the third edition of its Diagnostic and Statistical Manual, which is expected to go into effect in 1978 or 1979. In addition to contrasting this approach with previous ones and providing a rationale for this system, we include a provisional text of the mood disorder section of DSM-III.

Kraepelin's creative separation of the manic-depressive psychoses from dementia praecox (schizophrenia) in the 1890's is well known. In 1917 the first official classification system in this country was formulated by the American Medico-Psychological Association (later to become the American Psychiatric Association). It was largely Kraepelinian and was primarily designed for hospital use. Only two mood disorders were listed: manic-depressive psychosis and involutional melancholia. The category of "reactive depression," which reflected Meyerian influence, was added in the 1935 classification and was clearly separated from the psychotic mood disorders by its placement under the category of psychoneuroses. The term affective disorders was used first in 1951 in the Standard Veteran's Administration classification and included manic depressive reaction, psychotic depressive reaction and involutional melancholia. In addition, cyclothymic personality appeared for the first time under a section titled character and behavior disorders. The DSM-I classification of 1952 was essentially the same as the Veteran's Administration classification with only slight modifications. Affective disorders now became affective reactions, and involutional melancholia was reclassified in the general group of disorders of metabolism, growth, and nutrition or endocrine function. DSM-II, published in 1968, was greatly influenced by the eighth edition of the International Classification of Diseases. The DSM-I affective reactions became major affective disorders (corresponding to the ICD-8 term Affective Psychoses), which now included involutional melancholia as well as manic-depressive illness, but excluded psychotic depressive reaction which now was listed separately. This corresponded to the European emphasis on the endogenous-reactive distinction. The depressive reaction of DSM-I became depressive neurosis in DSM-II. Cyclothymic personality remained, even though the ICD-8 corresponding category of thymic personality was a broader concept which included individuals who were characterologically depressed without periods of hypomania.

In developing DSM-III, our first problem was to decide whether to continue the tradition of listing the mood disorders in several areas of the nomenclature. As the historical review indicates, the implication of the assignment of one milder form of the episodic disorder to the category of neurosis was that it was best understood as either reactive or as a defense against anxiety in contrast to the severe forms which were generally conceptualized as endogenous. Also, the implication of categorizing some mild mood swings as personality disorders assumed discontinuity with the severe forms (manic depressive illness) even though most observers have always believed that mild forms are probably related to severe forms in some way.

The general approach towards classification to be taken in DSM-III is to use etiology as a classification axis only if there is convincing evidence to support it. In the absence of such evidence, categories are grouped together if they share important clinical-descriptive features. This approach has the advantage that it groups disorders which share essential and common features without making assumptions as to their etiology. For this reason, we have decided to group together nearly all of the disorders which are characterized by a disturbance of mood. This includes all of the depressions and manias regardless of severity, chronicity, course, or apparent association with precipitating stress.

The category of schizo-affective disorders which was introduced first in the standard nomenclature in DSM-I as a subtype of schizophrenic reactions will not be included in the mood disorders. A burgeoning literature has developed recently which questions whether schizo-affective disorders should be considered subtypes of schizophrenia, variants of mood disorders, or a separate group of disorders entirely. Our assessment of this literature suggests that there is convincing evidence that at least some of the so-called schizo-affective disorders are probably atypical mood disorders (1, 2), whereas others may be schizophrenic (3, 4), and some may be neither. However, the lack of agreement as to how to define this group makes the interpretation of the research findings difficult, and has led us to the decision to continue to include these disorders as a subtype of schizophrenia until more definitive evidence is available. We believe that the provision of carefully defined operational criteria for schizo-affective disorders in DSM-III will facilitate such studies.

Major mood disorders frequently are accompanied by delusions or hallucinations which even may be prominent features of the illness. There are no features that are universally agreed upon as differentiating schizophrenia from the mood disorders. Nevertheless, we have chosen to use as exclusion criteria for a diagnosis of mood disorder certain forms of delusions and hallucinations which are highly suggestive of schizophrenia. Several of these features are called first rank symptoms, from the work of Kurt Schneider (5). An example is the experience of thought insertion or delusions of control. Although several American studies have questioned whether they actually are pathognomonic (5), the WHO International Pilot Study of Schizophrenia (6) and Wing and Nixon (7) have demonstrated that they are extremely useful for differential diagnosis.

Our next problem was to decide if we wished to continue the use of the term affective disorders to describe the section of the nomenclature under discussion. It is not clear to us why this term, rather than mood disorders, was used as the general term to describe these disorders beginning with the 1951 classification. This is particularly puzzling since the term affect is usually used in a broader sense than mood. Affect refers to an immediately observed emotion, such as anger, fear or sadness. Disturbances of affect thus are seen in a variety of psychiatric disorders, such as the flatness of affect which is characteristic of schizophrenia or the lability of affect which is characteristic of some organic brain disorders. In fact, disturbance of affect occurs with almost all medical as well as psychiatric disorders. On the other hand, mood usually is used in a more restricted sense to refer to a pervasive and sustained emotion which colors the individual's perception of the world. This definition of mood is consistent with Bleuler's use of the term: "If a definite affect persists and dominates for some time the whole personality, with all its experiences, we speak of a mood." In practice, the term mood disturbance usually is restricted to two specific types of emotion: depression and elation.

We believe that the distinction between a transient affective disturbance and a more pervasive and prolonged disturbance involving either depression or elation (mood) has clinical utility; in fact, this is the unifying principle which distinguishes all of the disorders discussed above from other conditions in which affect may be temporarily disturbed. Therefore, we have decided to group together all disorders involving the predominant disturbance of mood as defined above under the general rubric of mood disorders rather than affective disorders. We realize the difficulties in having to learn new terms for old concepts and advocate this change only because we believe that the long-term benefits of increased conceptual clarity outweigh the disadvantages of using a new term.

Our next task was to decide upon the most useful basis for subclassification of the mood disorders. A number of subclassifications, usually based on dichotomous subtypes, have been used or proposed. None of them has been entirely satisfactory for a variety of reasons. The DSM-II classification of these disorders used several, sometimes competing, principles. The major subdivision was between those disorders in which the "onset of the mood does not seem to be related directly to a precipitating life experience" (the major affective disorders) and those in which a life experience or internal conflict seemed to be a precipitant (psychotic depressive reaction and depressive neurosis). The problem with this approach is that it implies that stressful life events or internal conflicts are never a significant factor in manic depressive disorders, and it also implies the corollary that they are always involved in mild disorders. The research literature (8, 9, 10) on the relationship of life events and stress to the onset of depression indicates that there is no simple relationship. It is true that some evidence suggests that the absence of precipitating events has some predictive power regarding response to ECT. However, the unreliability of the judgment about the role of precipitating factors and the greater power of other bases for classification have led us to reject this dichotomy as a basis for subdivision.

DSM-II expanded the usual notion of psychotic (delusions, hallucinations, bizarre behavior) to include "mental functioning . . . sufficiently impaired to interfere grossly with (the) capacity to meet the ordinary demands of life," so that severe depression or mania without delusions or hallucinations could be justified as psychotic illnesses. However, by expanding the traditional definition of psychosis, DSM-II reduced it to a concept so vague as to limit its reliable usage. We have decided instead to restore the concept of psychotic to its traditional meaning, but have used it only as a qualifying phrase after more fundamental distinctions have been made.

DSM-II included involutional melancholia, a distinction based on age of onset of a first depressive episode. There has been vigorous discussion about whether this condition should be separated from others, which was acknowledged in the DSM-II text. Various authors have adopted different positions about the age limits of the involutional period itself, as well as about what the characteristic symptoms of a depression occurring for the first time during this period might be. Recently, some investigators (11, 12) have found little evidence to support its status as a separate diagnostic disorder, and therefore we have decided not to make the distinction in DSM-III.

A distinction that many research investigators have found useful is that of the primary-secondary dichotomy (13). A primary mood disorder is defined as one occurring without any antecedent psychiatric diagnosis, whereas a secondary mood disorder is defined as one occurring subsequent to the development of some other psychiatric disorder (not a mood disorder). The impetus for the development of this distinction was an effort to obtain relatively homogeneous subgroups of patients with mood disorder who did not manifest other conditions, such as alcoholism or antisocial personality. We believe that this distinction is important for research purposes and probably also for clinical reasons. However, the distinction could be expressed through the use of multiple diagnoses for con-

Table 1. — Comparison of Classification of Mood Disorders in DSM–II and III

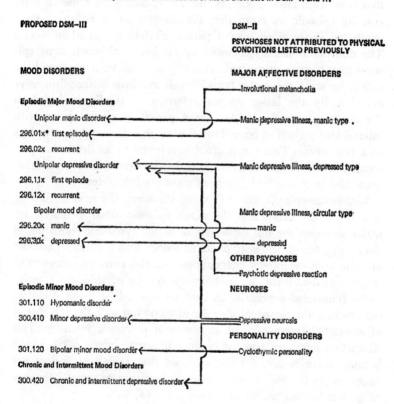

PROPOSED DSM–III	DSM–II
	PSYCHOSES NOT ATTRIBUTED TO PHYSICAL CONDITIONS LISTED PREVIOUSLY
MOOD DISORDERS	MAJOR AFFECTIVE DISORDERS
	Involutional melancholia
Episodic Major Mood Disorders	
Unipolar manic disorder	Manic depressive illness, manic type .
296.01x* first episode	
296.02x recurrent	
Unipolar depressive disorder	Manic depressive illness, depressed type
296.11x first episode	
296.12x recurrent	
Bipolar mood disorder	Manic depressive illness, circular type
296.20x manic	manic
296.30x depressed	depressed
	OTHER PSYCHOSES
	Psychotic depressive reaction
Episodic Minor Mood Disorders	NEUROSES
301.110 Hypomanic disorder	
300.410 Minor depressive disorder	Depressive neurosis
	PERSONALITY DISORDERS
301.120 Bipolar minor mood disorder	Cyclothymic personality
Chronic and Intermittent Mood Disorders	
300.420 Chronic and intermittent depressive disorder	

* An x as the sixth digit indicates that the current condition is further specified as 1 = psychotic, 2 = ill but not psychotic, and 3 = in remission.

current conditions or the listing of previous psychiatric disorders in a full diagnosis.

In the classification that we propose (Table 1), the first distinction is between mood disorders that are episodic and those that are not. By episodic we mean that the disorder has a relatively clear onset and is sustained over a period of time measured in weeks. The disorder is usually followed by remission, although some episodes may become protracted. This is contrasted with what we have called, for want of a better term, chronic and intermittent depressive disorder. By the latter we are referring to conditions in which the depressed mood persists over a period of several years with intermittent periods of normal mood which last from only a few days to a few weeks. This group often is referred to as depressive personality or depressive character, diagnostic terms which never have been used in a standard American classification system.

Within the episodic group of mood disorders, the next distinction is between the major and the minor episodic mood disorders. By major we mean the full depressive or manic syndrome consisting of the persistence of depressed or elated moods with a sufficient number of associated symptoms characteristic of the two syndromes. The major disorders often, but not invariably, are of sufficient severity to be considered psychotic. In contrast, the minor mood disorders demonstrate the persistent disorder of mood but lack the full cluster of associated symptoms and are never of psychotic intensity. This distinction has been adopted because it can be made reliably, and because there is considerable evidence that biological factors are important in the major mood disorders, response to somatic therapy or genetic loading within the family (14, 15, 16).

The DSM-II categories of manic-depressive psychosis, involutional melancholia, psychotic depressive reaction, and severe forms of neurotic depression all are included in the DSM-III category of major episodic mood disorders. The milder forms of DSM-II neurotic depression and cyclothymic personality would be included in the episodic minor mood disorders of DSM-III.

Within the episodic major mood disorder, the next distinction is between unipolar and bipolar, a distinction that Kraepelin himself was aware of and which was emphasized later by Leonhard (14, 15, 16, 17). Bipolar refers to the presence of both manic and depressive episodes (at least one of which was major); unipolar refers to major episodes of either manic or depressive illness alone. The unipolar-bipolar distinction has been validated by a number of studies that found differences in clinical variables such as age of onset, sex ratio, familial pattern of illness, and response to somatic treatment (14). Other studies have suggested differences in biochemical and neuro-physiological variables (18).

Within the unipolar and bipolar groups, the unipolars initially are subtyped as first episode or recurrent episode, and the bipolars as manic or depressed depending on the symptoms of the current or most recent episode.

We recognize that some investigators use the term unipolar in a more restricted sense, sometimes to refer to patients with at least three or more episodes, sometimes to refer only to depressive conditions. We have chosen the first episode vs. recurrent episode because it avoids the problem of classification of patients who have had only one or two episodes. At the same time, it discriminates between individuals who have had only one episode from those who have had more. We have chosen to restrict bipolar illness to those patients who have had both types to leave open the question of whether unipolar manic patients differ in some fundamental way from bipolar patients. A further consideration is that the proposed system is simpler and more logical in that patients diagnosed as bipolar will have manifested both poles of the illness.

The last distinction within the episodic major mood disorders is relegated to a sixth digit and characterizes the current condition as either psychotic (as defined above), ill but not psychotic, or in remission. The psychotic-not psychotic distinction is of practical importance in patient management, and there is some evidence suggesting it has a relationship to somatic treatment outcome (19). The notation "in remission" is of particular importance to psychiatrists now who have begun to treat some patients with lithium even when they are completely asymptomatic and in remission.

A diagnosis of episodic minor mood disorder would be given only to individuals who never have had an episode of major mood disorder. Thus, it is assumed that minor mood disturbances which occur in individuals who previously were ill with major mood disorders are attenuated forms of the more severe disorder. The episodic minor mood disorders are subtyped into three groups which correspond roughly to the major disorders: minor depressive disorder, hypomanic disorder and bipolar minor mood disorder. The latter is for individuals who have had at least one episode of both minor depressive disorder and hypomania (the equivalent of minor mania). Patients who would have been classified as cyclothymic personality in DSM-II (few ever were!) would be classified here.

It is recognized that many individuals with minor depressive disorders, and particularly those with hypomanic or bipolar minor mood disorders, may eventually develop a major mood disorder.

We believe that this proposed classification is consistent with the general goals of DSM-III: to develop a classification system that is as objective and reliable as possible, that takes into account the latest available research evidence in order to delineate categories that are useful (i.e., valid) for clinical, research and administrative purposes. We invite the profession to examine this classification critically so that we may make improvement in it prior to its inclusion in DSM-III. We neither expect nor wish this classification to endure forever. It is hoped that the provision of specific criteria for all of the categories will enable future research studies to supply data that will be useful in making improvements.

The proposed text for the mood disorder section of DSM-III follows.

V. MOOD DISORDERS

Episodic major mood disorders

Essential features, course, familial pattern, sex ratio, age at onset. A group of disorders characterized by episodes of illness in which there is a prominent and persistent disturbance in mood involving either the depressive or manic syndrome. Such episodes are referred to as major depressive or manic episodes. Major mood disorders include unipolar depressive disorders, unipolar manic disorders, and bipolar mood disorders. These conditions are often recurrent, and usually followed by a return to the premorbid level of function. Although some cases are chronic, there is rarely deterioration in general functioning or personality. During an episode, however, these conditions are often incapacitating. Relatives of patients with these conditions have a higher prevalence of mood disorder than occurs in the general population. These conditions are diagnosed more frequently in women than in men. Unlike most other psychiatric disorders, the age at onset is fairly evenly distributed throughout adult life, although manic conditions tend to begin in early adulthood.

Differential diagnosis. Several features distinguish these disorders from schizophrenia. Personality and general functioning are usually satisfactory prior to and after an episode of mood disorder, although mild disturbances in mood may occur. Although delusions, and more rarely hallucinations and disorders of thinking, may be present in the major mood disorders, schizo-affective schizophrenia should be diagnosed when these symptoms take certain specific forms (see exclusion criteria for each of the mood disorders).

Subclassification. A variety of subclassifications has been proposed for the episodic major mood disorders, usually based on dichotomous distinctions. The overall group has been divided into unipolar and bipolar while the depressive episodes have been divided into neurotic vs. psychotic, endogenous vs. reactive, agitated vs. retarded and primary vs. secondary. The subclassifications presented here separate the entire group into unipolar and bipolar based on whether or not both the manic and major depressive episodes are involved or only one of them. This distinction has considerable validity in terms of differential clinical and genetic features, as well as response to somatic therapy. The unipolar disorders are further classified at the fifth digit to indicate if the current episode is the first episode or a recurrence. The current condition is further classified at the sixth digit as either psychotic, ill but not psychotic, or in remission.

Major depressive disorder

Essential features. The essential feature of a major depressive episode is dysphoric mood which is prominent and relatively persistent and associated with other symptoms of the depressive syndrome. These symptoms may include loss of interest or pleasure, sleep disturbance, anorexia, weight loss, psychomotor agitation or retardation, cognitive disturbance, decreased energy, a feeling of worthlessness or guilt, and thoughts of death or suicide.

A person with the depressive syndrome will describe his mood as sad, hopeless, discouraged, down in the dumps, or some other colloquial variant. Sometimes, however, the mood disturbance may not be expressed as a synonym for depressive mood but rather as a complaint of not caring anymore, or a painful inability to experience pleasure. The loss of interest or pleasure is probably always present to some degree but sometimes the patient may not complain of this or even be aware of its existence except in retrospect. More typically there is withdrawal from friends and family, and avocations that used to be a source of pleasure are neglected. Early morning awakening is the most characteristic sleep disturbance, although initial insomnia, fitful sleep, or hypersomnia also occur. The anorexia may be accompanied by weight loss which can be severe. Psychomotor agitation may take the form of pacing, handwringing, inability to sit still, pulling or rubbing on hair, skin, clothing, or other objects, outbursts of complaining or shouting, or talking incessantly. The psychomotor retardation may take the form of slowed speech, increased pauses before answering, low or monotonous speech, slowed body movements, or when severe, markedly decreased amount of speech, or muteness.

The cognitive disturbance may manifest itself as inability to concentrate, indecisiveness, slowed thinking, or complaints of poor memory. The decrease in energy level is experienced as sustained tiredness or fatigue even in the absence of any physical exertion. The sense of worthlessness varies from mild feelings of inadequacy to completely unrealistic negative evaluation of one's worth. The smallest task may seem difficult or impossible. Minor failings may be exaggerated and the environment searched for cues confirming a negative self-evaluation. Guilt may be expressed as an excessive reaction to either current or past failings or as a delusional conviction of sinfulness or responsibility for some untoward or tragic event. Thoughts of death or suicide may involve fears of dying, the belief that the patient or others would be better off if they were dead, or suicidal desires or plans. Often the symptoms are worse when the patient wakes up but improve slightly as the day progresses. When the disturbance is mild, temporary improvement follows positive environmental stimuli. When the disturbance is severe, the syndrome is unrelentingly persistent despite any environmental change.

Associated features. Common associated features include depressed appearance, tearfulness, feelings of anxiety, irritability, or fearfulness, brooding, excessive concern with physical health, panic attacks, and phobias. Paranoid symptoms may be present and range from mild suspiciousness through ideas of reference and more rarely to frank delusions. Common paranoid delusions include the idea that one is being persecuted because of sinfulness or some inadequacy. Occasionally, however, paranoid delusions will be present in which there is no obvious connection with the depressive ideation. Other types of delusions which are more clearly consistent with the depressive ideation include nihilistic delusions of world destruction, hypochondriacal delusions of cancer or other serious illness, or delusions of poverty. Hallucinations are uncommon and when they occur are usually transient and the content is usually related to the depressed mood.

Onset and predisposing factors. The onset is variable with symptoms developing over a period of days to weeks. In some instances, prodromal symptoms, which include generalized anxiety, panic attacks, phobias, or mild depressive symptoms, may occur over a period of several months. Sometimes an episode develops immediately following a stressful life event, although other episodes, even in the same person, may occur without obvious precipitating factors. It is unclear whether episodes associated with stress are fundamentally different from those that are not.

Impairment and complications. The degree of impairment varies but there is always some interference in social or occupational functioning. If the depression is severe, incapacity may be marked and pervade all areas of functioning. The most serious complication is suicide, which occurs in approximately 15 percent of patients.

Differential diagnosis. Major depressive disorder must be distinguished from schizophrenia, schizo-affective, depressed type, and from minor depressive disorder. It differs from schizophrenia in that formal thought disorder is absent and delusions or hallucinations, when present, are usually consistent with the depressive mood. In addition, certain types of hallucinations or delusions are considered indicative of schizo-affective schizophrenia (see operational criteria). It differs from minor depressive disorder primarily in terms of severity. Many other psychiatric disorders, such as Briquet's disorder or antisocial personality, are accompanied by depressive mood. Major depressive disorder should be the basis of an additional diagnosis only when the full operational criteria are met.

Operational criteria for a major depressive disorder. A through C are required.

A. Dysphoric mood characterized by symptoms such as the following: depressed, sad, blue, hopeless, low, down in the dumps, "don't care anymore," irritable, worried. The mood disturbance must be prominent and relatively persistent but not necessarily the most dominant symptom. It does not include momentary shifts from one dysphoric mood to another dysphoric mood, e.g., anxiety to depression to anger, such are seen in states of acute psychotic turmoil.

B. At least 4 of the following symptoms:

    1) Poor appetite or weight loss or increased appetite or weight gain (change of 1 lb. a week over several weeks or 10 lbs. a year when not dieting).

    2) Sleep difficulty or sleeping too much.

    3) Loss of energy, fatigability, or tiredness.

    4) Psychomotor agitation or retardation (but not mere subjective feeling of restlessness or being slowed down).

    5) Loss of interest or pleasure in usual activities, or decrease

in sexual drive (do not include if limited to a period when delusional or hallucinating).

6) Feelings of self-reproach or excessive or inappropriate guilt (either may be delusional).

7) Complaints or evidence of diminished ability to think or concentrate such as slow thinking, or indecisiveness (do not include if associated with obvious formal thought disorder).

8) Recurrent thoughts of death or suicide, including thoughts of wishing to be dead.

C. Duration of at least 2 weeks.

D. None of the following which suggests schizophrenia is present.

1) Delusions of control or thought broadcasting, insertion, or withdrawal.

2) Hallucinations of any type throughout the day for several days or intermittently throughout a 1 week period unless all of the content is clearly related to depression or elation.

3) Auditory hallucinations in which either a voice keeps up a running commentary on the patient's behaviors or thoughts as they occur, or 2 or more voices converse with each other.

4) At some time during the period of illness had delusions or hallucinations for more than 1 month in the absence of prominent affective (manic or depressive) symptoms (although typical depressive delusions, such as delusions of guilt, sin, poverty, nihilism, or self-deprecation or hallucinations of similar content are permitted).

5) Preoccupation with a delusion or hallucinations to the relative exclusion of other symptoms or concerns (other than delusions of guilt, sin, poverty, nihilism, or self-deprecation, or hallucinations with similar content).

6) Definite instances of formal thought disorder.

E. Excludes grief reactions following loss of a loved one if all of the features are commonly seen in members of the subject's subcultural group in similar circumstances.

Manic episode

Essential features. The essential feature of a manic episode is a distinct period when the predominant mood is either elevated, expansive or irritable and is associated with other symptoms of the manic syndrome. These symptoms may include hyperactivity, excessive involvement in activities without recognizing the high potential for painful consequences, pressure of speech, flight of ideas, inflated self-esteem, decreased need for sleep, and distractibility. The elevated mood may be described as euphoric, unusually good, cheerful, or high, and often has an infectious quality to the uninvolved observer but is recognized as excessive by those who know the patient well. The expansive quality of the mood disturbance is characterized by unceasing and unselective enthusiasm for relating to people and other aspects of the environment. Although elevated mood is considered the classic symptom, the mood disturbance may primarily be one of irritability instead. The irritability may be most apparent when the patient is thwarted. The hyperactivity is generalized and often involves excessive planning and participation in multiple activities which may be sexual, occupational, political or religious. Almost invariably there is increased sociability, such as renewing old acquaintances or calling friends at all hours of the night. The intrusive, domineering, and demanding nature of these interactions is not recognized by the patient. Frequently the patient's expansiveness, grandiosity, and lack of judgment regarding possible consequences lead to such activities as buying sprees, reckless driving, foolish business investments, and sexual behavior unusual for the patient. Often the activities have a disorganized, flamboyant or bizarre quality; for example, dressing up in colorful and strange garments, wearing excessive and poorly applied make-up, and distributing bread, candy, money and advice to passing strangers.

Manic speech is typically loud, rapid, and difficult to interpret. Often it is full of jokes, puns, amusing irrelevancies, and it can become theatrical with singing and rhetorical mannerisms. If the mood is more irritable than expansive, there often are complaints, hostile comments and angry tirades. Frequently there are abrupt changes from topic to topic based on understandable associations, distracting stimuli or play on words (flight of ideas). Distractibility is usually present and manifests itself as changes in speech or activity as a result of attending to various irrelevant external stimuli, such as background noise, or clothing worn by a visitor.

Almost invariably there is inflated self-esteem ranging from uncritical self-confidence to marked grandiosity which often approaches delusional proportions. For instance, advice may be given on matters about which the patient has no special knowledge, such as how to run a psychiatric hospital or the federal government. In the absence of any particular talent a novel may be started, music composed, or a patent sought for some impractical invention. Common grandiose delusions involve a special relationship to God or some well-known figure from the political, religious or entertainment worlds.

Almost invariably there is a decreased need for sleep so that the patient awakens several hours before his usual time full of energy. When the sleep disturbance is severe, the patient may go for days without any sleep at all and yet feel well rested.

Associated features. Common associated features include lability of mood with rapid shifts to anger or depression. The depression, with tearfulness, suicidal threats and other depressive symptoms, may last moments, hours, or more rarely, days. Occasionally the depressive symptoms are intermingled with the manic symptoms while at other times they replace them temporarily. Hallucinations of any type may occur but the content is almost always clearly related to the mood. For example, God's voice may be heard explaining the patient's special mission. Persecutory or sexual delusions may occur, usually with an implicit grandiose theme, or related to the response of others to the disturbed behavior.

Impairment and complications. The degree of impairment varies from mild to severe. Mild forms of the manic syndrome, in which there is no gross impairment in judgment, functioning or ability to hold a meaningful conversation, are often referred to as hypomanic episodes. In the moderate to severe forms, incapacity is such that the patient is usually unable to function and requires protection from the consequences of his poor judgment or hyperactivity. In the past, this condition has sometimes resulted in death from physical exhaustion. During the manic episode there may be drug or alcohol abuse.

Onset and course. Manic episodes typically begin suddenly with a rapid escalation of symptoms over a few days. The episodes usually last from a few days to months, are briefer and have a more abrupt termination than major depressive episodes.

Differential diagnosis. The differential diagnosis of a manic episode chiefly involves distinguishing it from drug-induced mood disorders (e.g., amphetamines and steroids), some of the subtypes of schizophrenia, particularly schizo-affective, and paranoid subtypes. There is considerable controversy as to which clinical features can be used to separate manic disorders from schizophrenia. The guidelines suggested here are of necessity tentative and need to be tested to determine their ultimate validity. Manics may have disorganized speech which cannot be distinguished from the formal thought disorder of schizophrenia. However, in the untreated manic it is always accompanied by a disturbance in mood and, usually, hyperactivity. When formal thought disorder persists after the resolution of an episode of the manic syndrome, the diagnosis of schizophrenia should be made. The delusions of a manic may be bizarre. However, certain delusions, such as the experience of being controlled by external forces or of having one's thoughts taken away, should at this stage of knowledge preclude a diagnosis of mania. Manics may have hallucinations. However, if the content is unrelated to the disturbance in mood and the hallucinations dominate the clinical picture, the diagnosis of schizophrenia should be made.

It may be particularly difficult to distinguish the excited paranoid schizophrenic from the irritable and angry manic on a cross-sectional evaluation. In such instances it may be necessary to rely on features which, on a statistical basis, are associated differentially with the two conditions. Thus, the diagnosis of mania is more likely if there is a family history of affective disorder, good premorbid adjustment, and a previous episode from which there was complete recovery.

Operational criteria for a manic episode. A through C are required.

A. One or more distinct periods with a predominantly elevated, expansive or irritable mood. The elevated or irritable mood must be a prominent part of the illness and relatively persistent although it may alternate with depressive mood. Do not include if mood change is apparently due to alcohol or drug intoxication.

B. If mood is elevated or expansive, at least 3 of the following symptom categories must be definitely present to a significant degree (4 if mood is only irritable). (For past episodes, because of memory difficulty, one less symptom is required):

1) More active than usual—either socially, at work, sexually, or physically restless.
2) More talkative than usual or felt a pressure to keep talking.
3) Flight of ideas or subjective experience that thoughts are racing.
4) Inflated self-esteem (grandiosity, which may be delusional).
5) Decreased need for sleep.
6) Distractibility, i.e., attention is too easily drawn to unimportant or irrelevant external stimuli.
7) Excessive involvement in activities without recognizing the high potential for painful consequences, e.g., buying sprees, sexual indiscretions, foolish business investments, reckless driving.

C. None of the following which suggests schizophrenia is present:

1) Delusions of control or thought broadcasting, insertion, or withdrawal.
2) Hallucinations of any type throughout the day for several days or intermittently throughout a 1 week period unless all of the content is clearly related to depression or elation.
3) Auditory hallucinations in which either a voice keeps up a running commentary on the patient's behavior as it occurs, or 2 or more voices converse with each other.
4) At some time during the period of illness had delusions or hallucinations for more than 1 week in the absence of prominent mood (depressed or manic) symptoms.
5) At some time during the period of illness had more than 1 week when he exhibited no prominent manic symptoms but had several instances of formal thought disorder.

D. Overall disturbance is so severe that at least 1 of the following is present:

1) Meaningful conversation is impossible.
2) Serious impairment socially, with family, at home, at school, or at work.
3) In the absence of (1) or (2), hospitalization.

E. Duration of manic features at least 1 week (or any duration if hospitalized).

Unipolar manic disorder [Manic-depressive psychosis, manic type]

Essential features. The essential feature is one or more manic episodes (see description of manic episode above) in the absence of a prior major depressive episode.

Prevalence. This condition is extremely rare and the diagnosis usually must be changed to bipolar mood disorder because of a major depressive episode which occurs at some later time. Little information is available regarding this condition and whether or not it is a separate condition from bipolar mood disorder.

296.01X *Unipolar manic disorder, first episode*
296.02X *Unipolar manic disorder, recurrent*

Unipolar depressive disorder [Manic-depressive psychosis, depressed type]

Essential features. The essential feature is one or more major depressive episodes (see description of major depressive episode above) in the absence of a prior manic episode. At the present time, it is unclear whether individuals with a single major depressive episode who have had several episodes of minor depressive disorder should be considered first episode or recurrent unipolar depressive disorder.

In this classification, unipolar depressive disorder includes what was formerly referred to as manic-depressive, depressed type, involutional melancholia, and severe forms of neurotic depression. It also includes the research diagnosis primary mood disorder, unipolar type. Mild forms of depression which do not meet the suggested criteria should be categorized as minor depressive disorder.

Prevalence, sex ratio, course. This condition is rarely seen before adolescence. This condition is common with a reported lifetime prevalence of 5 percent. The female-male ratio is 2 to 1. Some of these patients will eventually have manic episodes and then be reclassified as bipolar mood disorder.

296.11X *Unipolar depressive disorder, first episode*

Essential features and prevalence. This diagnosis is for those patients who have had only one major depressive episode and have never had a manic episode. It is estimated that at least 50 percent of patients with an initial diagnosis of first episode unipolar depressive disorder will eventually have another episode of major depressive disorder.

296.12X *Unipolar depressive disorder, recurrent*

Essential features. This diagnosis is for those patients who have had two or more major depressive episodes and have never had a manic episode. When improvement in a depressive episode is short-lived, it may be difficult to know whether the patient has had a relapse or a new episode of illness. In such cases, the following arbitrary rule is suggested: for two periods of illness to be considered discrete episodes, they must be separated by at least a two month period of relatively complete remission of symptoms.

Prevalence. Patients with recurrent episodes have a higher probability of developing bipolar affective disorder, a more prominent family history of affective disorder, and perhaps a differential response to various forms of treatment.

Bipolar mood disorder [Manic-depressive psychosis, circular type, currently manic or depressed]

Essential features. The essential feature is one or more manic episodes and one or more major depressive episodes (see description above). This category should also be used if one of the episodes is minor (i.e., minor depressive episode or hypomanic episode) providing that the other pole has been major (i.e., major depressive

episode or manic episode). The disorder is subtyped according to
the current or more recent episode.

Age at onset and course. The onset is usually prior to age 30.
Both the manic and the major depressive episodes are more frequent and shorter than in either of the unipolar disorders. The
initial episode is usually manic. The course is variable, with some
patients having episodes separated by many years of normal functioning, others having clusters of episodes, while yet others have
an increased frequency of episodes as they grow older. Usually the
level of functioning between episodes returns to the premorbid level.
However, in approximately 20 percent of the cases, there is considerable residual impairment and the course is chronic. Frequently
a manic or major depressive episode will be followed immediately
by a short period of the other kind. In rare cases, over long periods
of time there is an alternation of the two kinds of episodes without
a normal interval period (cycling). There is some evidence that the
major depressive episodes associated with major bipolar mood disorder are more often of the retarded type than are those associated
with unipolar depressive disorder.

Premorbid personality. Usually the premorbid functioning is
normal. In the past, textbooks frequently mentioned cyclothymic
personality (now called bipolar minor mood disorder) as a common
premorbid personality in patients with bipolar mood disorder. This
belief is apparently based on the retrospective reports of patients
with bipolar mood disorder since prospective studies of cyclothymic
personality have not yet been conducted.

Prevalence and sex ratio. The prevalence of bipolar mood disorder has been reported as ranging from .5 to 1 percent, one fifth
to one tenth as common as reported for unipolar depressive disorder. The sex ratio is approximately equal. The prevalence of
mood disorder in relatives of patients with this disorder is higher
than that reported among relatives of patients with unipolar depressive disorder. The evidence of genetic factors in the transmission
of this condition is correspondingly greater than in unipolar depressive disorder.

296.20X *Bipolar mood disorder, manic* [Manic-depressive psychosis, circular but currently manic]

This category includes patients whose current or most recent episode was manic, as well as episodes in which both manic and depressive symptoms are intermingled (mixed episodes).

296.30X *Bipolar mood disorder, depressed* [Manic-depressive psychosis, circular but currently depressed]

This category includes patients whose current or most recent episode was depressed.

Episodic minor mood disorders

Essential features, impairment. The essential features of these disorders are, as with the major mood disorders, episodes with either depressed or manic mood. They differ from the major disorders in that the full manic or depressive syndrome of associated symptoms is absent, as well as any signs of psychosis (delusions, hallucinations, formal thought disorder, or grossly bizarre behavior). Patients who have previously had a major mood disorder should be classified as the appropriate major mood disorder even if they currently are having a minor episode of mood disorder. The term minor only refers to the absence of the full syndrome and does not imply that these disorders are always mild in terms of intensity of those symptoms that are present, functional impairment or suicidal risk.

The episodic minor mood disorders include hypomanic disorder, minor depressive disorder, and bipolar minor mood disorder. The relationship of these disorders to their major counterparts is unclear. Hypomanic disorder and bipolar minor mood disorder may have a closer relationship to their major counterparts (and to each other) than does minor depressive disorder to its major counterpart. It is expected that often patients with any of these disorders may subsequently develop an episode of a major mood disorder.

301.110 *Hypomanic disorder*

Essential features. This category is for describing nonpsychotic manic-like episodes that are less severe than manic episodes in terms of both the number of symptoms and functional impairment. It should not be used for individuals who have ever had a manic episode or a major or minor depressive episode. (They should be diagnosed as either unipolar manic, or recurrent bipolar mood disorder, manic.)

There is invariably an elevated, expansive or irritable mood with some accompanying symptoms of the core manic syndrome. These symptoms may include hyperactivity, overtalkativeness, inflated self-esteem, decreased need for sleep, excessive involvement in activities without recognizing the high potential for painful consequences (poor judgment), and distractibility. The manifestations of these are similar to those described in the section on manic episode except that they tend to be milder.

Impairment and differential diagnosis. By definition, there must be some impairment involving either judgment, relationships with people or ability to work, in order to distinguish this condition from simple periods of effective functioning accompanied by good mood. On the other hand, if the impairment in functioning is so severe that the patient is unable to work, or needs to be protected from the consequences of his own poor judgment or hyperactivity, then the diagnosis for the episode is most likely mania. Examples of impairment in hypomania disorder include intrusiveness with family, associates or coworkers, buying sprees, and indiscreet sexual behavior. The differential diagnosis also includes drug induced mood disorders, such as that seen with amphetamines and steroids.

Premorbid personality, prevalence, sex ratio, familial pattern. Since this is a new diagnostic category, there is no information available on the premorbid personality, prevalence, sex ratio and presence of a familial pattern. It is included in this nomenclature because of the possible treatment implications for recognizing early or mild forms of manic disorder.

Operational criteria for hypomanic disorder

A. One or more distinct periods with a predominantly expansive, elevated or irritable mood. Do not include if the mood change is apparently due to alcohol or drug intoxication.

B. If the mood is elevated or expansive, at least 2 of the symptoms listed under B of manic episode must be present (3 if mood is only irritable).

C. There is some impairment involving either judgment, relationships with people, or ability to work.

D. Duration of mood disturbance at least 2 days.

E. Excludes patients whose impairment is so severe that there is inability to work, a need to be protected from the consequences of poor judgment or hyperactivity. Excludes patients who meet the criteria for schizophrenia. Excludes patients who have ever had an episode of either manic or major depressive disorder.

300.410 *Minor depressive disorder* [Neurotic depression]

Essential features. This category is for nonpsychotic episodes of illness in which the major feature is a relatively persistent mood of depression without the full depressive syndrome that characterizes a major depressive disorder. It should not be used for individuals who have ever had a major depressive disorder or either a hypomanic or manic episode. The depressed mood is described as depressed, sad, blue, hopeless, low, down in the dumps, "don't care anymore," or some other colloquial variant. Anxiety may be present or even co-equal in intensity. In addition, there are some of the core symptoms that are present in the depressive syndrome as well as such symptoms as crying, a pessimistic attitude, brooding about past or current unpleasant events or preoccupation with feelings of inadequacy.

Onset and predisposing factors. The onset is variable with symptoms developing over a period of days to weeks. Often the onset of the disorder is associated with a stressful life event, such as a loss of a loved one or some other form of disappointment.

Impairment, complications. Although generally the incapacitation associated with minor depressive disorder is less than with major depressive disorder, sometimes the incapacitation is excessive in relation to the number of symptoms. The most serious complication is suicide, as it is with major depressive disorder. The frequency with which this occurs is not now known.

Prevalence, familial pattern. The frequency of this disorder relative to major depressive disorder is unknown. Likewise, the prevalence of depressive disorders among family members has not been ascertained.

Differential diagnosis. The relationship between minor and major depressive disorders is uncertain. In some instances, major depressive disorder may initially take the form of minor depressive disorder. An episode of minor depressive disorder may be superimposed on another pre-existing condition, for example, alcoholism, phobic or obsessive compulsive disorder. Since depressed mood is so common in almost all psychiatric disorders, this category should be given as an additional diagnosis only if the depressed mood, by virtue of its intensity or effect, can be clearly distinguished from the patient's usual condition.

It is distinguished from major depressive disorder primarily in terms of severity. It is distinguished from chronic and intermittent depressive disorder in which there is a chronic and intermittent course. It is distinguished from generalized anxiety disorder in which there is a clear predominance of anxious mood. It is distinguished from labile personality in which the symptoms are a life-long pattern. However, patients with labile personality can be given the additional diagnosis of minor depressive disorder if they develop a new episode of illness characterized by depressive mood that lasts more than two weeks.

Operational criteria for a minor depressive episode. A through C are required.

A. Relatively persistent depressed mood as described above.

B. Two or more of the symptoms listed below:

1) Poor appetite or weight loss or increased appetite or weight gain (change of 1 lb. a week or 10 lbs. a year when not dieting).
2) Sleep difficulty or sleeping too much.
3) Loss of energy, fatigability, or tiredness.
4) Psychomotor agitation or retardation (but not mere subjective feeling of restlessness or being slowed down).
5) Loss of interest or pleasure in usual activities, or decrease in sexual drive (do not include if limited to a period when delusional or hallucinating).
6) Feelings of self-reproach or excessive or inappropriate guilt (either may be delusional).
7) Complaints or evidence of diminished ability to think or concentrate, such as slow thinking or mixed-up thoughts (do not include if associated with obvious formal thought disorder).
8) Recurrent thoughts of death or suicide, including thoughts of wishing to be dead.
9) Crying.
10) Pessimistic attitude.
11) Brooding about past or current unpleasant events.
12) Preoccupation with feelings of inadequacy.

C. Duration at least 2 weeks.

D. Excludes grief reactions following the loss of a loved one if all the features are commonly seen in members of the subject's subcultural group in similar circumstances, and any form of delusions, hallucinations, or formal thought disorder.

301.120 *Bipolar minor mood disorder* [Affective personality]

Essential features. The essential feature is at least one minor depressive episode and one hypomanic episode, in the absence of a history of either a manic or a major depressive disorder. If there is a life-long pattern of recurrent episodes of depressed and elevated mood lasting at least a few days, with or without a normal interval period, the condition corresponds to the DSM-II category of cyclothymic personality.

Impairment and differential diagnosis. Impairment and differential diagnosis are similar to those for hypomanic disorder and minor depressive disorder.

Premorbid personality, prevalence, sex ratio, familial pattern. Since this is a new diagnostic category, there is no information available on the premorbid personality, prevalence, sex ratio and presence of a familial pattern. It is included in this nomenclature because of the possible treatment implications for recognizing early or mild forms of bipolar mood disorder.

Chronic and intermittent mood disorders

This category contains only one disorder, chronic and intermittent depressive disorder, because no parallel disorder involving manic features has been described. Some individuals have been characterized as hypomanic personalities because of their relatively persistent and unusually high energy level, good spirits, less need for sleep, and involvement in numerous activities. This condition is not included in this nomenclature because it is not associated with the negative consequences which are criteria for the definition of mental disorder used here.

300.420 *Chronic and intermittent depressive disorder*

Essential features, course, differential diagnosis. The essential feature of this disorder is a chronic nonpsychotic disturbance involving depressed mood and some associated symptoms lasting at least two years with intermittent periods of normal mood lasting from a few days to a few weeks. During the periods of depressed mood, the patient may or may not have the full depressive syndrome. If an individual has ever had either a manic or hypomanic episode, he should be diagnosed as either bipolar mood disorder, depressed, or bipolar minor mood disorder. The differential diagnosis mainly involves episodic major or minor depressive disorder, and labile personality. The cross-sectional clinical picture is the same as that seen in either minor or major depressive disorder. This disorder is distinguished by both its chronic and intermittent nature. The disorder is intermittent in that patients are bothered by depressed mood to a noticeably greater degree than most people much of the time. There are, however, frequent periods of interspersed normal mood lasting a few days or weeks. The intermittent mood is in contrast to the relatively clear-cut episodes of sustained depressed mood required for the diagnosis of the episodic (major or minor) mood disorders. The course is distinguished from that of labile personality in that in labile personality the depressed mood rarely lasts more than a few hours or days and the mood changes are abrupt in onset.

If chronic and intermittent depressive disorder follows an episode of major or minor depressive disorder, it should be noted as the current diagnosis and the previous condition noted as a past diagnosis.

Onset. Typically there is no clear onset and it begins in early adult life (often referred to as depressive character). However, in some cases it may begin later in adult life with or without a clear onset.

Associated features, impairment, complications. The associated features are similar to those of the other depressive disorders, except there are no psychotic symptoms (by definition). The impairment may be considerable because of the chronicity, rather than the severity, of the depressive syndrome. Therefore, hospitalization is rarely required unless there is a suicide attempt, or a superimposed major depressive disorder. The complications are similar to those of the other depressive disorders, although there may be a greater likelihood of developing alcoholism and drug abuse.

Predisposing factors. A predisposing factor is the presence of a chronic medical disorder, chronic life stresses, or another psychiatric disorder, such as unipolar depressive disorder, which does not completely remit and merges imperceptibly into this condition.

Prevalence, sex ratio, and familial pattern. This is a new diagnostic category so that the exact prevalence is not known. However, the condition probably is common amongst outpatients. The sex ratio is not known, but it is probably more common in females, as are the other unipolar depressive disorders. The presence of a familial pattern is not known.

Operational criteria for chronic and intermittent depressive disorder. A through E are required.

A. Has been bothered by depressed mood to a noticeably greater degree than most people much of the time.

B. Intermittently there are periods of normal mood for a few days to a few weeks.

C. Had at least two of the associated symptoms listed in criterion B of episodic minor depressive disorder when feeling depressed.

D. Duration of at least two years and still present or continuous with a superimposed present illness of some other disorder.

E. The depressed mood cannot be completely accounted for by any other psychiatric condition such as Briquet's disorder or schizophrenia.

REFERENCES

1. CLAYTON, P. J., RODIN, L. and WINOKUR, G.: Family history studies: III. Schizo-affective disorder, clinical and genetic factors including a one- to two-year follow-up. *Compr. Psychiat.*, 9: 31-49, 1968.
2. MCCABE, M. S., FOWLER, R. C., CADORET, R. J. and WINOKUR, G.: Symptom differences in schizophrenia with good and poor prognosis. *Am. J. Psychiat.*, 128:1239-1243, 1972.
3. WELNER, A., CROUGHAN, J. L. and ROBINS, E.: The group of schizoaffective and related psychoses—Critique, record, follow-up, and family studies. *Arch. Gen. Psychiat.*, 31:628-631, 1974.
4. CROUGHAN, J. L., WELNER, A. and ROBINS, E.: The group of schizoaffective and related psychoses—Critique, record, follow-up, and family studies. *Arch. Gen. Psychiat.*, 31:632-637, 1974.
5. CARPENTER, W. T., JR., STRAUSS, J. S. and MULEH, S.: Are there pathognomonic symptoms in schizophrenia? An empiric investigation of Schneider's first-rank symptoms. *Arch. Gen. Psychiat.*, 28:847-857, 1973.
6. WORLD HEALTH ORGANIZATION (Ed.): *International Pilot Study of Schizophrenia.* Vol. I. Geneva: World Health Organization Press, 1973.
7. WING, J. and NIXON, J. Discriminating symptoms in schizophrenia. *Arch. Gen. Psychiat.*, 32:853-862, 1975.
8. DOHRENWEND, B. S. and DOHRENWEND, B. P.: *Stressful Life Events. Their Nature and Effects.* New York: John Wiley and Sons, 1974.
9. CLAYTON, P. J., HALIKAS, J. A. and MAURICE, W. L.: The depression of widowhood. *Brit. J. Psychiat.*, 120:59-63, 1972.

10. PAYKEL, E. S., MYERS, J. K., DIENELT, M. N., KLERMAN, G. L., LINDENTHALL, J. J. and PEPPER, M. P.: Life events and depression. *Arch. Gen. Psychiat.*, 21:753-761, 1969.
11. KENDELL, R. E.: *The Classification of Depressive Illness*. Maudsley Monographs, Number 18. London: Oxford University Press, 1968.
12. POST, F.: *The Significance of Affective Symptoms in Old Age*. Maudsley Monographs, Number 10. London: Oxford University Press, 1962.
13. WOODRUFF, R. A., JR., GOODWIN, D. W. and GUZE, S. B.: *Psychiatric Diagnosis*. New York: Oxford University Press, 1974.
14. WINOKUR, G., CLAYTON, P. J. and REICH, T.: *Manic Depressive Illness*. St. Louis: The C. V. Mosby Co., 1969.
15. MENDLEWICZ, J., FLEISS, J. L. and FIEVE, R. R.: Evidence for X-linkage in the transmission of manic depressive illness. *J.A.M.A.*, 222:1624-1627, 1972.
16. GERSHON, E. S., DUNNER, D. L., STUART, L., et al.: Assortative mating in the affective disorders. *Biol. Psychiat.*, 7:63-73, 1973.
17. LEONHARD, K., KORFF, I. and SCHULZ, H.: Die Temperamente in de Familien der monopolaren and bipolaren phasischen Psychosen. *Psychiat. Neurol.*, 143:416, 1962.
18. DUNNER, D. L., COHN, C. K., GERSHON, E. S. and GOODWIN, F. K.: Differential catechol-o-methyltransferase activity in unipolar and bipolar affective illness. *Arch. Gen. Psychiat.*, 25: 348-353, 1971.
19. GLASSMAN, A. H., CANTOR, S. J. and SHOSTAK, M.: Depression, delusion and drug response. *Am. J. Psychiat.*, 132:716-719, 1975.

5

Genetics of Affective Disorders

Remi J. Cadoret, M.D. and
Vasantkumar L. Tanna, M.D.

INTRODUCTION

There is evidence for considerable heterogeneity of causes as well as outcomes of depression, one of the most common psychiatric disorders. This paper provides some evidence for heterogeneity obtained from studies employing techniques used by geneticists. The most widely used technique is the family pedigree study, in which types and patterns of psychiatric illness are noted in blood relatives of patients. Since most family members share extensively in similar environments, it is clear that correlations of type of illness between members of the same family could be attributable to common environmental factors (social, malnutrition, physical stress) as well as genetic inheritance. However, other techniques such as twin studies and genetic linkage provide more direct evidence of genetic factors. This is not to say that the genetic factor is a necessary or sufficient cause in affective disorder. However, we shall cite current evidence for a genetic factor in depression.

Our thesis is that depression represents a variety of conditions, and that genetic techniques can be used to obtain more homogeneous subgroups, which in turn can be examined more extensively. With more homogeneous subgroups, techniques such as genetic linkage might be more fruitful.

TABLE 1

Prevalence of Five Types of Psychiatric Illness in Parents of
Patients with Affective Disorder and of Control Patients*

| Illness | Patients with Affective Disorder ($N=366$) | | Control Patients ($N=180$) | |
	Mothers %	Fathers %	Mothers %	Fathers %
Alcoholism	1.1	9.5	0	1.7
Neurosis	3.6	1.4	1.1	0
Schizophrenia	0	0.5	0	0
Chronic brain syndrome	0.8	0.5	0.6	0
Affective disorder	22.9	13.6	1.1	2.2

* From Winokur & Pitts (4).

In the search for subgroups, the definition of depression is cardinal. Most studies we cite use depressive conditions which, in DSM-II terms, would be called "psychotic depression" or "manic depressive disease, depressed or circular type," or in Robins and Guze's (1) terminology, "primary affective disorder." By "affective illness or disorder" we mean a psychiatric condition in which a changed mood is the primary feature, and other symptoms are derived from the change in mood. In this paper, "depression" will refer to the depressive syndrome of primary affective disorder, and "mania" will refer to the manic syndrome of primary affective disorder as defined by Feighner et al. (2).

AFFECTIVE DISORDER — A FAMILIAL ILLNESS

For a long time it has been accepted that the incidence of affective illness is higher in families of patients with affective disorder. Over the years, a number of family studies from a variety of countries have shown that affective disorder is increased in families of such patients, generally significantly above population values (3). An example of such a study is that of Winokur and Pitts (4) shown in Table 1. This study, comparing parents of patients with primary affective disorder with parents of control medical patients who are matched on the basis of age and sex, showed that affective disorder was significantly increased in both parents of the patients with affective disorder. One other condition was also increased in these patients' families and that was alcoholism in the fathers. Alcoholism will be shown to be a statistically significant factor when we consider one type of affective disorder later in this paper. As discussed above, the increased affective disorder in these families is consistent with either genetic or environmental factors (or both).

A Unipolar-Bipolar Difference — Evidence for Heterogeneity of Affective Disorders from Family Studies

Studies of families of individuals with affective disorder provide strong evidence for heterogeneity within affective disorder. One of the earliest approaches to differentiating kinds of affective disordered individuals was to start with an affectively ill group thought to be homogeneous with respect to certain clinical characteristics and then to contrast its familial pattern of inheritance with remaining affective cases. This approach was used by Leonhard (5) and Perris (6) who separated affective disordered individuals into two groups on the basis of the presence or absence of mania or manic symptoms in the clinical picture or history. In one group, the bipolar, there is a history of a manic episode or at least current manic-like features in the clinical picture. The other larger group, termed unipolar, is characterized by a history of depressive episodes with no manic periods or symptoms.

One of the earliest differences reported between these two groups of families in Table 2 is that the percentage of families affected with psychosis is consistently higher in bipolar probands than in unipolar probands. This finding holds true in a number of studies (Table 2). In most of these studies the psychotically ill relative in both groups was found to be suffering from an affective disorder.

The strongest evidence for specificity of type of illness in families of bipolar patients was provided by Perris (6). He reported that affectively ill relatives of unipolar probands almost never were

TABLE 2

Incidence of Psychosis in One or More Relatives of Unipolar and Bipolar Probands*

Source of Data	Bipolar Probands Number of Probands	% Affected Families	Unipolar Probands Number of Probands	% Affected Families
Neele (8)	201	29.9	324	19.4
Kinkelin (9)	51	68.6	89	40.5
Leonhard (5)	238	39.9	288	25.7
Asano (10)	84	61.9	78	52.5
Dorzab, Baker Cadoret & Winokur (11)	89	52.0	100	26.0

* From Cadoret & Winokur (7).

TABLE 3

Concordance of Affective Disorder in Twins*

	M-Z Twins	D-Z Twins
Both unipolar depressive	22	8
Both bipolar	21	0
One bipolar and one unipolar	7	5
Incompletely concordant or discordant	33	43
Total	83	56

* After Zerbin-Rudin (16).

manic; but, in contrast, the risk of mania was significantly higher in the affectively ill relative of bipolar probands. This differentiation was less conclusive in three other series, one by Angst (12), the Stenstedt series (13), which was re-analyzed by Price (14), and the series reported by Winokur and Reich (15).

However, twin studies suggest that there is a specificity of type which may be genetic in origin. Zerbin-Rudin (16) contrasted mono-zygotic and dizygotic twins on the basis of concordance for the type of affective disorder, taking into account whether the twin was unipolar or bipolar. The results (Table 3) suggest that: 1) There is a higher concordance rate for monozygotic twins compared to dizygotic; 2) there appears to be a correlation between the illness of one twin and that of the other regarding the type of illness, unipolar versus bipolar. These results appear to confirm the specificity of type of illness and are consistent with a genetic factor with the higher concordance rate for monozygotic twins. Other twin studies in the literature, summarized by Price (14) and Allen (17), show concordance of monozygotic twins for affective disorder. A summary of published twin studies shows that, for affective disorder in general, monozygotic (MZ) concordance is 57 percent compared to a dizygotic (DZ) concordance of 14 percent, a statistically significant difference. In a number of series, it was possible to classify the affective disorders into unipolar and bipolar. Bipolar MZ concordance was 40 percent compared to 11 percent DZ. This significant difference for both unipolar and bipolar MZ-DZ rates of concordances is compatible with a genetic factor in both conditions. The lower MZ concordance in unipolar affective disorder suggests a lesser importance of a genetic factor in that condition.

The studies of Leonhard et al. (18) offer additional evidence for unipolar-bipolar familial differences. They found personality or temperament types to be correlated with unipolar and bipolar families (Table 4). The striking difference is the excess of hypomanic temperament in bipolar relatives and the higher incidence of subdepressive temperaments in relatives of unipolar probands.

One difficulty with the Leonhard study is the possible absence of a double blind method for diagnosing temperament of family members. This is an especially important consideration since temperament diagnoses might be expected to be affected by the investigator's knowledge of the diagnosis of the proband. However, significant data on personality types of children of affectively disordered probands were collected by Hoffmann (19). These temperament diagnoses were made before the distinction of the unipolar-bipolar dichotomy (Table 5). Here the incidence of hypomanic temperament is higher in children of bipolar patients, and the cyclothymic pattern (which appeared to include individuals with depressive mood

TABLE 4

Temperament in Relatives of Unipolar and Bipolar Ss*

Relative	N	Hypomanic N	%	Subdepressive N	%	Cyclothymic N	%	Total N	%
Bipolar illness in S									
Siblings	94	16	17	5	5.3	14	15	35	37
Parents	80	21	26	6	7.5	12	15	39	49
Total	174	37	21	11	6.3	26	15	74	43
Unipolar illness in S									
Siblings	143	13	9.1	19	13	11	7.7	43	30
Parents	120	17	14	27	23	13	10	57	48
Total	263	30	11	46	17	24	9.2	100	38
χ^2 difference (unipolar vs. bipolar)									
Total siblings & parents		7.10**		10.55***		2.95		0.71	

* Data on parents and siblings from Leonhard et al. (18).
** $p < .01$.
*** $p < .005$.

TABLE 5

Temperament in Relatives of Unipolar and Bipolar Ss*

Relative	N	Hypomanic N	%	Subdepressive N	%	Cyclothymic N	%	Total N	%
Bipolar illness in S Children	97	15	15	2	2.1	3	3.1	20	21
Unipolar illness in S Children	73	2	2.7	6	8.2	10	14	18	25
χ^2 difference (unipolar vs. bipolar) Children		6.15**		2.28		5.22**		0.19	

* Data on children from Hoffmann (19).
** $p < .025$.

TABLE 6

Morbidity Risk for Affective Disorder in Relatives
of Unipolar and Bipolar Probands*

| | Unipolar | | Bipolar | |
	Proband Male	Proband Female	Proband Male	Proband Female
Mother	12.2	16.9	26.6	23.3
Father	14.2	11.8	6.8	17.1
Sister	11.7	13.1	18.0	23.4
Brother	15.8	7.4	28.9	6.7
Daughter	8.8	25.5	14.8	23.7
Son	6.6	8.8	15.4	22.9

* From Cadoret, Winokur, Clayton (20).

swings) is higher in the children of unipolars. These earlier data appear to substantiate the findings of Leonhard in part.

There are other data from family studies suggesting that unipolar and bipolar affective families differ in the pattern of "inheritance" shown by different family members. Table 6 shows the morbidity risk for affective disorder in relatives of unipolar and bipolar probands from a number of family studies. The patterns shown by the unipolar and bipolar families differ in two important ways. The most evident is that male and female children of bipolar females show an equal incidence of affective disorder while three times more daughters than sons of female unipolar probands are at risk. In addition, there is a relative lack of sick father-to-son pairs in bipolar families in contrast to the equal incidence of illness in parents of the unipolar families.

These findings suggest different modes of inheritance for the unipolar and bipolar conditions. Slater (21) developed a computational model to distinguish between a major dominant gene transmission and a multigenic type of transmission. In some studies (22) the pattern of inheritance in bipolar illness suggests a dominant type of transmission. However, the Slater model does not confirm such a difference between unipolar and bipolar conditions.

In summary, family studies have shown that there are differences between unipolar and bipolar affective disorders in a number of characteristics: 1) Bipolar families have a higher incidence of members with psychosis than do unipolar; 2) there is evidence that there is specificity of type of illness in the family; 3) there are significant temperament differences between members of unipolar and bipolar families; 4) the patterns of ill members in family pedigrees vary significantly between unipolar and bipolar families.

EVIDENCE FOR X-LINKAGE OF BIPOLAR ILLNESS

The significant familial differences between unipolar and bipolar families suggest a dominant X-linked transmission, though there are some inconsistent features (22). For example, in X-linked transmission, more females than males should be affected, and this is what is found in studies of most series of bipolar patients. Another consequence of X-linked dominant inheritance is that ill males should have an equal number of affected brothers and sisters, and ill females should have more ill sisters than brothers. This is found in a series by Winokur, Clayton, and Reich (22).

A critical consequence of X-linked dominant condition is, of course, no father-to-son transmission of illness. This important distinguishing point has formed the focus for much research effort. Approximately eight series dealing with the father-to-son transmission of bipolar affective disorder are reported in the literature (Table 7). Only two report no ill father-to-son transmission. Obviously, the maternal side of the family is a critical consideration in those series which report ill father-to-son pairs. If the maternal side were tainted with affective disorder, then an apparent father-to-son transmission might result. However, in several of the series reported in Table 7, the maternal side of the family tree was extensively investigated, and no evidence of affective disorder was found. These pedigree studies indicate that father-to-son transmission does occur in some families.

Other evidence connecting the X chromosome with bipolar illness is available in the marker traits known to be carried on the X chromosome of man: red-green color blindness and the Xg^a antigen

TABLE 7

Father-to-Son "Transmission" of Bipolar Affective Disorder*

Series Compatible with X-linked Transmission	Results
1. Winokur, Clayton & Reich (22)	In 89 families no ill father-son pairs.
2. Taylor & Abrams (24)	In 55 families no ill father-son pairs.

Series Not Compatible with X-linked Transmission as the Sole Transmission Possibility	
1. Perris (25)	In series of 138 bipolar probands, 13 ill father-son pairs.
2. Dunner, Gershon & Goodwin (26)	In 23 bipolar male patients, 4 had affectively ill fathers.
3. Green et al. (27)	In 35 bipolar families, 4 ill father-son pairs (no illness on maternal side).
4. Fieve et al. (28)	In 120 bipolar probands, 13 ill father-son pairs (9 pairs no evidence of illness on maternal side).
5. Helzer & Winokur (29)	Of 30 male manics, 8 affectively ill mothers (41%), and 1 affectively ill father (5%); in another ill father-ill son pair, considerable affective disorder existed on the maternal side of the family.
6. Von Greiff, McHugh & Stokes (30)	In 16 male probands, 4 ill father-son pairs with no illness on maternal side; 3 ill father-son pairs did have illness on maternal side.
7. Loranger (31)	In 69 male probands (who met criteria for mania used by Winokur, Clayton, Reich (22)) 3 father-son pairs without maternal illness; 4 mother-son, 2 father-daughter, and 5 mother-daughter combinations (66 female probands).

* From Cadoret & Winokur (23).

(Table 8). Significant linkage has been demonstrated for bipolar illness with both the red-green blindness (both protan and deutan types) and the Xg^a locus. Linkage has been demonstrated by two different techniques. The first two studies in Table 8 employed the sib-pair method for the analysis, while the method of the latter two studies was a maximum likelihood method, utilizing data from more than one generation in a family. Both methodologies have been consistent in demonstrating linkage.

The picture which the linkage studies give is an unusual one: The manic depressive locus shows linkage with both Xg^a and the color blindness loci. However, Xg^a and color blindness loci, although on the same chromosome, do not ordinarily show linkage because, presumably, the long chromosome distance between them allows for frequent crossing over. Thus, the manic depressive locus would appear to be unique in bridging a gap between Xg^a and color blindness. The question as to whether the distance between Xg^a and color blindness is sufficient to allow a condition such as manic depressive illness to appear between them and yet not show linkage is unresolved.

How can this evidence from the linkage studies that at least one factor for bipolar illness is transmitted on the X-chromosome be reconciled with the well documented cases of father-to-son transmission? A reasonable interpretation is that transmission of bipolar illness in families is probably heterogeneous, as occurs in retinitis pigmentosa, which can be inherited in some families in an X-linked fashion but in others is inherited as an autosomal type condition. The importance of the several positive linkage studies lies in the fact that they constitute the most direct evidence which we have at the present time for genetic inheritance in the affective disorders.

There are a few studies that attempt to demonstrate heterogeneity within bipolar affective disorder. One inconsistent finding is for early onset bipolar probands to have higher incidence of sick relatives than later onset probands (24). However, other studies fail to find this difference (20).

Recently, Dunner and Fieve (35) have described two clinically distinguishable types of bipolar illness which they designate bipolar

TABLE 8

Linkage Studies in Bipolar Affective Disorder*

Study	Genetic Marker	Results
1. Winokur & Tanna (32)	Xgᵃ	Report 3 pedigrees informative for linkage. In these, 10 children were compatible with X-linked transmission, one was incompatible. This difference is significant (2 of the 3 families suggest specific linkage with Xgᵃ blood system. This was not significant, however).
2. Reich, Clayton & Winokur (33)	red-green color blindness	Report 2 pedigrees, one with protan, the other with deutan color blindness. In each pedigree significant evidence of linkage with color blindness was found. Pedigrees suggest dominant inheritance.
3. Fieve et al. (28)	red-green color	Report 8** pedigrees—4 with protan and 4 with deutan color blindness. Total of protan and deutan families gave significant evidence for linkage. Pedigrees fit a dominant inheritance.
4. Mendlewicz, Fleiss & Fieve (34)	Xgᵃ	Report 12** pedigrees for Xgᵃ. Significant linkage reported.

* From Cadoret & Winokur (23).
** Since publication of these results, 9 additional families with red-green blindness and 11 more families informative for Xga and affective disorder have been examined, and the cumulative results found consistent with X-linkage (Mendlewicz & Fleiss, 34a).

I and bipolar II. Bipolar I refers to a patient hospitalized for mania and Bipolar II, a patient with hypomanic symptoms and hospitalized for depression (but never for mania). Unfortunately, for our present impasse regarding two types of inheritance, it appears that clear-cut father-to-son inheritance occurs with both bipolar I and II probands (35).

EVIDENCE FOR HETEROGENEITY OF UNIPOLAR
AFFECTIVE DISORDER

Studies of patterns of illness within families of unipolar depressed probands have revealed a number of differences which have led to the conclusion that unipolar affective disorder is a heterogeneous condition. A survey of published data of unipolar and bipolar family illnesses (20) showed that, in unipolar families, there was higher risk for affective disorder when the proband became ill prior to the age of 40. Further family studies confirmed this difference related to age of onset of illness in the proband. In a study of 100 unipolar affectively ill depressives Winokur et al. (36) found that younger onset probands had more affectively ill first-degree relatives. In addition, there were other important differences related to age of onset of illness in the probands (Table 9). Relatives of early onset probands also showed increased rates for both alcoholism and antisocial personality when contrasted with relatives of late onset probands. Further, antisocial personality and alcoholism were characteristic of the male relatives while more female relatives suffered from depressive illness.

Table 9 contains several additional features of importance which suggest heterogeneity. The first is that male and female relatives of male probands with later onset illness appear to have more equal risk for affective disorder. In contrast, the other proband groups (and especially the early onset female probands) show a preponderance of affectively ill female relatives. This pattern of findings has been essentially confirmed in five independently collected series comprising over 1,250 probands. Despite the variability in the collection of the five series and the sources of the probands, the following results have been confirmed: 1) there is more affective disorder in families of individuals with early onset illness than late onset (all six series have shown this difference); 2) alcoholism is increased in male relatives of early onset probands (all six series have shown this difference); these additional series contain little information about antisocial behavior, so conclusions about sociopathy in relatives cannot be made; 3) male and female relatives of late onset male probands showed equal risks for affective disorder (five out of six series showed this type of difference); 4) the risk of affective disorder in female relatives of early onset female probands was greater than the risk in male relatives (five out of six series are consistent in this finding).

On the basis of these differences, Winokur and his coworkers have postulated that there are at least two types of depressive illness. One, depressive spectrum disease, has considerable alcoholism among male relatives but more depression in female than male relatives. In the other type of unipolar illness, pure, depressive disease, depression occurs more equally in male and female relatives, and there is no familial increase in alcoholism over ordinary expectation.

Only recently have linkage studies of unipolar depressive illness been undertaken. Mendlewicz and Fleiss (37) not only failed to detect linkage with the loci of Xg^a blood group or protan type of color blindness, but also ruled out X-linked inheritance as the mode of transmission in unipolar illness. However, they did not divide unipolar depression further into more homogeneous groups. Tanna, Winokur, Elston, and Go (38) studied linkage in depressive spectrum disease, in which familial alcoholism and/or antisocial personality were used as disease markers to separate depressive spectrum disease families from other unipolar depressive families. That is, probands were selected on the basis that one first-degree relative had a unipolar depression and at least one other first-degree relative had an alcoholic or an antisocial personality. Depressive spectrum disease, defined in this way, was found in 13 families. One additional family with depression in a grandparent was included, making a total of 14 sibships comprising a total of 155 sib-pairs for the linkage analysis. Twenty genetic markers were analyzed in blood samples. Each individual in the sample was personally interviewed using a structured psychiatric interview, and diagnoses were made, blind as to the results of blood analyses. Preliminary analyses of a substantial number of sib-pairs, using a version of sib-pair method of Penrose, suggests the possibility of linkage ($p < 0.005$ with two genetic marker loci, viz., Haptoglobin [L-Hp] and Third Complement component [C3]). These results indicate that more definitive

TABLE 9

Risks for Depression, Alcoholism, and Sociopathy in Primary Relatives of 100 Depressive Probands Separated by Sex and Age of Onset (All Sources Data)*

| | Male Probands** | | | | Female Probands** | | | |
| | Early Onset (N=14) | | Late Onset (N=17) | | Early Onset (N=40) | | Late Onset (N=29) | |
	Male Relatives	Female Relatives	Male Relatives	Female Relatives	Male Relatives	Female Relatives	Male Relatives	Female Relatives
Risk for depression	(2/13) 16%	(5/14) 37%	(10/53) 19%	(5/43) 12%	(5/56) 9%	(16/55) 29%	(5/82) 6%	(16/87) 19%
Risk for sociopathy	(1/19) 5%	(0/23) —	(0/62) —	(0/51) —	(8/86) 9%	(3/83) 4%	(0/97) —	(0/102) —
Risk for alcoholism	(3/16) 19%	(1/17) 6%	(1/61) 2%	(0/48) —	(7/72) 10%	(1/66) 2%	(3/93) 3%	(1/94) 1%
Risk for alcoholism or sociopathy	24%	6%	2%	—	19%	6%	3%	1%
Total risk for alcoholism, sociopathy, or depression	40%	43%	21%	12%	28%	34%	9%	20%

* From Winokur, Cadoret, Dorzab et al. (36).
** Within the parenthesis, the numerator of the fraction is the number of family members ill and the denominator is the number at risk. This fraction refers to the morbid risk percentage below.

methods of linkage detection, such as the lod score method (39) be used to further investigate this promising lead. The same investigators are studying possible linkage in pure depressive disease (later age of onset in male probands with no family members having a diagnosis of alcoholism or of antisocial personality). Results of linkage analysis would be expected to be different if pure depressive disease were a genetically different entity.

SUMMARY

The linkage evidence indicates a genetic factor in at least one type of primary affective disorder—bipolar illness. This conclusion must be further qualified as occurring in certain, but not all, families with this condition. Evidence of a genetic factor from linkage studies in unipolar illness is suggestive, but confirmation awaits further analyses. Twin studies are compatible with a genetic factor in both unipolar and bipolar illness. There is also evidence that the mode of genetic transmission of bipolar illness is different from that in unipolar and in some families involves an X-linked gene.

REFERENCES

1. ROBINS, E. and GUZE, S.: Classification of affective disorders: The primary-secondary, the endogenous reactive, and the neurotic-psychotic concepts. In M. M. Katz & J. Shield, Jr. (Eds.), Recent Advances in the Psychobiology of the Depressive Illness: Proceedings of a Workshop sponsored by NIMH. Washington, D. C.: U.S. Government Printing Office, 1972.
2. FEIGHNER, J. P., ROBINS, E., GUZE, S. B., WOODRUFF, R. A., JR., WINOKUR, G. and MUNOZ, R.: Diagnostic criteria for use in psychiatric research. Arch. Gen. Psychiat., 26:57, 1972.
3. ZERBIN-RUDIN, E.: Manisch-depressive psychosen Involutions psychosen. In P. E. Becher (Ed.), Humangenetik, Vol. V/2. Stuttgart: Thieme Verlag, 1967.
4. WINOKUR, G. & PITTS, F. N., JR.: Affective disorder: VI. A family history study of prevalences, sex differences and possible genetic factors. J. Psychiat. Res., 3:113, 1965.
5. LEONHARD, K.: Aufteilung der endogenen Psychosen. Berlin: Akademie, 1966.
6. PERRIS, C.: A study of bipolar (manic-depressive) and unipolar recurrent depressive psychoses. Acta Psychiat. Scand., Suppl., 194:1, 1966.

7. CADORET, R. J. and WINOKUR, G.: Genetic principles in the classifi-
    cation of affective illnesses. *Int. J. Ment. Health*, 1:159, 1972.
8. NEELE, E.: *Die phasischen Psychosen nach ihrem Erscheinungs
    und Erbbild.* Leipzig: Johann Ambrosius Barth, 1949.
9. KINKELIN, M.: Verlauf und Prognose des Manisch-depressiven
    Irreseins. *Schweiz. Arch. Neurol. Psychiat.*, 75:100, 1954.
10. ASANO, N.: Study of manic-depressive psychosis. *In* H. Mitsuda
    (Ed.), *Clinical Genetics in Psychiatry.* Tokyo: Igaku Shoin,
    1967.
11. DORZAB, J., BAKER, M., CADORET, R. J. and WINOKUR, G.: De-
    pressive disease: Familial psychiatric illness. Paper presented
    at the Annual Meeting of the American Psychiatric Association,
    San Francisco, May, 1970.
12. ANGST, J.: *Zur Antiologie und Nosologie endogener depressiver
    Psychosen.* Berlin: Springer (*Monogr. Gesamtgeb. Neurol.
    Psychiat.*, No. 112), 1966.
13. STENSTEDT, A.: A study of manic depressive psychoses. *Acta Psy-
    chiat. Scand.*, Suppl., 79:1, 1952.
14. PRICE, J.: The genetics of affective disorder. *In* A. Coppen & A.
    Walk (Eds.), *Recent Developments in Affective Disorders
    (Brit. J. Psychiat.*, special publication No. 2), 1968.
15. WINOKUR, G. and REICH, T.: Two genetic factors in manic-de-
    pressive disease. *Com. Psychiat.*, 11:93, 1970.
16. ZERBIN-RUDIN, E.: Zur Genetik der depressiven Erkrankungen.
    Paper presented at symposium on "Das depressive Syndrom,"
    held at the Psychiatric and Neurologic Clinic of the Free Uni-
    versity of Berlin, Feb. 16-17, 1968.
17. ALLEN, M. G.: Twin studies of affective illness. Paper presented
    at 128th Annual Meeting APA, Anaheim, California, May,
    1975.
18. LEONHARD, K., KORFF, I. and SCHULZ, H.: Die Temperamente in
    der Familien der monopolaren und bipolaren phasischen Psy-
    chosen. *Psychiat. Neurol.* (Basel), 143:416, 1962.
19. HOFFMANN, H.: Die Nachkommenschaft bei endogenen Psychosen.
    In Rudin (Ed.), *Studien uber Vererbung und Entstehung
    Geistiger Storungen.* Berlin, 1921.
20. CADORET, R. J., WINOKUR, G. and CLAYTON, P. Family history
    studies: VI. Manic-depressive disease versus depressive disease.
    Brit. J. Psychiat., 116:625, 1970.
21. SLATER, E.: Expectation of abnormality on paternal and maternal
    sides: A computation model. *J. Med. Genet.*, 3:159, 1966.
22. WINOKUR, G., CLAYTON, P. and REICH, T.: *Manic Depressive
    Disease.* St. Louis: C. V. Mosby, 1969.
23. CADORET, R. J. and WINOKUR, G. X-Linkage in manic-depressive
    illness. *Ann. Rev. Med.*, 26:21, 1975.
24. TAYLOR, M. and ABRAMS, R.: Manic states: A genetic study of
    early and late onset affective disorders. *Arch. Gen. Psychiat.*,
    28:656, 1973.

25. PERRIS, C.: Abnormality on paternal and maternal sides: Observations in bipolar (manic-depressive) and unipolar depressive psychoses. *Brit. J. Psychiat.*, 118:207, 1971.
26. DUNNER, D., GERSHON, E. and GOODWIN, F. K.: Heritable factors in the severity of affective illness. Presented at 123rd Annual Meeting APA, San Francisco, 1969.
27. GREEN, R., GOETZE, V., WHYBROW, P. and JACKSON, R.: X-linked transmission of manic-depressive illness. *J. Am. Med. Assoc.*, 223:1289, 1973.
28. FIEVE, R., MENDLEWICZ, J., RAINER, J. and FLEISS, J.: Linkage studies in affective disorders, II. Color blindness and manic depressive illness. *In* R. Fieve, D. Rosenthal & H. Brill (Eds.), *Genetics and Psychopathology.* Baltimore: Johns Hopkins University, 1974.
29. HELZER, J. and WINOKUR, G.: A family interview study of male manic-depressives. *Arch. Gen. Psychiat.*, 31:73, 1974.
30. VONGREIFF, H., MCHUGH, P. R. and STOKES, P.: The familial history in sixteen males with bipolar manic-depressive disorder. Presented at 63rd Annual Meeting APA, New York, 1973.
31. LORANGER, A. W.: X-Linkage and manic-depressive illness. *Brit. J. Psychiat.*, 127:482, 1975.
32. WINOKUR, G. and TANNA, V. L.: Possible role of X-linked dominant factor in manic depressive disease. *Dis. Nerv. Syst.*, 30: 89, 1969.
33. REICH, T., CLAYTON, P. and WINOKUR, G.: Family history studies: V. The genetics of mania. *Am. J. Psychiat.*, 125:1358, 1969.
34. MENDLEWICZ, J., FLEISS, J. and FIEVE, R.: Linkage studies in affective disorders, I. Xg blood group and manic-depressive illness. *In* R. Fieve, D. Rosenthal & H. Brill (Eds.), *Genetics and Psychopathology.* Baltimore: Johns Hopkins University, 1974.
34a. MENDLEWICZ, J. and FLEISS, J.: Linkage studies with X-chromosome markers in bipolar (manic-depressive) and unipolar (depressive) illness. *Biol. Psychiatry*, 9(3):261-294, 1974.
35. DUNNER, D. and FIEVE, R. Psychiatric illness in fathers of men with bipolar primary affective disorder. *Arch. Gen. Psychiat.*, 32:1134, 1975.
36. WINOKUR, G., CADORET, R. J., DORZAB, J. and BAKER, M.: Depressive disease: A genetic study. *Arch. Gen. Psychiat.*, 24:135, 1971.
37. MENDLEWICZ, J. and FLEISS, J.: Linkage studies with X-chromosome markers in bipolar (manic-depressive) and unipolar (depressive) illnesses. *Recent Advan. Biol. Psychiat.*, 9:261, 1974.
38. TANNA, V. L., WINOKUR, G., ELSTON, R. C. and GO, R. C. P.: A linkage study of depression spectrum disease: The use of the sib-pair method. *Neuropsychobiology* (in press).
39. MORTON, N. E.: Sequential tests for the detection of linkage. *Am. J. Hum. Genetics*, 7:277, 1955.

6

Psychoneuroendocrinology: Fundamental Concepts and Correlates in Depression

Robert T. Rubin, M.D. and Kenneth S. Kendler, M.D.

Abbreviations used in this article:

1. Pituitary hormones
   ACTH—adrenocorticotropic hormone; corticotropin
   GH—growth hormone; somatotropin
   LH—luteinizing hormone; lutropin
   FSH—follicle stimulating hormone; follitropin
   PRL—prolactin
   TSH—thyroid stimulating hormone; thyrotropin
   MSH—melanocyte stimulating hormone; melanotropin

2. Hypothalamic-hypophyseal hormones
   CRF—corticotropin releasing factor; corticoliberin
   GRF—growth hormone releasing factor; somatoliberin
   GIF—growth hormone inhibiting factor; somatostatin
   LRF—gonadotropin releasing factor; luliberin
   PRL—prolactin releasing factor; prolactoliberin
   PIF—prolactin inhibiting factor; prolactostatin
   TRF—thyrotropin releasing factor; thyroliberin

Supported in part by ONR Contract N00014-73-C-0127 and NIMH Research Scientist Development Award K1-MH47363 (to R.T.R.).

Neuroendocrinology, the field of study concerned with the interactions of the nervous system and the endocrine glands, and psychoneuroendocrinology, the interrelationship between neuroendocrinology and psychological functioning, are closely related fields of research that have undergone rapid growth in the last decade. The importance of the central nervous system in the control of endocrine function is now widely recognized (1). Many endocrine systems have been found to respond to changes in psychological states (2).

In this paper we will present some general concepts of neuroendocrine function and will review briefly the relevant anatomy of the hypothalamo-pituitary system. We will survey each hormonal axis, using its pituitary hormone as the focus, by discussing the actions of the pituitary hormone, the pattern of its release including its biorhythm, and what is known of the brain neurochemistry involved in its control. Finally, we will review briefly the effects of psychological factors on each hormone system, with particular emphasis on hormonal changes associated with depression (3).

In recent years, two facets of neuroendocrinology have been recognized as increasingly important: the "open loop" control of pituitary function and the circadian rhythms of several of the pituitary hormones. Formerly, physiological systems were wedded to the concept of a constant internal milieu (homeostasis), which implied that the levels of hormones must be controlled by a thermostat-like mechanism to produce steady-state levels ("closed loop" control). It is now clear that central nervous system driving causes the pituitary hormones to be secreted in rapid bursts alternating with periods of little or no secretion (1). Also, many hormones have consistent major fluctuations in blood levels during the 24-hour period (4-6). Figure 1 illustrates typical secretion patterns of three anterior pituitary hormones, ACTH, GH, and LH, over the full 24-hour period in a normal young adult. Episodic bursts of hormone secretion occur for all three hormones; 24-hour rhythmic changes in baseline plasma hormone concentration are evident for ACTH and GH. These rhythmic changes will be discussed in more detail for the individual hormones in subsequent sections.

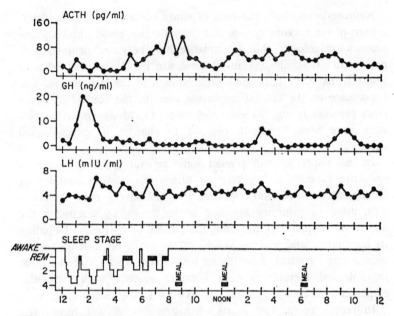

Fig. 1. Representation of the typical secretion patterns of three anterior pituitary hormones, adrenocorticotropic hormone (ACTH), growth hormone (GH), and luteinizing hormone (LH), during 24 hours in a young adult subject, as reflected by plasma hormone concentrations. Secretion of all three hormones is episodic; ACTH and GH have prominent circadian rhythms, the latter being linked to stage 3-4 sleep, as shown at the bottom of the figure.

ANATOMY AND PHYSIOLOGY

Figure 2 depicts the relationship among the central nervous system, the anterior and posterior pituitary glands, the target endocrine glands, and the peripheral tissues influenced by the pituitary and target organ hormones. The hypothalamus is a small area of the brain located below the thalamus, behind the crossing of the optic nerves (optic chiasm), and above the pituitary, being connected to it by a stalk, as shown in the lower part of Figure 2. The hypothalamus is a nodal point for multiple limbic system and midbrain circuits involved with emotive functions. The brain areas with important hypothalamic connections include the amygdala, hippocampus, septal region, midbrain, and, via the thalamus, cingulate gyrus and frontal lobes, as shown in the upper part of Figure 2. Besides its endocrine functions, the hypothalamus is involved in the control of blood pressure, heart rate, bowel function, temperature regulation, and food and water intake.

We will focus on the endocrine functions of the hypothalamus. Within this structure are cells that are neuroendocrine transducers. These neurosecretory cells are modified neurons that receive information via synapses (chemical neurotransmission) from other nerve cells, but their products are hormones. One group of neurosecretory cells secretes small polypeptide hormones into an area of the hypothalamus (the median eminence), whence portal blood vessels carry them to the anterior pituitary. These hypothalamic-hypophysiotropic hormones interact with pituitary cells to control the secretion of the anterior pituitary hormones, which are larger polypeptides that either affect peripheral tissues directly or cause target organ glands to secrete other hormones (7). These target organ hormones in turn affect metabolic processes, as shown at the bottom of Figure 2. The second type of neurosecretory cells in the hypothalamus has long axon terminals that go to the posterior pituitary, where they secrete their hormones into the general circulation, as also shown in Figure 2.

Thus, the pituitary has two lobes—anterior (adenohypophysis) and posterior (neurohypophysis)—that are related to the hypothalamus in different ways. The whole pituitary weighs only 0.7 gm, but in the adenohypophysis are six different identified populations of cells, secreting six different hormones.

ACTH

ACTH stimulates the adrenal cortex to secrete corticosteroid hormones, particularly cortisol. It recently has been shown to have extra-adrenal effects, including effects on the central nervous system, but the normal physiologic significance of these latter effects is as

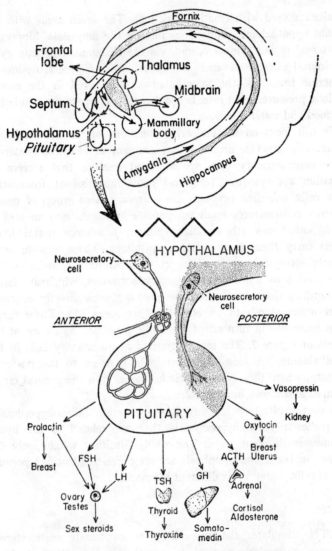

Fig. 2. Limbic brain circuits and their relationship to the hypothalamo-pituitary unit (top); the anterior and posterior pituitary, their functional relationships to the median emi-nence of the hypothalamus, their pituitary hormones, and their target organ effects (bottom).

yet unknown. ACTH is secreted by a distinct cell population in the anterior pituitary, the corticotrophs.

Though ACTH may inhibit its own secretion by a "short-loop" feedback to the hypothalamus, the predominant influences of ACTH release appear to be stimulatory, by CRF secreted by the hypothalamus, and inhibitory, by circulating cortisol. The locus of action of the negative feedback of circulating cortisol appears to be at both the hypothalamic and pituitary levels.

The neurochemical control of ACTH release via CRF is quite complex and far from being completely understood. A catecholaminergic (norepinephrine) pathway in the hypothalamus inhibits CRF release, and it has been postulated that this neurotransmitter system is the one involved in the negative feedback of cortisol on CRF release. Serotonin pathways appear to be involved in the ACTH response to stress and the negative feedback of cortisol. There is also evidence implicating acetylcholine as a stimulatory influence on ACTH release (8).

Clinicians long have known that cortisol excess or deficiency, as in Cushing's and Addison's disease respectively, can have profound effects on psychological functioning (9). Conversely, in recent years there has been a growing interest in the relationship between psychological states and the activation of the adrenal cortex via CRF and ACTH. This area of research, focusing particularly on the relationship of psychological stress to adrenal activation, is the largest and oldest in psychoneuroendocrinology. The adrenal cortical axis has been shown to be sensitive to such diverse psychological stresses as the anticipation of surgery, war movies, examinations for medical students, and the relapse of leukemic children for their parents (2).

ACTH is secreted episodically, and it has a pronounced circadian rhythm in blood. Its levels are lowest from about four hours prior to three hours after sleep onset, and peak levels are attained from about two hours prior to one hour after awakening (4-6). ACTH secretion is not directly related to sleep stages and has considerable inertia in its circadian rhythm. After an acute reversal of the sleep-wake cycle, as might occur in changing from a day to a night work shift, the cortisol rhythm is completely dissociated from the sleep-wake cycle, and only after two or three weeks does the ACTH rhythm return to being in phase with the new sleep schedule.

The more specific inquiry into the relationship of depression to the adrenal axis also has a long history. Early studies showed adrenal activation in depression. Some workers postulated that this was related to the general breakdown of ego defenses with experiencing of anxiety (10), while others felt that the interaction between depression and adrenal activation could be a more specific neurochemical one (3, 11).

Recent studies have uncovered several abnormalities of the ACTH axis that may be specific for depression (3). It has been demonstrated that the adrenal activation in depression is caused by increased central nervous system release of CRF and not by altered peripheral metabolism of cortisol. Using multiple sampling techniques, several investigators have noted significant alterations in the circadian rhythm of cortisol. There is an increased number of secretory episodes during each 24-hour period in some severely endogenously depressed patients, with active cortisol secretion during sleep in the late evening and early morning hours, a time when secretion normally is minimal (12). The disordered secretion during sleep has been considered as an argument against a non-specific psychoendocrine stress response in depression; rather it suggests a specific hypothalamic and/or limbic system dysfunction. Also, the normal negative feedback suppression of the pituitary-adrenal axis by the potent synthetic glucocorticoid, dexamethasone, is altered in a significant percentage of severely depressed patients (13). Some evidence suggests that patients may show a graded series of responses to the dexamethasone suppression test that approach normality as clinical improvement occurs.

GH

GH is secreted by the somatotrophs of the anterior pituitary. It has a number of important metabolic actions including stimulating cartilage and bone growth, increasing circulating levels of free fatty acids and blood sugar, and enhancing protein synthesis. The growth effects of GH, and possibly some other effects as well, appear to be mediated by somatomedin, a polypeptide hormone synthesized in the liver under the influence of GH.

Though GH has been shown to inhibit its own secretion, it appears that hypothalamic neural influences are predominant in its control, via the secretion of both GRF and GIF. The neurochemical control of GH release in man appears to be under α-adrenergic stimulatory and β-adrenergic inhibitory influences. Dopamine, and possibly serotonin, are stimulatory (8, 14). L-dopa increases GH levels in man, and chlorpromazine blockage of catecholamine receptors inhibits GH secretion.

Given the widespread metabolic actions of GH, it is not surprising that metabolic changes such as hypoglycemia, fasting and exercise are potent stimuli of GH release. GH is secreted episodically, with a well-delineated circadian rhythm. During most of the day, GH levels are very low, except for small increases several hours after meals. However, GH is secreted in large amounts in direct association with entry into slow-wave or deep (stage 3-4) sleep in the first hour or two of the night (4-6). The relationship between slow-wave sleep and GH release is a direct one, because if slow wave sleep does not occur, GH release does not occur either. GH also will be released if slow wave sleep occurs during a daytime nap.

In man GH has been shown to rise with a number of psychological stresses, such as surgery (15) and arterial puncture. Studies of the GH system in endogenous depression (16) suggest that basal GH levels are normal; however, the GH surge with slow wave sleep may be abnormal, and an impaired GH surge may occur in response to L-dopa and hypoglycemia challenge. Also, there is preliminary evidence of an impaired GH response to 5-hydroxytryptophan, the immediate precursor of serotonin, in some depressed patients.

A fascinating psychoneuroendocrine condition that may be related to depression is the so-called maternal deprivation syndrome (17). In this syndrome, children with disturbed family situations have growth retardation and low GH levels, both of which return to normal with environmental change. The improvement in growth in these children has yet to be specifically linked to the increased GH secretion, however, since improvement in diet and general psychosocial milieu can have effects on metabolism that are not mediated via GH.

FSH and LH

FSH and LH are both gonadotropins. In the female FSH stimulates early follicular development in the ovary, while LH supports final follicular maturation and ovulation. In the male, FSH, aided by LH and testosterone, stimulates sperm production, and LH, perhaps aided by PRL and FSH, stimulates testicular Leydig cells to secrete testosterone.

The control of the secretion of FSH and LH from their distinct cell populations in the anterior pituitary is complex and not fully understood. LRF, a hypothalamic hormone that stimulates the release of both LH and FSH, has been characterized and synthesized. There is a controversy as to whether LRF controls both LH and FSH under normal circumstances, or whether a separate FSH releasing hormone exists. Feedback of the steroid hormones stimulated by FSH and LH—progesterone and estrogens in the female and testosterone in the male—plays an important role in the control of FSH and LH. This feedback is both to the hypothalamus and to the pituitary, and is both negative and at times positive, as with the estradiol triggering of the LH ovulatory surge in the female. In the male, testosterone inhibits LH secretion, but the peripheral factor regulating FSH secretion is unclear. LH also may inhibit its own secretion.

The neurochemical control of the gonadotropins involves both the catecholamines, norepinephrine and dopamine, in a stimulatory role, and serotonin as an inhibitory influence (7, 8). Most research in this area has been done on animals, and its applicability to humans is as yet unclear. One fascinating aspect of the hypothalamic control of the pituitary-gonadal axis involves the evident "setting" of the relevant neural circuits into a male or a female pattern by perinatal exposure to sex steroids. This setting includes not only the characteristic male (tonic) vs. female (cyclic) gonadotropin release pattern, but other behavioral parameters as well, including sexual behavior and levels of aggressiveness. These findings in animals appear to apply in some measure to humans (18).

Both FSH and LH are secreted episodically. There is an ontogenetic variation in the circadian rhythm of LH, with low LH prepubertally and elevated levels beginning in puberty during the hours of sleep. However, in adults active secretion of FSH and LH occurs throughout the full 24 hours, with no apparent circadian rhythm of these hormones. In the adult male, testosterone has a well-documented rhythm, with peak levels around the time of awakening, suggesting other influences on its secretion besides FSH and LH.

In humans, FSH and LH secretion have been shown to be unresponsive to acute stress. In men, however, several studies have demonstrated a decreased secretion of testosterone (probably due to decreased LH) with chronic stress. The often postulated relationship in women between changing gonadotropin and sex steroid levels and the affective changes associated with the menstrual cycle and pregnancy has yet to be definitively demonstrated. Psychogenic amenorrhea, anorexia nervosa, and pseudocyesis (19) are three disorders in which both profound changes in pituitary-gonadal function and significant depressive features can occur. In specific studies of endogenous depression, plasma testosterone levels in men have been found to be unchanged, but LH levels in post-menopausal women have been found to be decreased (20). Because of the decreases in sexual appetite and general levels of drive and aggressiveness that can accompany depression, further studies of the pituitary-gonadal axis in depression are warranted in order to elucidate the contribution of sex hormone changes to symptomatology.

PRL

PRL, secreted by the lactotroph cells of the anterior pituitary, acts in the adult female to initiate and maintain lactation after the breasts are primed by estrogen, progesterone, and glucocorticoids. In large concentrations PRL has metabolic effects similar to GH, but this is of doubtful normal physiologic significance. In the adult male, PRL circulates in almost the same concentration as in the adult female, and it may play a role in stimulating the secretion of testosterone (21).

The major control of prolactin secretion is via the hypothalamic hormone PIF. PRF most likely also exists, although it has not been identified. PRL also may feed back to inhibit its own secretion. The major physiological stimuli of PRL release are pregnancy and manipulation of the female breast. TRF also is a potent stimulus of PRL secretion, but it may not play a role in the normal physiologic regulation of PRL.

The evidence that central dopamine inhibits PRL secretion is very strong. Antipsychotic drugs which are dopamine antagonists uniformly elevate PRL levels and can produce galactorrhea. Although dopamine itself may be PIF, it is more likely that dopamine controls PIF secretion. Serotonin stimulates PRL release, possibly via PRF. There is conflicting evidence concerning the role of norepinephrine and acetylcholine in PRL secretion (7, 8).

Like the other anterior pituitary hormones, PRL is secreted in a pulsatile fashion. It has a consistent circadian rhythm in the blood, with levels rising during sleep and peaking just before awakening (4-6). In general, PRL levels are increased with stress. An interesting example of interactions between hormone systems is that estrogens apparently sensitize the PRL system to numerous stimuli. Thus, the PRL response of the female to surgery is greater than that of the male (15). There is preliminary evidence that PRL may be secreted with orgasm in some women (15). Because of the dopamine hypothesis of schizophrenia and the close relationship between PRL and central dopamine, PRL physiology is being studied in this disorder. The only study of PRL in depression has been the measurement of basal PRL levels, which were slightly elevated, perhaps as a stress effect (16). The suppression of PRL with L-dopa has been reported to be normal in depression.

TSH

TSH is secreted by the thyrotrophs of the anterior pituitary and acts on the thyroid hormone. Two major controls exist for TSH secretion. The first is TRF, and the second is feedback inhibition of thyroid hormone to the pituitary to shut off TSH release. The neurotransmitters involved in TRF control have not yet been clearly elucidated. Both the catecholamines, dopamine and norepinephrine, and the indoleamine, serotonin, have been implicated (7, 8).

TSH is secreted intermittently throughout the day, with some studies reporting peak levels occurring between 10:00 P.M. and 2:00 A.M. (4, 5). It is believed that the central nervous system, via TRF, is responsible for both the pulsatile release and the circadian rhythm of TSH. A stimulus that releases TSH in infants, again via TRF, is cold. The hypothalamic areas that control temperature regulation and TRF secretion are in close proximity. In animals, stress tends to lower TSH secretion.

It has long been appreciated that if thyroid hormone either is in excess, as in Graves' disease, or is deficient, as in myxedema, profound effects on psychological functioning can result (10). Specific disorders of the thyroid axis in depression, however, have been limited to the finding that the pituitary secretion of TSH in response to a TRF infusion may be blunted.

The thyroid axis may be involved in depression also in another way. Both the thyroid hormone triiodothyronine and TSH have been shown to accelerate the clinical response to tricyclic antidepressants when given to depressed patients (22). This may have its neurochemical basis in an increased sensitivity of the postsynaptic neurotransmitter receptors produced by the thyroid hormone. This increased receptor sensitivity would complement the increased synaptic levels of neurotransmitters produced by the antidepressants. Some workers also have found a short-lived primary antidepressant effect of TRF, although this finding has not been consistently confirmed.

Vasopressin and Oxytocin

Unlike the hormones of the anterior pituitary, the posterior pituitary hormones vasopressin (antidiuretic hormone) and oxytocin are hypothalamic hormones, synthesized by hypothalamic neuroendocrine cells but stored and released in the posterior pituitary. Both vasopressin and oxytocin are small polypeptides. The main action of vasopressin is on the renal collecting tubules to increase the resorption of water from the urine, though in pharmacological doses it has a vasoconstrictor effect. The physiological role of oxytocin is to cause milk ejection from the female breast and to aid in labor by causing contraction of uterine muscle. The major stimuli for vasopressin release are hypertonicity of body fluids and decreased circulating blood volume. Oxytocin is released by nipple and cervical stimulation.

The neurochemical control of the posterior pituitary hormones is not well understood. Animal work suggests that acetylcholine, dopamine and norepinephrine all may be involved in vasopressin secretion. Both vasopressin and oxytocin are secreted in pulses, but little is known about their circadian rhythms. Preliminary evidence suggests that vasopressin secretion may increase during sleep, although its episodic secretion is not related to sleep staging (23).

Some animal studies have shown vasopressin secretion to be increased with pain, but other studies have not shown this hormone to be stress-responsive. Vasopressin secretion may be increased in certain psychotic states, but to our knowledge no work specifically investigating vasopressin physiology in depression has been done. Furthermore, almost nothing is known of the specific psychoneuroendocrinology of oxytocin, although milk let-down in response to stress or a baby's cry are well known phenomena.

Other Hormone Systems

One pituitary hormone we have not discussed is MSH, secreted by the intermediate lobe of the pituitary (a modified portion of the anterior pituitary). There are actually two MSH's, α and β. Though their chemistry and the chemistry of their hypothalamic factor, MSH inhibiting factor, are known, neither their function, neurochemical control, nor response to psychological stimuli in man is understood. Some animal studies have shown that MSH secretion does respond to certain stresses.

In this brief review we have had to neglect the area of neuro-endocrinology involving interactions between several peripherally secreted hormones and the autonomic nervous system. There is good evidence that the CNS is involved in the renin-angiotensin system and possibly in gastrointestinal hormone systems as well. Of course, epinephrine and norepinephrine are hormones secreted by the adrenal medulla that have long been known to be under direct control of the sympathetic nervous system. Other than for the adrenal catecholamines, few psychoneuroendocrinologic studies have been done on these systems, though preliminary evidence suggests that one of the pancreatic hormones (glucagon) may respond to stress.

A new area of interest that should be mentioned is the presence of hypothalamic releasing and inhibiting hormones, such as TRF, in parts of the brain other than the hypothalamus. Some workers have suggested that these small peptides may have a function, such as neurotransmission, completely separate from their actions on the piuitary. There is presently some evidence to support this claim (24).

CONCLUSIONS

Now that we have reviewed basic psychoneuroendocrinology and its application to depression, we can discuss three areas of potential relevance of this field to the psychiatric clinician (one theoretical and two practical).

The theoretical relevance is that neuroendocrine responses are excellent tools for testing various neurochemical hypotheses about psychiatric disease. Since our knowledge of the neurochemical control of the pituitary hormones is increasing, it is now possible, given an established neuroendocrine abnormality in a psychiatric illness, to postulate to what degree the activity levels of neurotransmitters might be altered to cause that abnormality. For example, the documented neuroendocrine disorders in some severe endogenous depressions include overactivity of the adrenal cortical axis with poor response to dexamethasone suppression, poor response of GH to hypoglycemia, and low LH levels (in post-menopausal women).

Norepinephrine is a hypothalamic neurotransmitter thought to be involved in inhibiting ACTH secretion and stimulating LH and GH secretion; a norepinephrine deficiency might explain the neuroendocrine findings in depression.

The first practical relevance that neuroendocrinology holds for clinical psychiatry is in the area of diagnosis and prognosis. Psychiatric diagnosis is now based on such parameters as clinical symptoms and signs, premorbid functioning, family history and sometimes (retrospectively) response to medication. Often, however, these parameters are not sufficient to diagnose and treat patients with great confidence. Neuroendocrine techniques may aid clinicians in this dilemma. For example, there is a case report of a young woman who presented as a differential diagnosis between a neurotic condition and an agitated depression. Though some clinicians felt that the depression was not an important part of her problem, her dexamethasone suppression test was quite abnormal. It was then decided to treat the patient with an antidepressant, and she responded quite well. Had it not been for the neuroendocrine test, she might never have received the appropriate antidepressant medication (B. J. Carroll, personal communication).

Neuroendocrine techniques also may be useful in another practical problem in clinical psychiatry. Often the specific type and dose of a psychopharmacologic agent are difficult to choose with adequate assurance of clinical response. This is especially true for those drugs where there may be an expected delay between the beginning of therapy and clinical response. Monitoring blood levels of drugs will provide some objective measure of response potential, since the absorption and metabolism of many psychopharmacologic agents are so variable from patient to patient. But even this will not tell the clinician how much drug is active in the brain. Since a number of psychopharmacologic agents have been demonstrated to affect neuroendocrine systems, the monitoring of neuroendocrine responses to drugs may provide an index of the CNS neurochemical effect of treatment. Thus, the PRL system has been suggested for monitoring therapy with antipsychotic drugs which block dopamine receptors

(25); PRL levels in blood may reflect how much medication is penetrating the brain and how it is interacting with neurotransmitter systems.

REFERENCES

1. REICHLIN, S.: Neuroendocrinology. *In* R. H. Williams (Ed.), *Textbook of Endocrinology*, Fifth Edition. Philadelphia: W. B. Saunders, 1974, pp. 774-828.
2. MASON, J. W.: Organization of psychoendocrine mechanisms. *Psychosom. Med.*, 30:565-808, 1968.
3. CARROLL, B. J. and MENDELS, J.: Neuroendocrine regulation in affective disorders. In E. J. Sachar (Ed.), *Hormones, Behavior and Psychopathology*. New York: Raven Press, 1976, 193-224.
4. RUBIN, R. T., POLAND, R. E., RUBIN, L. E. and GOUIN, P. R.: The neuroendocrinology of human sleep. *Life Sci.*, 14:1041-1052, 1974.
5. RUBIN, R. T.: Sleep-endocrinology studies in man. *In* W. H. Gispen, Tj, B. van Wimersma Greidanus, B. Bohus, and D. de Wied (Eds.), *Hormones, Homeostasis and the Brain, Progress in Brain Research*, Volume 42. Amsterdam: Elsevier, 1975, pp. 73-80.
6. WEITZMAN, E. D., BOYAR, R. M., KAPEN, S. and HELLMAN, L.: The relationship of sleep and sleep stages to neuroendocrine secretion and biological rhythms in man. *Rec. Prog. Horm. Res.*, 31:399-446, 1975.
7. DAUGHADAY, W. H.: The adenohypophysis. *In* R. H. Williams (Ed.), *Textbook of Endocrinology*, Fifth Edition. Philadelphia: W. B. Saunders, 1974, pp. 31-79.
8. DE WIED, D. and DE JONG, W.: Drug effects and hypothalamic-anterior pituitary function. *Ann. Rev. Pharmacol.*, 14:389-412, 1974.
9. SMITH, C. K., BARISH, J., CORREA, J. and WILLIAMS, R. H.: Psychiatric disturbance in endocrinologic disease. *Psychosom. Med.*, 34:69-86, 1972.
10. SACHAR, E. J., KANTER, S. S., BUIE, D., ENGLE, R. and MEHLMAN, R.: Psychoendocrinology of ego disintegration. *Amer. J. Psychiat.*, 126:1067-1078, 1970.
11. RUBIN, R. T., GOUIN, P. R. and POLAND, R. E.: Biogenic amine metabolism and neuroendocrine function in affective disorders. *In* R. de la Fuente and M. N. Weisman (Eds.), *Psychiatry*. Proc. V World Congr. Psychiatry, Mexico City, 1971, Part II. Amsterdam: Excerpta Medica, 1973, pp. 1036-1039.
12. SACHAR, E. J., HELLMAN, L., ROFFWARG, H. P., HALPERN, F. S., FUKUSHIMA, D. K. and GALLAGHER, T. F.: Disrupted 24-hour patterns of cortisol secretion in psychotic depression. *Arch. Gen. Psychiat.*, 28:19-24, 1973.

13. CARROLL, B. J., MARTIN, F. I. R., and DAVIES, B.: Resistance to suppression by dexamethasone of plasma 11-OHCS levels in severe depressive illness. *Brit. Med. J.*, 3:285-287, 1968.
14. FROHMAN, L. A. and STACHURA, M. E.: Neuropharmacologic control of neuroendocrine function in man. *Metabolism*, 24:211-234, 1975.
15. NOEL, G. L., SUH, H. K., STONE, G. and FRANTZ, A. G.: Human prolactin and growth hormone release during surgery and other conditions of stress. *J. Clin. Endocrinol. Metab.*, 35:840-851, 1972.
16. SACHAR, E. J., FRANTZ, A. G., ALTMAN, N. and SASSIN, J.: Growth hormone and prolactin in unipolar and bipolar depressed patients: Responses to hypoglycemia and L-Dopa. *Amer. J. Psychiat.*, 130:1362-1367, 1973.
17. POWELL, G. F., BRASEL, J. A. and BLIZZARD, R. M.: Emotional deprivation and growth retardation simulating idiopathic hypopituitarism, Parts I and II. *New Engl. J. Med.*, 276:1271-1283, 1967.
18. MONEY, J. and EHRHARDT, A. A.: *Man and Woman, Boy and Girl.* Baltimore: Johns Hopkins University Press, 1972.
19. BROWN, E. and BARGLOW, P.: Pseudocyesis: A paradigm for psychophysiological interactions. *Arch. Gen. Psychiat.*, 24:221-229, 1971.
20. ALTMAN, N., SACHAR, E. J., GRUEN, P. H., HALPERN, F. S. and ETO, S.: Reduced plasma LH concentration in postmenopausal depressed women. *Psychosom. Med.*, 37:274-276, 1975.
21. RUBIN, R. T., GOUIN, P. R., LUBIN, A., POLAND, R. E. and PIRKE, K. M.: Nocturnal increase of plasma testosterone in men: Relation to gonadotropins and prolactin. *J. Clin. Endocrinol. Metab.*, 40:1027-1033, 1975.
22. PRANGE, A. J., WILSON, I. C., KNOX, A., McCLANE, T. K. and LIPTON, M. A.: Enhancement of imipramine by thyroid stimulating hormone: Clinical and theoretical implications. *Amer. J. Psychiat.*, 127:191-199, 1970.
23. RUBIN, R. T., POLAND, R. E., RAVESSOUD, F., GOUIN, P. R. and TOWER, B. B.: Antidiuretic hormone: Episodic nocturnal secretion in adult men. *Endocr. Res. Comm.*, 2:459-469, 1975.
24. MARTIN, J. B., RENAUD, L. P. and BRAZEAU, P.: Hypothalamic peptides: New evidence for "peptidergic" pathways in the C.N.S. *Lancet*, 2:393-395, 1975.
25. RUBIN, R. T., POLAND, R. E., O'CONNOR, D., GOUIN, P. R. and TOWER, B. B.: Selective neuroendocrine effects of low-dose haloperidol in normal adult men. *Psychopharmacol.*, 47:135-140, 1976.

7

Neuropharmacological Aspects of Affective Disorders

Jack D. Barchas, M.D., Robert L. Patrick, Ph.D., Joachim Raese, M.D., and Philip A. Berger, M.D.

This chapter presents a picture of the central nervous system (CNS) from a neuropharmacological point of view, with special emphasis on basic concepts concerning the regulation of neurotransmitter synthesis, storage, and release and the potential sites of interaction with drugs used in the treatment of affective (manic-depressive) disorders.

The focus on neurotransmitters is based on the conviction that since a good deal of intercellular communication in the central nervous system depends upon the release and receptor interaction of these chemical transmitters, disorders in central nervous system functioning may be related to disorders in neurotransmitter processes. This suggests that clinically effective drugs utilized in psychiatry should be acting, at least in part, through their interactions

Supported by NIMH Program Project Grant, MH 23861. JDB is recipient of Research Scientist Development Award, MH 24161.

We should like to thank Dr. Thomas A. Gonda of Stanford for his encouragement of this chapter and Dr. Earl Usdin of the NIMH for his helpful comments on an early draft.

with central nervous system neurotransmitter systems. This chapter will discuss the neuropharmacological aspects of the catecholamine and serotonin systems in the central nervous system since these have been the most extensively studied in relation to the affective disorders. We will discuss these neurotransmitters with regard to regulation of synthesis, release, receptor interaction and inactivation; evidence that these transmitters may be involved in affective disorders will be evaluated, and some concepts concerning the mechanism of action of clinically effective drugs will be presented. A number of reviews concerning more specifically the clinical aspects of affective disorders have been published recently (1-4).

NEUROTRANSMITTERS IN THE CENTRAL NERVOUS SYSTEM

Dopamine, norepinephrine, epinephrine, serotonin, histamine, acetylcholine, and gamma-aminobutyric acid, as well as several amino acids, have been suggested as neurotransmitters in the central nervous system. This list of putative neurotransmitters will undoubtedly grow larger with time. The criteria for determining whether or not a compound may be acting as a neurotransmitter usually involve trying to satisfy as many of the following properties as possible: 1) the compound should be found localized in the synaptic region being studied; 2) the enzymes necessary for its synthesis should be localized in this region, or at least in a region where transport from the site of synthesis to the site of release can be demonstrated; 3) some means of inactivation of the compound should be demonstrated that would terminate its action, either by enzymatic destruction and/or removal from the synaptic cleft, for instance by reuptake back into the nerve; 4) neuronal stimulation should be demonstrated to lead to release of the compound; 5) the exogenous administration of the compound should mimic the effects of neuronal stimulation; 6) agents that block the effects of neuronal stimulation should also block the effect of exogenous administration of the compound; and 7) the prevention of the normal removal of the compound by inhibiting its enzymatic breakdown or its reuptake may be expected to lead to a potentiation of its action.

How well do the catecholamines and serotonin fulfill these requirements in the central nervous system? 1) Specific neuronal tracts containing catecholamines or serotonin have been identified and mapped using the technique of histofluorescence (5). 2) Immuno-histofluorescent techniques have also indicated the neuronal localization of the enzymes necessary for the formation of these compounds (6). Treatments which cause nerve terminal destruction, such as electrolytic lesions or administration of the catecholaminergic-toxic substance 6-hydroxydopamine cause parallel losses of catecholamines and their synthetic enzymes (7). 3) The enzymes necessary for inactivation of these compounds are found in the central nervous system, as well as an active nerve-ending reuptake process (8). 4) Depolarization-induced release of these compounds can be demonstrated in central nervous system tissue (9). 5) In some systems, such as cerebellar Purkinje cells, the application of norepinephrine can mimic the inhibitory effects of neuronal stimulation (10). However, since, in general, the precise effects of neuronal stimulation in the central nervous system attributable to one specific transmitter are not known, satisfying requirements (5-7) has proved quite difficult.

Catecholamine and Serotonin Formation in the
Central Nervous System

The basic synthetic pathways for catecholamine and serotonin formation are shown in Figure 1. The first steps in both systems involve a ring hydroxylation reaction which requires oxygen and a reduced pteridine cofactor. Both tyrosine and tryptophan hydroxylations are considered to be the rate-limiting reaction in their respective overall synthetic pathways. Decarboxylation of the newly formed hydroxylated compounds occurs very rapidly to form either dopamine from dopa or serotonin from 5-HTP. Catecholaminergic neurons that contain the enzyme dopamine-β-hydroxylase can convert dopamine to norepinephrine and those that contain the enzyme phenylethylamine-N-methyltransferase (PNMT) can catalyze the conversion of norepinephrine to epinephrine. Both the catecholamines and serotonin are believed to be localized predominantly in storage vesicles, from which they can be released upon neuronal depolarization. Based,

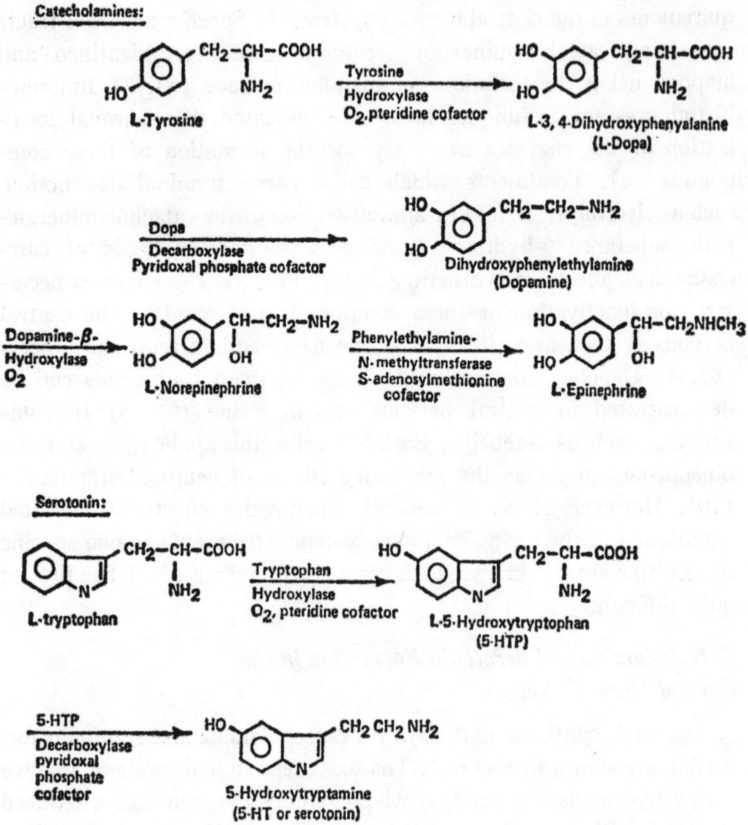

Catecholamines:

Serotonin:

Figure 1.

in part, on studies of the adrenal medulla, dopamine-β-hydroxylase is believed to be localized in the catecholaminergic storage vesicles. Adrenal medullary studies suggest that dopamine must be taken up into the vesicles before it can be converted to norepinephrine, since reserpine, a rauwolfia alkaloid that blocks the uptake of catecholamines into vesicles, inhibits the conversion of dopamine to norepinephrine in intact vesicle preparations, but not in lysed vesicle preparations (where the enzyme and substrate would have free access to each other) (11). The decarboxylase enzymes, PNMT, and tryptophan hydroxylase are considered soluble enzymes since most of the activity is found in the supernatant fraction after homogenization in hypotonic medium and high speed centrifugation. The fraction that tyrosine hydroxylase will be found in can depend on the exact composition of the homogenizing medium (12) with a good deal of the activity usually being found in the supernatant fraction. Evidence has been presented, however, for the existence of a soluble and particulate form in rat brain, with the particulate form exhibiting a lower K_m for pteridine cofactor (13).

The activity of tyrosine hydroxylase can be markedly inhibited by dopamine, norepinephrine, or epinephrine. This finding has prompted the suggestion that one mode of regulation of catecholamine synthesis may involve end-product inhibition so that when there is an increase in end-product, the synthesis rate will decrease and, conversely, that when the end-product decreases, the synthesis rate will increase (14). Numerous studies have indicated, in fact, a significant increase in the activity of tyrosine hydroxylase *in vivo*, following treatments (such as exercise or cold stress) that may lead to increased sympathetic neuronal activity and increased release of catecholamine transmitters (15, 16). This increase in synthesis can also be observed *in vitro*, utilizing preparations that maintain a certain level of cellular organization such as intact nerves, tissue slices, or synaptosomes (nerve-ending preparations that are formed upon homogenization in isotonic sucrose). *In vitro* studies make use of either direct electrical stimulation, elevated extracellular potassium concentrations, or agents such as veratridine (an alkaloid capable of increasing sodium permeability) in order to study more directly the effects of depolarization on catecholamine synthesis and release. The fact that the depolarization-induced increase in catecholamine synthesis in central nervous system preparations, such as cortex slices or striatal synaptosomes, is calcium-dependent (17, 18) suggests that this increase may in some way be linked to transmitter release.

Tyrosine hydroxylase can be shown to be activated by cyclic AMP (19, 20), calcium (21, 22), or phospholipids (23, 24) in free enzyme preparations (preparations in which the homogenization technique has been purposefully vigorous enough to disrupt the cellular organization). These findings greatly expand concepts of tyrosine hydroxylase regulation beyond merely the relief of feedback inhibition by removal of end-product and offer further approaches for studying the relationships between catecholaminergic neuronal firing rate and transmitter synthesis.

Numerous studies have also indicated that the rate of serotonin synthesis can be increased by various agents *in vivo* (such as increased environmental temperature, reserpine and electroconvulsive shock) (25) as well as by direct electrical stimulation of the raphe nuclei, which contain serotonergic cell bodies (26, 27). The amount of tryptophan available for tryptophan hydroxylase may normally be non-saturating and consequently the amount of serotonin in the brain can be increased by tryptophan injections (28). Whether or not this increase in serotonin content significantly alters the effects of serotonergic neuronal firing remains to be determined.

Although the addition of serotonin to tissue slices (29) and synaptosomes (30) can decrease the serotonin synthesis rate, serotonin has been reported to have no direct effect on tryptophan hydroxylase activity in free enzyme preparations (31, 32). Thus, the increase in serotonin synthesis rate observed after electrical stimulation of the raphe does not appear to be due simply to removal of end-product inhibition, nor is there any measurable change in tryptophan content of the tissue to account for the increased synthesis rate. The recent findings that free enzyme preparations of tryptophan hydroxylase can be activated by calcium (33, 34) offer one possible explanation for these observations, since an increased uptake of calcium has been observed to occur following neuronal depolarization (35).

Besides regulation of transmitter synthesis by alterations in the activities of the synthetic enzymes, alterations in the actual amounts of enzyme can also occur. This phenomenon has been most extensively studied with regard to the induction of catecholamine synthesizing enzymes such as tyrosine hydroxylase and dopamine-β-hydroxylase in the adrenal medulla. In this system, treatments such as insulin-induced hypoglycemia, reserpine administration, or immobilization stress, which can increase sympathetic discharge, produce a trans-synaptic, protein synthesis-dependent increase in the levels of tyrosine hydroxylase (25). Reserpine has also been found to increase the amount of tyrosine hydroxylase in specific brain areas, such as the locus coeruleus (36, 37). The importance of these inductive changes remains to be determined, but in the adrenal medulla there is some evidence that they may play a role in affecting the ability of the gland to restore its catecholamine supply following drug-induced depletion (38).

Neurotransmitter Release and Inactivation

Nerve terminal depolarization is accompanied by an increase in sodium permeability followed by an increase in calcium uptake and release of transmitter at the synaptic cleft (35). The released transmitter is then capable of interacting with the postsynaptic receptor to bring about a change in membrane permeability that will produce either an inhibitory or excitatory effect on the post-synaptic neuron. The transmitter release process is calcium-dependent, although the exact mode of action of calcium is not yet known. Inactivation of the transmitter can occur either enzymatically (as in the breakdown of acetylcholine to acetate and choline by acetylcholinesterase) or by removal of the transmitter from the synaptic cleft. *In vitro* studies of central nervous system nerve-ending preparations show that they possess the ability to take up and store many biogenic amine putative neurotransmitters, such as dopamine, norepinephrine, and serotonin, suggesting that reuptake of transmitter may be quite important in the inactivation of these compounds (39).

In addition to the reuptake process, the biogenic amines are also subject to enzymatic degradative action. The basic pathways for norepinephrine, dopamine and serotonin metabolism are shown in Figure 2.

Neurotransmitter-Receptor Interactions

Of crucial importance, of course, in considering synaptic transmission is the nature of the interaction between the transmitter and

Fig. 2. ADR = Aldehyde reductase; ADH = Aldehyde dehydrogenase; COMT = Catechol-O-Methyltransferase; MAO = Monoamine oxidase; NE = Norepinephrine; DA = Dopamine; DPG = Dihydroxyphenylglycol; NMN = Noremetanephrine; DMA = Dihydroxymandelic acid; VMA = Vaniyllmandelic acid; MHPG = 3-methoxy-4-hydroxyphenylglycol; DOPAC = Dihydrophenylacetic acid; HVA = Homovanillic acid; 5-HIAA = 5-Hydroxyindoleacetic acid.

its receptor. It is possible that neurotransmitter receptors may be located both pre- and post-synaptically. The amount and/or sensitivity of the receptor may be subject to alteration, as is seen, for instance, in the case of skeletal muscle which undergoes the phenomenon of denervation supersensitivity, that is, the area of muscle that is sensitive to acetylcholine increases following denervation (40, 41). The frequency and nature of interaction between transmitter and receptor can thus be a key event through which cells can transmit information which may affect not only the receptors themselves but also could affect the pre-synaptic firing rate, the rate of pre-synaptic transmitter synthesis, and a host of other metabolic processes both pre- and post-synaptically.

One potentially very important metabolic alteration that can take place in the post-synaptic neuron in response to biogenic amine release is an increase in intracellular levels of cyclic AMP, due to an activation of a biogenic amine-sensitive adenyl cyclase. Thus, tissue slices from various brain regions can be demonstrated to show an increase in cyclic AMP formation in response to biogenic amines such as dopamine, norepinephrine, or histamine (42). Depolarizing agents have also been shown to increase the levels of cyclic AMP, and in some cases also cyclic GMP, in central nervous system tissue slice preparations (43, 44). It has been suggested that the stimulation-induced increase in cyclic AMP, acting through protein kinase activation, may be of great significance in mediating the change in membrane permeability that occurs as a result of transmitter-receptor interaction (45).

Neurotransmitters and Affective Disorders

The observations that iproniazid, a monoamine oxidase inhibitor, could produce mood elevation in tuberculosis patients and that reserpine could produce mood depression in hypertensive patients, suggested that catecholamine functioning in the central nervous system is capable of influencing mood. The findings that the tricyclic antidepressants could inhibit catecholamine uptake led to suggestions that depression was characterized by subnormal catecholamine functioning which could be improved either by inhibiting catecholamine breakdown with monoamine oxidase inhibitors or by prolonging catecholamine synaptic action by preventing its reuptake with tricyclics. Serotonin is affected similarly by these medications. Thus, the concept of subnormal functioning has been extended to include the serotonergic system as well. Another treatment used in the treatment of depression, electroconvulsive therapy, has been found to increase the central nervous system catecholamine turnover rate (46), a finding which would also be consistent with the hypothesis that subnormal catecholamine activity plays a role in depression.

Neurotransmitters and Their Metabolites in Patients
with Affective Disorders

The hypothesis of altered biogenic amine activity in affective disorders would predict that the levels of the main catecholamine and serotonin metabolites, either in the urine or cerebral spinal fluid (CSF), might be different in depressed or manic patients compared to normal controls. In fact, studies of catecholamine and serotonin and their metabolites in biological fluids have produced remarkably inconsistent results. Dopamine and norepinephrine and the catecholamine metabolites normetanephrine and vanillyl mandelic acid have been reported to be decreased in the urine of depressed patients and increased in the urine of manic patients by some investigators (47-49). However, other investigators find no consistent differences in catecholamine excretion between patients and controls (50). The variable results may in part reflect the significant peripheral sources of these substances.

Urinary 3-methoxy-4-hydroxyphenylglycol (MHPG) is the catecholamine metabolite which has been suggested to reflect central nervous system catecholamine metabolism. This hypothesis is based on double norepinephrine isotope labeling studies in the dog and the use, in non-human primates, of 6-hydroxydopamine, which destroys central norepinephrine neurons (51, 52). These studies suggest that from a third to a half of urinary MHPG may reflect central metabolism in these animals. However, the proportion of urinary MHPG which reflects central norepinephrine metabolism in man remains controversial (53, 54).

Several investigators report decreased urinary excretion of MHPG in depression (55, 56) and increased excretion in mania (56, 57), but one group of investigators could not confirm these reports (58). Particularly interesting is the recent suggestion by three groups of researchers that urinary MHPG excretion may predict the response of depressed patients to the tricyclic antidepressants, imipramine and amitriptyline (59-62).

Another approach to the study of catecholamines in affective disorders has been the examination of plasma levels. However, resting concentrations of plasma catecholamines in 13 drug-free, depressed patients were reported to be significantly increased, rather than decreased, when compared to 47 normal controls in a recent study (63). No significant differences between normal subjects and depressed patients were found in two earlier studies of plasma catecholamine levels (64, 65). Again, the large peripheral sources of catecholamines decrease the relevance of these results for the catecholamine hypothesis of affective disorders. Further, there is very little information as to the normative processes involving plasma catecholamines including circadian rhythms, pulsatile release and effects of behavior, including social behavior, that would be necessary to interpret these findings (66, 67).

Another approach to the study of neurotransmitter metabolites has been the assay of spinal fluid levels. Cerebrospinal fluid MHPG has been reported to be within the normal range in depressed patients by two groups of investigators (58, 68). However, a shift of cerebrospinal fluid MHPG in the direction of mood change in bipolar patients has been reported (47, 58).

The spinal fluid levels of the dopamine metabolite homovanillic acid (HVA) has been found to be both normal and low in patients with depression, while both high and normal levels have been reported in mania (69-76). The probenecid technique has recently added a new dimension to studies of acid metabolites of neurotransmitters in the spinal fluid. Probenecid inhibits the active transport of organic acids from the spinal canal. It has been suggested that the accumulation of HVA after probenecid administration may give a more accurate measure of dopamine metabolism than baseline levels (77).

In depressed patients decreased levels of HVA accumulation after probenecid have been found in several studies (69, 75, 78). However, higher probenecid HVA accumulation was reported in depressed patients in one study (79). In manic patients results have been more variable. Thus, HVA accumulation has been reported to be both higher and lower than in controls or depressives (69, 75).

The serotonin metabolite 5-hydroxyindoleacetic acid (5-HIAA) has also been studied in the CSF of patients with affective disorders. 5-HIAA has been reported to be lower in depressed patients than in controls by some investigators (70, 80-82), while others find no differences from controls (75, 78, 83). A bimodal distribution of baseline spinal fluid 5-HIAA has recently been reported and may partially explain the variable results in earlier studies (84). However, 5-HIAA has been reported to be both lower and higher than controls in mania (75, 80, 81, 83).

The probenecid technique has also been used with cerebrospinal fluid 5-HIAA. The results have been fairly consistent. When probenecid is given to depressed patients the accumulation of 5-HIAA has been lower than controls in several reports (69, 76, 79, 85), but in one study this decrease was not statistically significant (86).

Inconsistent results in cerebrospinal fluid and urinary metabolite studies have several possible explanations. There are many methodological problems in these studies. The possible diurnal variation of metabolites, the effects of diet and psychomotor activity, the possible existence of a cerebrospinal fluid concentration gradient for metabolites (87) and the possibility of individual variation in rates of metabolite removal from cerebrospinal fluid or blood must be considered. The specificity of some of the assays used has also been questioned (88). Probenecid adds further complications. It is possible that probenecid may produce variable levels of metabolite transport inhibition in different patients. Finally, and perhaps most important, patients with affective disorders are probably a metabolically heterogeneous group. Thus, it is possible that only subgroups of patients would demonstrate specific metabolic abnormalities.

The problems encountered in human urinary and cerebrospinal fluid metabolite studies make it difficult to establish a biochemical basis for the affective disorders. However, these studies have produced promising leads which may allow the division of patients into subgroups with different metabolic abnormalities. The urinary excretion of MHPG and the spinal fluid accumulation of 5-HIAA after probenecid administration seem to be the most promising methods for the subdivision of depressed patients currently available. These methods may also represent the best current techniques for the clinical assessment of central catecholamine and indoleamine metabolism.

Attempts to Alter Neurotransmitter Functioning in Patients with Affective Disorders

A second major approach to the study of the neuropharmacology of affective disorders attempts to alter the activity of brain neurotransmitter amine systems in patients. It was hoped that this method would increase our knowledge of the role of neurotransmitters in affective disorders and perhaps lead to new therapies for patients with depression and mania. Several approaches have been used. The "precursor loading strategy," is an attempt to increase neurotransmitter synthesis by increasing the amount of precursors available. Thus, L-tryptophan (L-TP) and 5-hydroxytryptophan (5-HTP) have been used in attempts to increase brain serotonin, while L-dopa has been administered to increase central catecholamine synthesis. Enzyme inhibitors have also been used. Inhibition of serotonin synthesis is attempted using p-chlorophenylalanine (PCPA), an inhibitor of the enzyme tryptophan hydroxylase, while α-methyl-p-tyrosine (AMPT) decreases catecholamine synthesis by inhibiting tyrosine hydroxylase. Fusaric acid inhibits dopamine-β-hydroxylase (DBH) and should decrease the formation of norepinephrine in norepinephrine neurons.

Precursor loading therapies with L-tryptophan and L-dopa have been largely unsuccessful. Some investigators report L-tryptophan as effective as imipramine in the treatment of depression (79-81), but most investigators find no significant antidepressant effect (82-84). The report by two investigators that L-tryptophan reduced symptoms in mania is interesting but contrary to the hypothesis that serotonin activity is increased in mania (85, 86). L-dopa in both low (less than 1 gram) (85, 86) and high (up to 7 grams) (82, 87) doses had no significant antidepressant activity in most studies. However, L-dopa has been found to produce hypomanic symptoms in some depressed patients with a history of previous hypomanic episodes (90).

5-HTP has been reported to be an effective treatment for some depressed patients by several groups of investigators (94, 95). In a study with patients refractory to other treatments, however, 5-HTP was effective in only one of six patients (96). This result might be explained by the suggestion that only depressed patients with decreased 5-HIAA accumulation after probenecid respond to 5-HTP (59).

Enzyme inhibitors have produced disappointing results in patients with affective disorders. The tryptophan hydroxylase inhibitor, PCPA, in doses up to 4 g/day, did not decrease manic symptoms in three patients (91). The tyrosine hydroxylase inhibitor, AMPT, may have decreased symptoms in five of seven patients with mania in one study, but only two of these five patients relapsed on placebo (92). Fusaric acid which inhibits the enzyme DBH may also have caused a slight improvement in some patients with hypomania, but these effects were not dramatic (93).

Thus, attempts to alter central neurotransmitter activity, like studies of neurotransmitter metabolites, have produced surprisingly inconsistent results. These studies have not yet produced a clinically useful pharmacological treatment for depression or mania. However, the studies have produced some hypotheses that are worthy of further study. The suggestion that 5-HTP is only effective in the subgroup of depressed patients with evidence of altered central serotonin metabolism is perhaps the most important of these hypotheses.

In addition, the recent demonstrations of different forms of monoamine oxidase exhibiting differential substrate and inhibitor specificities (97) and also the development of more specific biogenic amine uptake blockers (98) may aid in determining more specifically the role of each biogenic amine in affective disorders.

NEUROPHARMACOLOGY AND AFFECTIVE DISORDERS

As mentioned above, the appearance of depression during reserpine treatment and the treatment of depression with monoamine oxidase inhibitors first suggested the relationship between neurotransmitters and affective disorders. Reserpine was suggested to produce depression by depleting serotonin, norepinephrine, and dopamine from the central nervous system (99, 100). The monoamine oxidase inhibitors, as their name suggests, were postulated to improve depression by preventing neurotransmitter breakdown by inhibiting the enzyme monoamine oxidase (101, 102).

The tricyclic antidepressants are also proposed to act through central nervous system neurotransmitters. The tricyclic antidepressants are thought to prevent the reuptake of catecholamines and serotonin in the nerve ending, theoretically increasing their concentration at postsynaptic receptors. This hypothesis is based on studies which show that the prototype tricyclic antidepressant imipramine inhibits the uptake of tritiated norepinephrine by tissues innervated by adrenergic nerves (103, 104) and decreases the uptake of intraventricularly administered tritiated norepinephrine by the rat brain *in vivo* (105). Serotonin reuptake has also been shown to be blocked by the action of tricyclic antidepressants (106).

Lithium carbonate is an effective treatment for mania (107-109). The mechanism of action of lithium has also been suggested to involve brain neurotransmitters. Lithium is reported to inhibit the electrically stimulated release of serotonin and norepinephrine from rat brain slices (110), although there is not complete agreement on this point (111). The uptake of metaraminol, a catecholamine-like drug, and serotonin seems to be enhanced in the platelets of patients treated with lithium (112). Lithium is also reported to decrease the excretion of normetanephrine and increase the appearance of deaminated metabolites in studies on the metabolism of tritiated norepinephrine in the rat brain (113). These studies, taken together, suggest that lithium would tend to reduce the quantities of the catecholamines and serotonin at the receptor.

Thus, the original hypothesis of action of reserpine, monoamine oxidase inhibitors, tricyclic antidepressants and lithium carbonate proposed altered catecholamine and serotonin activity in the central nervous system. Reserpine depletes central nervous system neurotransmitters and may cause depression in some individuals. Tricyclic antidepressants and monoamine oxidase inhibitors are thought to increase neurotransmitter activity; both classes of drugs are useful in clinical depression. Finally, lithium carbonate may reduce the quantity of catecholamines and serotonin at the synapse.

These hypotheses seem to fit together nicely. However, there are many problems with these suggested mechanisms of action. Reserpine causes a syndrome in animals that includes sedation and motor retardation (114). This syndrome has been suggested to be a model for human depression. However, there is evidence that this reserpine syndrome in animals can be reversed by L-dopa (115, 116). As described in this chapter, L-dopa is not an effective antidepressant in human patients.

The effects of the monoamine oxidase inhibitors may also be more complicated than originally thought. One group of investigators suggests that inhibition of catecholamine reuptake may be more important than monoamine oxidase inhibition (117). These investigators report that the comparative clinical efficacy of monoamine oxidase inhibitors more closely corresponds to their comparative ability to inhibit the uptake of metaraminol in rat cortical slices than to their relative potency as inhibitors of monoamine oxidase (117). Thus, it is possible that both the monoamine oxidase inhibitors and tricyclic antidepressants act by blocking catecholamine reuptake.

There are also problems with this suggested mechanism. Iprindole is a tricyclic antidepressant related to imipramine that does not inhibit the *in vivo* uptake of tritiated norepinephrine (118); however, it has been found to be an effective antidepressant (119, 129). Cocaine is a potent inhibitor of catecholamine reuptake at the synapse, yet in a recent study, cocaine did not have significant antidepressant activity (121).

The delay in clinical activity of the tricyclic antidepressants also poses a problem for the suggestion that reuptake blockade is responsible for their antidepressant action. Inhibition of catecholamine reuptake is evident after acute tricyclic antidepressant administration; however, it takes two to three weeks for antidepressant activity to become clinically evident.

The proposed mechanism of action of lithium carbonate seems appropriate for its antimanic activity. Lithium should reduce the postulated overactive catecholamine and serotonin neurotransmitter activity in mania. However, there is increasing evidence that lithium carbonate may be useful in the treatment and prevention of depressive episodes, particularly in patients with a history of both mania and depression (122).

Thus, the mechanism of pharmacological action of reserpine, monoamine oxidase inhibitors and tricyclic antidepressants may not be as simple as originally proposed. However, it is still likely that these agents act through brain neurotransmitters. For this reason it will be important to study the dynamic interactions between these pharmacological agents and aspects of neurotransmitters. In the first section of this chapter, basic concepts of neurotransmitter synthesis, storage, release, receptor interaction and inactivation were reviewed. Study of the chronic effects of pharmacological agents on each of these aspects of neurotransmitter processes is a most important goal for future research. Recent studies on the chronic effects of lithium on several neurotransmitter processes are an example of this type of research.

Chronic lithium administration in rats has been found to produce an initial increase in striatal synaptosomal tryptophan uptake and serotonin formation, followed by an apparent reduction in either the amount or activity of tryptophan hydroxylase isolated from these synaptosomes, so that the rate of serotonin formation is similar to controls, while tryptophan uptake is still increased (123). In addition, the usual decrease in synaptosomal serotonin formation produced by amphetamine administration was prevented by chronic lithium administration, as was the usual amphetamine-induced increase in locomotor activity (124). Whether or not this lithium-induced "stability" to amphetamine-induced alterations in biogenic amine synthesis and behavior is related to lithium's "stabilizing" action in the treatment of manic-depressives is, of course, quite speculative, but it is indicative of some of the types of neurochemical alterations that lithium has the potential to produce.

Chronic lithium administration has been reported to increase the activity of tyrosine hydroxylase in cell-free nigro-striatal and caudate homogenates after 8 days of treatment (124) but to decrease the rate of dopamine synthesis in rat striatal slices after 14 days of treatment (125). These apparently contradictory results may be due either to a different time-course of treatment or to the different types of preparations studied. Thus, studies examining both free enzyme preparations and preparations retaining cellular organization will be important.

The clinical and pharmacological observations summarized above suggest that drugs that are clinically effective in treating affective disorders may not be acting simply by increasing or decreasing biogenic amine availability. This could be because an alteration in biogenic amine availability may be only a first step (and not necessarily the only possible first step) in triggering some sort of adaptive response from the neurotransmitter systems. Some drugs that are clinically ineffective, such as cocaine, may alter availability in what would appear to be the right direction, but may have other actions that could counter this adaptive response. Conversely, some drugs that are clinically effective, such as iprindole, may be able to trigger this response without altering amine availability at all. What this hypothetical adaptive response may turn out to be will, of course, have to await the results of further basic research on the neurotransmitter processes, their chronic alteration by pharmacological agents and the interactions between biogenic amines, pharmacological agents and behavior (126). It is hoped that some of the biochemical adaptive mechanisms outlined earlier in this chapter may serve as useful models for this research.

REFERENCES

1. GERSHON, S.: Lithium salts in the management of the manic-depressive syndrome. *Ann. Rev. Medicine*, 23:439-452, 1972.
2. SCHILDKRAUT, J. J.: Neuropharmacology of the affective disorders. *Ann. Rev. Pharmacol.*, 13:427-454, 1973.

3. SCHILDKRAUT, J. J.: Biogenic amines and affective disorders. *Ann. Rev. Medicine*, 25:333-348, 1974.
4. BALDESSARINI, R. J.: The basis for amine hypotheses in affective disorders. *Arch. Gen. Psychiat.*, 32:1087-1093, 1975.
5. LINDVALL, O. and BJORKLUND, A.: The organization of ascending catecholamine neuron systems in the rat brain as revealed by glyoxylic acid fluorescence method. *Acta Physiol. Scand. Suppl.*, 411, 1974.
6. HARTMAN, B. K.: Immunofluorescence of dopamine-β-hydroxylase: Application of improved methodology to the localization of the peripheral and central noradrenergic nervous system. *J. Histochem. Cytochem.*, 21:312-332, 1973.
7. IVERSEN, L. L. and URETSKY, N. J.: Biochemical effects of 6-hydroxydopamine on catecholamine-containing neurones in the rat central nervous system. *In* T. Malmfors and H. Thoenen (Eds.), *6-Hydroxydopamine and Catecholamine Neurons*. New York: American Elsevier Publishing Co., 1971, p. 171.
8. IVERSEN, L. L.: Uptake processes for biogenic amines. *In* L. L. Iversen, S. D. Iversen, and S. H. Snyder (Eds.), *Handbook of Psychopharmacology*, Vol. 3. New York: Plenum Press, 1975.
9. BALDESSARINI, R. J.: Release of catecholamines. *In* L. L. Iversen, S. D. Iversen, and S. H. Snyder (Eds.), *Handbook of Psychopharmacology*, Vol. 3. New York: Plenum Press, 1975, p. 37.
10. SIGGINS, G. R., BATTENBERG, E. F., HOFFER, B. J., and BLOOM, F. E.: Noradrenergic stimulation of cyclic adenosine monophosphate in rat Purkinje neurons: An immunocytochemical study. *Science*, 179:585-588, 1973.
11. KIRSHNER, N.: Uptake of catecholamines by a particulate fraction of the adrenal medulla. *J. Biol. Chem.*, 237:2311-2317, 1962.
12. WURZBURGER, R. J. and MUSACCHIO, J. M.: Subcellular distribution and aggregation of bovine adrenal tyrosine hydroxylase. *J. Pharmacol. Exp. Therap.*, 177:155-168, 1971.
13. KUCZENSKI, R. T. and MANDELL, A. J.: Regulatory properties of soluble and particulate rat brain tyrosine hydroxylase. *J. Biol. Chem.*, 247:3114-3122, 1972.
14. SPECTOR, S., GORDON, R., SJOERDSMA, A. and UDENFRIEND, S.: End-product inhibition of tyrosine hydroxylase as a possible mechanism for regulating of norepinephrine synthesis. *Mol. Pharmacol.*, 3:549-555, 1967.
15. GORDON, R., SPECTOR, S., SJOERDSMA, A. and UDENFRIEND, S.: Increased synthesis of norepinephrine and epinephrine in the intact rat during exercise and exposure to cold. *J. Pharmacol. Exp. Ther.*, 153:440-447, 1966.
16. WEINER, N.: Regulation of norepinephrine biosynthesis. *Ann. Rev. Pharmacol.*, 10:273-290, 1970.
17. HARRIS, J. E. and ROTH, R. H.: Potassium-induced acceleration

of catecholamine biosynthesis in brain slices. *Mol. Pharmacol.,* 7:593-604, 1971.
18. PATRICK, R. L., SNYDER, T. E. and BARCHAS, J. D.: Regulation of dopamine synthesis in rat brain striatal synaptosomes. *Mol. Pharmacol.,* 11:621-631, 1975.
19. MORGENROTH, V. H., III, HEGSTRAND, L. R., ROTH, R. H., and GREENGARD, P.: Evidence for involvement of protein kinase in the activation of adenosine 3':5'-monophosphate of brain tyrosine hydroxylase. *J. Biol. Chem.,* 250:1946-1948, 1975.
20. LOVENBERG, W., BRUCKWICK, E. A. and HANBAUER, I.: ATP, cyclic AMP, and magnesium increase the affinity of rat striatal tyrosine hydroxylase for its cofactor. *Proc. Natl. Acad. Sci. U.S.A.,* 72:2955-2958, 1975.
21. GUTMAN, Y. and SEGAL, J.: Effect of calcium, potassium and sodium on tyrosine hydroxylase activity in different regions of the rat brain. *Biochem. Pharmacol.,* 22:865-868, 1973.
22. MORGENROTH, V. H., III, BOADLE-BIBER, M. C. and ROTH, R. H.: Activation of tyrosine hydroxylase from central noradrenergic neurons by calcium. *Mol. Pharmacol.,* 11:427-435, 1975.
23. LLOYD, T. and KAUFMAN, S.: The stimulation of partially purified bovine caudate tyrosine hydroxylase by phophatidyl-L-serine. *Biochem. Biophys. Res. Comm.,* 59:1262-1269, 1974.
24. RAESE, J., PATRICK, R. L. and BARCHAS, J. D.: Phospholipid-induced activation of tyrosine hydroxylase from rat brain triatal synaptosomes. *Biochem. Pharmacol.,* 25:2245-2250, 1976.
25. COSTA, E. and MEEK, J. L.: Regulation of biosynthesis of catecholamines and serotonin in the CNS. *Ann. Rev. Pharmacol.,* 14:491-511, 1974.
26. SHIELDS, P. J. and ECCLESTON, D.: Effects of electrical stimulation of rat midbrain on 5-hydroxytryptamine synthesis as determined by a sensitive radioisotope method. *J. Neurochem.,* 19:265-272, 1972.
27. HERR, B. E., GALLAGHER, D. W. and ROTH, R. H.: Tryptophan hydroxylase: Activation *in vivo* following stimulation of central serotonergic neurons. *Biochem. Pharmacol.,* 24:2019-2023, 1975.
28. FERNSTROM, J. D. and WURTMAN, R. J.: Brain serotonin content: Physiological dependence on plasma tryptophan levels. *Science,* 173:149-152, 1971.
29. HAMON, M., BOURGOIN, S., MOROT-GAUDRY, Y. and GLOWINSKI, J.: End product inhibition of serotonin synthesis in the rat striatum. *Nature New Biol.,* 237:184-187, 1972.
30. KAROBATH, M.: Serotonin synthesis with rat brain synaptosomes. *Biochem. Pharmacol.,* 21:1253-1263, 1972.
31. JEQUIER, E., ROBINSON, D. S., LOVENBERG, W. and SJOERDSMA, A.: Further studies on tryptophan hydroxylase in rat brainstem and beef pineal. *Biochem. Pharmacol.,* 18:1071-1081, 1969.

32. YOUDIM, M. B. H., HAMON, M. and BOURGOIN, S.: Properties of partially purified pig brain stem tryptophan hydroxylase. *J. Neurochem.*, 25:407-414, 1975.

33. BOADLE-BIBER, M-C.: Effect of calcium on tryptophan hydroxylase from rat hind brain. *Biochem. Pharmacol.*, 24:1455-1460, 1975.

34. KNAPP, S., MANDELL, A. J. and BULLARD, W. P.: Calcium activation of brain tryptophan hydroxylase. *Life Sci.*, 16:1583-1594, 1975.

35. RUBIN, R. P.: The role of calcium in the release of neurotransmitter substances and hormones. *Pharmacol. Rev.*, 22:389-428, 1970.

36. ZIGMOND, R. E., SCHOU, E. and IVERSON, L. L.: Increased tyrosine hydroxylase activity in the locus coeruleus of rat brain stem after reserpine treatment and cold stress. *Brain Res.*, 70:547-552, 1974.

37. REIS, D. J., JOH, T. H., ROSS, R. A. and PICKEL, V. M.: Reserpine selectively increased tyrosine hydroxylase and dopamine-β-hydroxylase enzyme protein in central noradrenergic neurons. *Brain Res.*, 81:380-386, 1974.

38. PATRICK, R. L. and KIRSHNER, N.: Acetylcholine-induced stimulation of catecholamine recovery in denervated rat adrenals after reserpine-induced depletion. *Mol. Pharmacol.*, 7:389-396, 1971.

39. DE BELLEROCHE, J. S. and BRADFORD, H. F.: The synaptosome: An isolated, working, neuronal compartment. *Progr. Neurobiol.*, 1:275-298, 1973.

40. AXELSSON, J. and THESLEFF, S.: A study of supersensitivity in denervated mammalian skeletal muscle. *J. Physiol.*, 147:178-193, 1959.

41. MILEDI, R.: Acetylcholine sensitivity of partially denerved frog muscle fibres. *J. Physiol.*, 147:45P-46P, 1959.

42. PERKINS, J.: Adenyl cyclase. *In* P. Greengard and G. A. Robison (Eds.), *Advances in Cyclic Nucleotide Research*, Vol. 3. New York: Raven Press, 1973, pp. 1-64.

43. SHIMIZU, H., CREVELING, C. R. and DALY, J. W.: Cyclic adenosine 3',5'-monophosphate formation in brain slices: Stimulation by batrachotoxin ouabain, veratridine, and potassium ions. *Mol. Pharmacol.*, 6:184-188, 1970.

44. FERRENDELLI, J. A., KINSCHERF, D. A. and CHANG, M. M.: Regulation of levels of guanosine cyclic 3',5'-monophosphate in the central nervous system: Effects of depolarizing agents. *Mol. Pharmacol.*, 9:445-454, 1973.

45. JOHNSON, E. M., VEDA, T., MAENO, H. and GREENGARD, P.: Adenosine 3',5'-monophosphate-dependent phosphorylation of a specific protein in synaptic membrane fractions from rat cerebrum. *J. Biol. Chem.*, 247:5650-5653, 1972.

46. KETY, S. S., JAVOY, F., THIERRY, A., JULOU, L. and GLOWINSKI, J.: A sustained effect of electroconvulsive shock on the turnover of norepinephrine in the central nervous system of the rat. *Proc. Natl. Acad. Sci. U.S.A.*, 58:1249-1254, 1967.

47. BUNNEY, W. E., JR., MURPHY, D. L. and GOODWIN, F. K.: The switch process from depression to mania: Relationship to drugs which alter brain amines. *Lancet*, 1:1022-1027, 1970.

48. GREENSPAN, K., SCHILDKRAUT, J. J., GORDON, E. K., LEVY, B., and DURELL, J.: Catecholamine metabolism in affective disorders: II. Norepinephrine, normetanephrine, epinephrine, metanephrine, and VMA excretion in hypomanic patients. *Arch. Gen. Psychiat.*, 21:710-716, 1969.

49. TAKAHASHI, R., NAGAO, Y., TSUCHIYA, K., TALCAMIZAWA, T., TORU, M., KOBOYASHI, K. and KARIYU, T.: Catecholamine metabolism of manic depressive illness. *J. Psychiat. Res.*, 6:185-199, 1968.

50. BERGSMAN, A.: Urinary excretion of adrenaline and noradrenaline in some mental diseases: Clinical and experimental study. *Acta Psychiat. Neurol. Scand. Suppl.*, 54:5-107, 1959.

51. MAAS, J. W. and LANDIS, D. H.: *In vivo* studies of the metabolism of norepinephrine in the central nervous system. *J. Pharmacol. Exp. Ther.*, 163:147-162, 1968.

52. MAAS, J. W., DEKIRMENJIAN, H., GARVER, D., REDMOND, D. E. and LANDIS, D. H.: Excretion of catecholamine metabolites following intraventricular injection of 6-hydroxydopamine in the macaca speciosa. *Eur. J. Pharmacol.*, 23:121-130, 1973.

53. SHOPSIN, B., WILK, S., GERSHON, S., ROFFMAN, M. and GOLDSTEIN, M.: Collaborative psychopharmacologic studies exploring catecholamine metabolism in psychiatric disorders. *In* E. Usdin and S. Snyder (Eds.), *Frontiers in Catecholamine Research.* New York: Pergamon, 1974, pp. 1173-1179.

54. WILK, A. and MONES, R.: Cerebrospinal fluid levels of 3-methoxy-4-hydroxy-phenylethylene glycol in Parkinsonism before and after treatment with L-dopa. *J. Neurochem.*, 18:1771-1773, 1971.

55. MAAS, J. W., FAWCETT, J. and DEKIRMENJIAN, H.: 3-Methoxy-4-hydroxyphenylglycol (MHPG) excretion in depressive states. A pilot study. *Arch. Gen. Psychiat.*, 19:129-134, 1968.

56. BOND, P. A., JENNER, F. A. and SAMPSON, G. A.: Daily variations of the urine content of 3-methoxy-4-hydroxyphenylglycol in two manic depressive patients. *Psychol. Med.*, 2:81-85, 1972.

57. GREENSPAN, K., SCHILDKRAUT, J. J., GORDON, E. K., BAER, L., ARANOFF, M. S. and DURELL, J.: Catecholamine metabolism in affective disorders: III. MHPG and other catecholamine metabolites in patients treated with lithium carbonate. *J. Psychiat. Res.*, 7:171-183, 1970.

58. SHOPSIN, B., WILK, S., SUTHANANTHAN, G., GERSHON, S. and DAVIS, K.: Catecholamines and affective disorders revised: A critical assessment. *J. Nerv. Ment. Dis.*, 158:369-383, 1974.
59. MAAS, J. W., FAWCETT, J. A. and DEKIRMENJIAN, H.: Catecholamine metabolism, depressive illness, and drug response. *Arch. Gen. Psychiat.*, 26:252-262, 1972.
60. FAWCETT, J., MAAS, J. W. and DEKIRMENJIAN, H.: Depression and MHPG excretion: Response to dextroamphetamine and tricyclic antidepressants. *Arch. Gen. Psychiat.*, 26:246-251, 1972.
61. SCHILDKRAUT, J. J.: Norepinephrine metabolites as biochemical criteria for classifying depressive disorders and predicting responses to treatment: Preliminary findings. *Am. J. Psychiat.*, 130:695-699, 1973.
62. BECKMANN, H. and GOODWIN, F. K.: Antidepressant response to tricyclics and urinary MHPG in unipolar patients: Clinical response to imipramine and amitriptyline. *Arch. Gen. Psychiat.*, 32:17-21, 1975.
63. WYATT, R., PORTNOY, B., KUPFER, D., SNYDER, F. and ENGELMAN, K.: Resting plasma catecholamine concentrations in patients with depression and anxiety. *Arch. Gen. Psychiat.*, 24:65-70, 1971.
64. MANGER, W. M., SCHAZ, B. E. and BAARS, C. W.: Epinephrine and arterenol (norepinephrine) in mental disease. *Arch. Neurol. Psychiat.*, 78:396-412, 1957.
65. REILLY, J. and REGAN, P. F., III: Plasma catecholamines in psychiatric patients. *Proc. Soc. Exp. Biol. Med.*, 95:377-380, 1957.
66. BARCHAS, P. R. and BARCHAS, J. D.: Physiological sociology: Endocrine correlates of status behaviors. *In* D. A. Hamburg and H. K. H. Brodie (Eds.), *American Handbook of Psychiatry—Research Frontiers in Psychiatry*. New York: Basic Books, 1975, pp. 623-640.
67. BARCHAS, P. R. and BARCHAS, J. D.: Social behavior and adrenal medullary function in relation to psychiatric disorders. *In* E. Usdin, H. Hamburg, and J. Barchas (Eds.), *Neuroregulators of Psychiatric Disorders*. New York: Oxford University Press (in press).
68. COPPEN, A. J.: The chemical pathology of the affective disorders. *In: The Scientific Basis of Medicine Annual Reviews*. London: Athone, 1970, pp. 189-210.
69. VAN PRAAG, H. M., KORF, J. and SCHUT, D.: Cerebral monoamines and depression: An investigation with the probenecid technique. *Arch. Gen. Psychiat.*, 28:827-831, 1973.
70. MENDELS, J., FRAZER, A., FITZGERALD, R. G., RAMSEY, T. A., and STOKES, J. W.: Biogenic amine metabolites in the cerebrospinal fluid of depressed and manic patients. *Science*, 175:1380-1382, 1972.

71. PAPESCHI, R. and McCLURE, D. J.: Homovanillic and 5-hydroxy-indoleacetic acid in cerebrospinal fluid of depressed patients. *Arch. Gen. Psychiat.*, 25:354-358, 1971.

72. POST, R. M., KOTIN, J., GOODWIN, F. K. and GORDON, E. K.: Psychomotor activity and cerebrospinal fluid amine metabolites in affective illness. *Am. J. Psychiat.*, 130:67-72, 1973.

73. NORDIN, G., OTTOSSON, J. O. and ROOS, B. E.: Influence of con-vulsive therapy on 5-hydroxyindoleacetic acid and homovanillic acid in cerebrospinal fluid in endogenous depression. *Psycho-pharmacologia*, 20:315-320, 1971.

74. WILK, S., SHOPSIN, B., GERSHON, S. and SUHL, M.: Cerebro-spinal fluid levels of MHPG in affective disorders. *Nature*, 235:440-441, 1972.

75. GOODWIN, F. K., POST, R. M., DUNNER, D. L. and GORDON, E. K.: Cerebrospinal fluid amine metabolites in affective illness: The probenecid technique. *Am. J. Psychiat.*, 130:73-79, 1973.

76. SJOSTROM, R. and ROOS, B. E.: 5-Hydroxyindoleacetic acid and homovanillic acid in cerebrospinal fluid in manic-depressive psychosis. *Eur. J. Clin. Pharmacol.*, 4:170-176, 1972.

77. NEFF, N. H., TOZER, T. N. and BRODIE, B. B.: Application of steady-state kinetics to studies of the transfer of 5-hydroxy-indoleacetic acid from brain to plasma. *J. Pharmacol. Exp. Ther.*, 158:214-218, 1967.

78. ROOS, B. E. and SJOSTROM, R.: 5-Hydroxyindoleacetic acid (and homovanillic acid) levels in the cerebrospinal fluid after pro-benecid application in patients with manic-depressive psychosis. *Pharmacol. Clin.*, 1:153-155, 1969.

79. BOWERS, M. B., JR.: Cerebrospinal fluid 5-hydroxyindoleacetic acid (5-HIAA) and homovanillic acid (HVA) following pro-benecid in unipolar depressives treated with amitriptyline. *Psychopharmacologie* (Berl.), 23:26-33, 1972.

80. ASHCROFT, G. W., CRAWFORD, T. B. B., ECCLESTON, D. F., SHAR-MAN, D. F., MacDOUGALL, E. J., STANTON, J. B. and BINNS, J. K.: 5-Hydroxyindole compounds in the cerebrospinal fluid of patients with psychiatric or neurological diseases. *Lancet*, 2:1049-1052, 1966.

81. DENCKER, S. J., MALM, U., ROOS, B. E. and WERDINIUS, B.: Acid monoamine metabolites of cerebrospinal fluid in mental depression and mania. *J. Neurochem.*, 13:1545-1548, 1966.

82. VAN PRAAG, H. M., KORF, J. and PUITE, J.: 5-Hydroxyindole-acetic acid levels in the cerebrospinal fluid of depressive pa-tients treated with probenecid. *Nature*, 225:1259-1260, 1970.

83. BOWERS, M. B., JR., HENIGER, G. R. and GERBODE, F.: Cerebro-spinal fluid 5-hydroxyindoleacetic acid and homovanillic acid in psychiatric patients. *Int. J. Neuropharmacol.*, 8:255-262, 1959.

84. ASBERG, M., BERTILSSON, L., TUCK, D., CRONHOLM, B. and SJO-QVIST, F.: Indoleamine metabolites in the cerebrospinal fluid

of depressed patients before and during treatment with nor-triptoline. *Clin. Pharmacol. Ther.*, 14:277-287, 1973.

85. VAN PRAAG, H. M. and KORF, J.: Monoamine metabolism in depression: Clinical application of the probenecid test. *In* J. D. Barchas and E. Usdin (Eds.), *Serotonin and Behavior.* New York: Academic Press, 1973, pp. 457-468.

86. GOODWIN, F. K. and POST, R. M.: The use of probenecid in high doses for the estimation of central serotonin turnover in affective illness and addicts on methadone. *In* J. D. Barchas and E. Usdin (Eds.), *Serotonin and Behavior.* New York: Academic Press, 1973, pp. 469-480.

87. SEIVER, L., KRAEMER, H., SACK, R., ANGWIN, P., PERGER, P. A., ZARCONE, V., BARCHAS, J. and BRODIE, H. K. H.: Gradients of biogenic amine metabolites in cerebrospinal fluid. *Dis. Nerv. Syst.*, 36:13-16, 1975.

88. WILK, S. and GREEN, J. P.: On the measurement of 5-hydroxyindoleacetic acid in cerebrospinal fluid. *J. Neurochem.*, 19: 2893-2895, 1975.

89. COPPEN, A., WHYBROW, P. C., NOGUERA, M. B. R., MAGGS, R. and PRANGE, A. J.: The comparative antidepressant value of L-tryptophan and imipramine with and without attempted potentiation by triiodothyronine. *Arch. Gen. Psychiat.*, 26:234-241, 1972.

90. KLINE, N. S. and SHAH, B. K.: Comparative therapeutic efficacy of tryptophan and imipramine: Average therapeutic ratings versus "true" equivalence: An important difference. *Curr. Ther. Res.*, 15:484-487, 1973.

91. BROADHURST, A. D.: L-tryptophan versus E.C.T. *Lancet*, 1:1392, 1970.

92. CARROLL, B. M., MOWBRAY, R. M. and DAVIS, B. M.: Sequential comparison of L-tryptophan with ECT in severe depression. *Lancet*, 1:967-969, 1970.

93. MURPHY, D. L., BAKER, M., KOTIN, J. and BUNNEY, W. E., JR.: Behavioral and metabolic effects of L-tryptophan in unipolar depressed patients. *In* J. Barchas and E. Usdin (Eds.), *Serotonin and Behavior.* New York: Academic Press, 1973, pp. 529-537.

94. MENDELS, J., STINNETT, J. L., BURNS, D. and FRAZER, A.: Amine precursors and depression. *Arch. Gen. Psychiat.*, 32:22-30, 1975.

95. PRANGE, A. J., JR., WILSON, I. C., LYNN, C. W., ALLSOP, L. B., and STIKELEATHER, R. A.: L-tryptophan in mania. *Arch. Gen. Psychiat.*, 30:56-62, 1974.

96. MURPHY, D. L., BAKER, M., GOODWIN, F. K., MILLER, H., KOTIN, J. and BUNNEY, W. J., JR.: L-tryptophan in affective disorders: Indoleamine changes and differential clinical effects. *Psychopharmacologia*, 34:11-20, 1974.

97. YOUDIM, M. B. H.: Multiple forms of mitochondrial monoamine oxidase. *Brit. Med. Bull.*, 29:120-122, 1973.

98. WONG, D. T., BYMASTER, F. P., HORNG, J. S. and MOLLOY, B. B.: A new selective inhibitor for uptake of serotonin into synaptosomes of rat brain: 3-(p-trifluoromethylphenoxy)-N-methyl-3-phenylpropylamine. *J. Pharmacol. Exp. Ther.*, 193:804-811, 1975.

99. PLETSCHER, A., SHORE, P. A. and BRODIE, B. B.: Serotonin as a mediator of reserpine action in brain. *J. Pharmacol. Exp. Ther.*, 116:84-89, 1956.

100. HOLZBAUER, M. and VOGT, M.: Depression by reserpine of the noradrenaline concentration in the hypothalamus of the cat. *J. Neurochem.*, 1:1-7, 1956.

101. ZELLER, E. A. and FOUTS, J. R.: Enzymes as primary targets of drugs. *Ann. Rev. Pharmacol.*, 3:9-32, 1963.

102. BRODIE, B. B., SPECTOR, S. and SHORE, P. A.: Interaction of monoamine oxidase inhibitors with physiological and biochemical mechanisms in brain. *Ann. N.Y. Acad. Sci.*, 80:609-616, 1959.

103. DENGLER, H. J., SPIEGEL, H. E. and TITUS, E. O.: Effects of drugs on uptake of isotopic norepinephrine by cat tissues. *Nature*, 191:816-817, 1961.

104. AXELROD, J., HERTTING, G. and POTTER, L.: Effect of drugs on the uptake and release of 3H-norepinephrine in the rat heart. *Nature*, 194:297, 1962.

105. GLOWINSKI, J. and AXELROD, J.: Inhibition of uptake of tritiated noradrenaline in intact rat brain by imipramine and related compounds. *Nature*, 204:1318-1319, 1964.

106. CARLSSON, A., CORRODI, D., FUXE, K. and HOKFELT, T.: Effect of antidepressant drugs on the depletion of intraneuronal brain 5-hydroxytryptamine stores caused by 5-methyl-α-ethyl-meta-tyramine. *Eur. J. Pharmacol.*, 5:357-366, 1969.

107. SCHOU, M., JUEL-NIELSON, N., STROMGREN, E. and VOLDBY, H.: The treatment of manic psychoses by the administration of lithium salts. *J. Neurol. Neurosurg. Psychiatr.*, 17:250-260, 1954.

108. BUNNEY, W. E., JR., GOODWIN, F. K., DAVIS, J. M. and FAWCETT, J. A.: A behavioral-biochemical study of lithium treatment. *Am. J. Psychiat.*, 125:499-512, 1968.

109. STOKES, P. E., STOLL, P. M., SHAMOIAN, C. A. and PATTON, M. J.: Efficacy of lithium as acute treatment of manic-depressive illness. *Lancet*, 1:1319-1325, 1971.

110. KATZ, R. I., CHASE, T. N. and KOPIN, I. J.: Evoked release of norepinephrine and serotonin from brain slices: Inhibition by lithium. *Science*, 162:466-467, 1968.

111. SALDATE, C. and ORREGO, F.: Electrically induced release of [3H]5-hydroxytryptamine from neocortical slices *in vitro*: in-

fluence of calcium but not of lithium ions. *Brain Res.*, 99:184-188, 1975.
112. MURPHY, D. L., COLBURN, R. W., DAVIS, J. M. and BUNNEY, W. E., JR.: Imipramine and lithium effects on biogenic amine transport in depressed and manic-depressed patients. *Am. J. Psychiat.*, 127:339-344, 1970.
113. SCHANBERG, S. M., SCHILDKRAUT, J. J. and KOPIN, I. J.: The effects of psychoactive drugs on norepinephrine-^{3}H metabolism in brain. *Biochem. Pharmacol.*, 16:393-399, 1967.
114. BEIN, H. J.: Zur Pharmakologie des Reserpin, eines neuen Alkaloids aus Rauwolfia serpentina Benth. *Experientia*, 9:107-110, 1953.
115. CARLSSON, A. and LINDQVIST, M.: Metatyrosine as a tool for selective protection of catecholamines stores against reserpine. *Eur. J. Pharmacol.*, 2:192-197, 1967.
116. PARE, C. M. B.: Some clinical aspects of antidepressant drugs. *In* J. Marks and C. M. B. Pare (Eds.), *The Scientific Basis of Therapy in Psychiatry*. New York: Pergamon Press, 1965, pp. 103-113.
117. HENDLEY, E. D. and SNYDER, S. H.: Relationship between the action of monoamine oxidase inhibitors on the noradrenaline uptake system and their antidepressant efficacy. *Nature*, 220: 1130-1131, 1968.
118. GLUCKMAN, M. I. and BAUM, T.: The pharmacology of iprindole, a new antidepressant. *Psychopharmacologia*, 15:169-185, 1969.
119. DANEMAN, E. A.: Treatment of depressed patients with iprindole. *Psychosomatics*, 8:216-221, 1967.
120. EL-DEIRY, N. K., FORREST, A. D. and LITTMAN, S. K.: Clinical trial of a new antidepressant (WY. 3263). *Brit. J. Psychiat.*, 113:999-1004, 1967.
121. POST, R. M., KOTIN, J. and GOODWIN, F. K.: The effects of cocaine on depressed patients. *Am. J. Psychiatry*, 131:511-517, 1974.
122. DAVIS, J. M.: Overview: Maintenance therapy in psychiatry II. Affective disorders. *Am. J. Psychiatry*, 133:1-13, 1976.
123. KNAPP, S. and MANDELL, A. J.: Effects of lithium chloride on parameters of biosynthetic capacity for 5-hydroxytryptamine in rat brain. *J. Pharmacol. Exp. Ther.*, 193:812-823, 1975.
124. SEGAL, D. S., CALLAGHAN, M. and MANDELL, A. J.: Alterations in behavior and catecholamine biosynthesis induced by lithium. *Nature*, 254:58-59, 1975.
125. FRIEDMAN, E. and GERSHON, S.: Effect of lithium on brain dopamine. *Nature*, 243:520-521, 1973.
126. HAMBURG, D. A., HAMBURG, B. and BARCHAS, J.: Anger and depression in perspectives of behavioral biology. *In* L. Levi (Ed.), *Parameters of Emotion*. Oxford, England: Oxford University Press, 1975, pp. 235-278.

8

Biochemical Research in Affective Disorders

Joseph J. Schildkraut, M.D.

The introduction of drugs such as the monoamine oxidase inhibitors, the tricyclic antidepressants, and lithium salts in the treatment of the affective disorders has had a major impact on clinical psychiatric practice and on biological research in psychiatry. The neuropharmacology of these agents has been studied by many investigators who have suggested that the effects of these drugs on biogenic amine metabolism may be related to their clinical effects (1). Considerable biochemical research in the affective disorders has, therefore, concentrated upon studies of the biogenic amines which include the catecholamines norepinephrine and dopamine, and the indoleamine serotonin.

The clinical and biological heterogeneity of the affective disorders has long been recognized, and the possibility that depressive subtypes might be distinguished by differences in the metabolism of one or another monoamine was suggested a number of years ago (2). This possibility is now supported by a number of recent findings which suggest that biochemical measures related to biogenic amine metabolism may soon provide clinically useful criteria for

This work was supported in part by USPHS grant number MH 15413.

classifying depressive disorders and perhaps for predicting responses to individual treatment modalities.

METABOLISM, PHYSIOLOGY AND NEUROPHARMACOLOGY OF THE BIOGENIC AMINES*

The term biogenic amine is generally used to refer to three compounds—norepinephrine and dopamine, which are catecholamines, and serotonin, which is an indoleamine. All of these compounds have a single amine group on the side chain and are therefore referred to as monoamines.

The neuroanatomy of specific monoamine-containing neurons in the brain has recently been mapped using the techniques of histochemical fluorescence microscopy. While these studies have provided evidence for discrete monoaminergic neuronal systems within the brain, they have also indicated that these systems may be neuroanatomically, as well as physiologically, interconnected. Moreover, it must be noted that these monoaminergic neuronal systems account for only a very small fraction of the neurons within the central nervous system. Thus, while it has been strategic in pharmacological or clinical studies to focus on one or another of the monoamines, physiological interactions among the monoaminergic neuronal systems or other neurotransmitter systems are generally recognized, and it appears that biochemical, as well as physiological, processes involving one neurotransmitter may be modulated or regulated by another.

Catecholamine biosynthesis in noradrenergic neurons proceeds along the following pathway starting with the amino acid tyrosine:

$$\text{Tyrosine} \xrightarrow[\text{hydroxylase}]{\text{tyrosine}} \underset{\text{(Dopa)}}{\text{Dihydrophenylalanine}} \xrightarrow[\text{decarboxylase}]{\substack{\text{aromatic} \\ \text{amino acid}}}$$

$$\text{Dopamine} \xrightarrow[\beta\text{-hydroxylase}]{\text{dopamine}} \text{Norepinephrine}$$

---

* This material is reviewed in greater detail in Chapter 7 on Neuropharmacological Aspects of Affective Disorders by Barchas et al. in this volume.

In dopaminergic neurons, the synthesis of catecholamines proceeds only up to dopamine since these neurons lack the enzyme dopamine-beta-hydroxylase which converts dopamine to norepinephrine.

Norepinephrine which is stored in the presynaptic noradrenergic neuron may be discharged into the synaptic cleft by nerve impulses. Most of the discharged norepinephrine is thought to be removed from the synaptic cleft by a process of reuptake into the presynaptic neuron, where it may be retained by the storage granules or undergo deamination by monoamine oxidase. A small fraction of discharged norepinephrine is inactivated in the region of the postsynaptic neuron by the enzyme catechol-O-methyl transferase (COMT) to normetanephrine.

This O-methylated metabolite may then in turn be deaminated by monoamine oxidase (MAO), and, in brain, the major metabolite of normetanephrine appears to be 3-methoxy-4-hydroxyphenylglycol (MHPG). Considerable interest has recently been focused on MHPG in clinical studies since it appears to be the final major metabolite of norepinephrine originating in the brain, and since it may provide the best available index of norepinephrine synthesis and metabolism in the central nervous system.

Within the presynaptic neuron, some norepinephrine may diffuse or leak from the storage granules into the cytoplasm and onto mitochondrial monoamine oxidase without this norepinephrine exerting an extraneuronal physiological effect at receptors. Monoamine oxidase converts norepinephrine into deaminated catechol metabolites, dihydroxymandelic acid and dihydroxyphenylglycol. These metabolites subsequently may be O-methylated by catechol-O-methyl transferase to form 3-methoxy-4-hydroxymandelic acid (vanillylmandelic acid or VMA) and 3-methoxy-4-hydroxyphenylglycol (MHPG).

Dopamine may also be metabolized by monoamine oxidase and catechol-O-methyl transferase. The major dopamine metabolite of interest in clinical studies is the deaminated O-methylated metabolite homovanillic acid (HVA).

The biosynthesis and metabolism of serotonin proceed along the following pathway, starting with the amino acid tryptophan:

Tryptophan $\xrightarrow[\text{hydroxylase}]{\text{tryptophan}}$ 5-Hydroxytryptophan $\xrightarrow[\text{decarboxylase}]{\substack{\text{aromatic} \\ \text{amino acid}}}$

Serotonin $\xrightarrow[\text{oxidase}]{\text{monoamine}}$ 5-Hydroxyindoleacetic Acid (5-HIAA)

The major serotonin metabolite of interest in clinical studies is the deaminated metabolite 5-hydroxyindoleacetic acid (5-HIAA).

Psychoactive drugs may alter the physiological activity of monoamines by interfering with any of the processes involved in synthesis, in storage, in release, in metabolism, or in controlling the sensitivity of receptors to one or another monoamine. In general, the drugs used in the treatment of depressive and manic disorders have been found to cause alterations in the metabolism or physiological disposition of one or another of the monoamines, and these biochemical effects may be related to the effects of these drugs on affective states in man (1).

Approximately 20 years ago it was recognized that reserpine, a drug originally used as an antihypertensive, could in some individuals cause depressions that appeared to be clinically indistinguishable from certain naturally occurring depressions. In studies in animals it was found that reserpine impaired the capacity of neurons to retain monoamines in storage granules (leading to intraneuronal deamination) and that brain levels of the biogenic amines, norepinephrine, dopamine and serotonin, were depleted after the administration of reserpine.

At about the same time, it was observed that monoamine oxidase inhibitors, which were initially used in the treatment of tuberculosis, could cause euphoria, and exert antidepressant effects in at least some patients. By inhibiting the enzyme monoamine oxidase, drugs of this class prevent the deamination of monoamines and increase the levels of norepinephrine, dopamine, and serotonin in the brain.

The tricyclic antidepressants in turn appear to increase the physiological effects of one or another of the monoamines at receptors, and have been found to potentiate the peripheral effects of norepinephrine and serotonin in a number of physiological systems. A mechanism for the potentiation of norepinephrine by the tricyclic antidepressants was suggested by the finding that imipramine interfered with the reuptake of norepinephrine in peripheral and central neurons. Such inhibition of reuptake of norepinephrine by presynaptic neurons may prevent the physiological inactivation of norepinephrine at the synapse and may consequently increase the level of norepinephrine at receptors.

The results of more recent studies indicate that certain other tricyclic antidepressant drugs (e.g., desmethylimipramine, nortriptyline and protriptyline) may also inhibit the uptake of norepinephrine in presynaptic neurons. Some other tricyclics, such as amitriptyline, are considerably weaker inhibitors of norepinephrine uptake. Amitriptyline has, however, been found to be a relatively potent inhibitor of serotonin uptake, while drugs such as desmethylimipramine or protriptyline are much weaker in this regard. These differences may account for some of the differences in clinical properties observed among the individual tricyclic antidepressant drugs.

Various studies have indicated that tricyclic antidepressants may also prevent the deamination of norepinephrine by mitochondrial monoamine oxidase. This might be explained by the findings from *in vitro* studies that high concentrations of tricyclic antidepressants may inhibit the enzyme monoamine oxidase. However, it is also possible that these drugs may act at intraneuronal membranes (such as the mitochondrial membranes) to prevent norepinephrine from interacting with monoamine oxidase, just as they act at neuronal membranes to prevent the reuptake of norepinephrine into presynaptic neurons.

These effects of the tricyclic antidepressants have all been observed after acute administration in animal studies. One may therefore wonder whether these changes are relevant to the clinical antidepressant effects of these drugs, since clinical antidepressant effects are not observed acutely but generally require chronic administration. Recent studies of the effects of chronic administration of a variety of tricyclic antidepressants on norepinephrine turnover and metabolism have indicated that, in addition to the above mentioned effects observed after acute administration, other changes (e.g., in turnover) occur with more prolonged administration of the drugs. These changes (in conjunction with the effects observed acutely) may help to account for the clinical antidepressant effects. Like the antidepressant drugs, electroconvulsive therapy also produces alterations in the turnover and metabolism of biogenic amines in the brain. In studies in animals, acutely administered electroconvulsive shock has been found to increase the turnover of norepinephrine, dopamine, and serotonin in the brain. After a series of chronic electroconvulsive shocks, increased turnover of norepinephrine was found to persist for at least one day after the last shock. It should be pointed out, however, that other forms of prolonged stress appear to cause similar changes in the turnover of monoamines in the brain.

Numerous studies have examined the effects of lithium on the turnover and metabolism of biogenic amines in the brain, but it is difficult to draw simple generalizations from these findings. Studies in animals and man suggest that, under some conditions, lithium produces alterations in catecholamine disposition and metabolism. In several studies, during acute or short-term administration of lithium, the turnover of norepinephrine in brain appeared to be increased; but it appears that this increase may not persist with more prolonged drug administration. Moreover, lithium also appears to alter the metabolism of norepinephrine in animal brain by increasing its intraneuronal release and its deamination by mitochondrial monoamine oxidase. Lithium may, thereby, decrease the amount of norepinephrine available for discharge onto receptors, and in this regard, its effects on norepinephrine metabolism appear to be opposite to those of many antidepressant or stimulant euphoriant drugs.

STUDIES OF BIOGENIC AMINE METABOLISM IN PATIENTS WITH AFFECTIVE DISORDERS

The observation that drugs which altered affective state in man had profound effects on biogenic amine disposition and metabolism in the brain prompted the study of biogenic amine metabolism in affective disorders more than a decade ago. This literature will be reviewed with particular reference to the recent body of data pointing toward the emergence of biochemical criteria for classifying the depressive disorders.

A. Catecholamines and Normetanephrine in Urine and Blood

In a number of studies of manic-depressive* patients, the urinary excretion of norepinephrine or dopamine (and, less consistently, epinephrine) has been found to be relatively lower during periods of depression than during periods of mania or after recovery (3-9). In one of these studies (7), a regular cycle of norepinephrine excretion was observed in cyclothymic manic-depressive patients, with increases starting during the transition phases preceding manias and decreases commencing during the transition phases preceding depressions.

In another study which examined the transition from depression into mania in a small number of subjects, an increase in urinary norepinephrine was observed on the day prior to the onset of mania when patients exhibited a brief transition period of normal behavior. This increase of urinary norepinephrine continued during the manic period. Although elevated dopamine levels were also observed during the manic phase, the increase in dopamine excretion, in contrast to that of norepinephrine, did not appear to precede the onset of mania (4). Other investigators have also found increased dopamine excretion in manic patients (8, 10).

In a large series of manic patients, the excretion of both norepinephrine and epinephrine was elevated above the corresponding values in control subjects. Norepinephrine and epinephrine levels in a heterogeneous group of depressed patients were not different

---

* Throughout this review, the terms "manic-depressive" and "bipolar" are used synonymously to refer to patients with disorders characterized by having had at least one hypomanic or manic episode as well as one or more depressive episodes. These are to be distinguished from unipolar depressions in which there is no history of a prior hypomanic or manic episode.

from control values; however, these depressed patients did have a lowered catecholamine response to insulin stress (11). Increased catecholamine excretion has been observed in some depressed patients (12), but mainly in those with agitated or anxious depressions (8, 13, 14).

In a recent study, elevated levels of plasma epinephrine and norepinephrine were observed in a group of patients with depression and anxiety, most of whom were diagnosed as depressive or anxiety neuroses. The correlation in this group between the concentration of plasma catecholamines and the degree of anxiety was highly significant. The correlation between plasma catecholamines and the degree of depression was not significant (15). Depressed patients with delusions or hallucinations have been found to excrete higher levels of catecholamines (and some metabolites) than patients who did not manifest these psychotic symptoms (16, 17).

A gradual rise in the excretion of normetanephrine, the O-methylated metabolite of norepinephrine which may reflect noradrenergic activity (18-20), was observed during the period of definitive clinical improvement in our own studies of patients with endogenous depressions who were treated with the tricyclic antidepressant, imipramine (21); this was subsequently confirmed by other investigators (22, 23). Patients with retarded depressions had lower levels of normetanephrine excretion before treatment than after discontinuation of imipramine during clinical remission (21). In some, but not all, patients with agitated depressions, normetanephrine, as well as norepinephrine and epinephrine, were higher during the depression than after improvement (13).

In longitudinal studies, the excretion of normetanephrine has been observed to be relatively higher during manias or hypomanias than during depressions, with intermediate values observed in periods of remission. The magnitude of the normetanephrine elevation appears to be related to the clinical severity of the hypomanic symptoms (5, 9, 21, 24).

Muscular activity may produce significant changes in catecholamine excretion (25). However, the alterations in the excretion of the catecholamines or metabolites in association with changes in the affective state did not appear to be a consequence of changes in motor activity in one study designed to measure these particular parameters (9). Moreover, the increases in urinary norepinephrine appeared to precede the onset of mania in two studies (4, 7). Nevertheless, one cannot exclude the possibility that these increases in norepinephrine excretion might have been secondary to subtle behavioral or postural changes. Normetanephrine and metanephrine excretion has been reported to be elevated in association with agitated and unstable behavior in depressed patients and in other subjects (26).

After infusion with radioactive norepinephrine, patients with retarded depressions, which were classified as manic-depressive, were found to have an elevated ratio of radioactive amines to deaminated metabolites in the urine when compared with normal controls or patients with agitated unipolar depressions (27, 28). Many factors could account for this finding, including an alteration in the disposition of the infused radioactive norepinephrine as well as a decrease in the deamination of norepinephrine or normetanephrine in the manic-depressive depressed group.

Since all studies have not employed a uniform system for classifying the depressions, it is difficult to summarize the findings reviewed here. In longitudinal studies, norepinephrine and normetanephrine excretion appears to be relatively decreased in patients with retarded (endogenous) depressions and increased in patients with manias when compared with values observed in these same patients during clinical remissions. The findings in patients with agitated or anxious depressions are less consistent. Some of these patients seem to show an increased excretion of norepinephrine, normetanephrine, epinephrine, and metanephrine.

While these findings do provide information concerning aspects of the biochemical pathophysiology of affective disorders, it should be stressed that urinary norepinephrine, normetanephrine, epinephrine, metanephrine, and VMA principally derive from catecholamines originating in the peripheral sympathetic nervous system or the adrenal medulla. Thus, at best, their levels are only very indirect reflections of physiologic events in the brain.

B. *MHPG in Urine*

A number of lines of evidence suggest that 3-methoxy-4-hydroxy-phenylglycol (MHPG) or its sulfate conjugate is the major final metabolite of norepinephrine in the human brain as in a number of other species (29-36). It is generally recognized that urinary MHPG may also derive in part from the peripheral sympathetic nervous system as well as from the brain itself (35, 37). The fraction of urinary MHPG which does, in fact, derive from norepinephrine originating in the brain remains problematic (33, 38-40). However, recent data suggest that in man the contribution from the brain may be substantial—i.e., greater than 50 percent (41).

The findings from a number of longitudinal studies of individual patients with naturally occurring or amphetamine-induced manic-depressive alternations indicate that levels of urinary MHPG are relatively lower during depressions and are higher during manic or hypomanic episodes than they are after clinical remissions (13, 24, 42-45). However, all findings do not agree (46, 47).

In such studies, administration of psychoactive drugs must be controlled, since some of these drugs (e.g., imipramine) are known to cause pharmacologically induced alterations in MHPG excretion which may be independent of effects on the clinical state. While urinary excretion of MHPG has been shown to increase in response to various forms of stress (48, 49) and may also vary in response to changes in motor activity (50), it is unlikely that these factors account for the changes in MHPG excretion which have been observed in manic-depressive patients.

In several of the studies demonstrating the relationship between MHPG excretion and affective state in patients with manic-depressive episodes, the changes in MHPG excretion appeared to precede the changes in the clinical state and the peaks in MHPG excretion did not appear to coincide with the peaks in motor activity (43, 44). In another of these studies, reduced MHPG excretion was observed during agitated depressions in a small series of patients with manic-depressive disorders (13).

Thus, it appears that MHPG excretion does vary with changes

in the clinical status in patients with bipolar manic-depressive disorders. However, all depressions are not clinically or biologically homogeneous, and all depressed patients do not excrete comparably low levels of MHPG (22, 51-53). A number of recent studies have, therefore, examined MHPG excretion as a possible biological criterion for classifying the depressive disorders and for predicting the responses to specific forms of antidepressant pharmacotherapy.

In a study of a small group of patients with various clinically defined subtypes of depressive disorders studied prior to treatment, my colleagues and I (53) initially reported that MHPG excretion was significantly lower in patients with manic-depressive depressions (i.e., bipolar disorders with histories of hypomanias or manias) than in patients with unipolar chronic characterological depressions (i.e., unipolar dysphoric depressive syndromes). These differences could not be explained by differences in the levels of agitation, retardation, or anxiety in these two groups (54). The urinary excretion of norepinephrine tended to be lower in bipolar manic-depressive depressions than in unipolar chronic characterological depressions, but this difference did not attain statistical significance, and there were no differences in normetanephrine, epinephrine, metanephrine or VMA excretion between these two groups. Thus, of the urinary catecholamines and metabolites measured, only MHPG showed significant differences when values in bipolar manic-depressive and unipolar chronic characterological depressions were compared (54).

We have subsequently replicated these findings in a larger series of patients (55), and these findings of differences in MHPG excretion in different clinically defined subtypes of depressive disorders have also been supported by the work of two other groups of investigators, although somewhat different systems of classification were used in each of these studies. Goodwin and his associates (45) have reported lower MHPG excretion in bipolar depressions than in unipolar depressions, and similar findings of low MHPG excretion in patients with bipolar depressions have been reported by Maas and his associates (56).

These findings thus suggest that there may be a biologically distinct group of depressive disorders with relatively low MHPG excretion (of which bipolar manic-depressive depressions represent a clinically identifiable subgroup) and a biologically distinct group of depressive disorders with relatively higher MHPG excretion (of which unipolar chronic characterological depressions represent a clinically identifiable subgroup).

The relationship between MHPG excretion and the clinical diagnosis of primary depressive disorders (57) was also examined by Maas and his associates (56), who reported that MHPG excretion was reduced not only in bipolar depressions but also in patients with unipolar primary depressive disorders. However, Goodwin and his associates (45) did not observe a reduction in MHPG excretion in patients with unipolar primary depressive disorders. Further studies will be required to clarify this.

MHPG excretion has been examined as a biochemical criterion for predicting the clinical response to antidepressant drugs in several studies. Maas and his associates (22) found that patients who excreted relatively low levels of MHPG prior to treatment with imipramine or desmethylimipramine responded better to treatment with these antidepressants than did patients who excreted relatively higher levels of MHPG. This finding was confirmed by Beckmann and Goodwin (58) but not by Prange and his associates (23).

In another preliminary study of a small group of depressed patients (52, 59), my colleagues and I observed favorable responses to treatment with amitriptyline in patients with relatively high levels of urinary MHPG, but not in patients with lower levels of MHPG. These findings have recently been confirmed by Beckmann and Goodwin (58). Their work lends support to the hypothesis that MHPG might serve as a biochemical criterion for choosing between amitriptyline and imipramine in the treatment of patients with depressive disorders (59).

In summary, a number of recent findings suggest that the urinary excretion of MHPG varies in relation to clinical state in patients with bipolar manic-depressive disorders, and that urinary MHPG may provide a biochemical criterion for classifying some types of depressive disorders and possibly also for predicting their differential responses to pharmacotherapy with one or another tricyclic anti-depressant drug.

C. MHPG in Cerebrospinal Fluid

Both free and conjugated MHPG has been identified in human cerebrospinal fluid (CSF) (35, 60, 61), and several studies have recently examined the levels of MHPG in the lumbar cerebrospinal fluid of patients with affective disorders. However, lumbar CSF MHPG does not necessarily provide a better index of norepinephrine metabolism in the brain than does urinary MHPG since MHPG measured in the lumbar cerebrospinal fluid probably reflects nore-pinephrine metabolism in the spinal cord as well as in the brain (62). Moreover, CSF levels of MHPG are determined by the rate of efflux of MHPG from the CSF, as well as by its rate of produc-tion in the central nervous system. Several investigators have reported a poor correlation between measurements of CSF and urinary MHPG (45, 63, 64).

In a small number of depressed patients (not classified with re-spect to diagnostic subtypes), Gordon and Oliver (60) reported that CSF MHPG levels were significantly lower than in control subjects. Further studies from that laboratory have confirmed this decrease in CSF MHPG levels in a larger series of depressed patients (65). CSF levels were not different from control values in a small group of manic patients. In this study, the levels of CSF MHPG in depressed patients were not related to the presence or absence of a history of mania (65).

Other investigators (63) have recently reported that levels of MHPG in the cerebrospinal fluid of patients with unipolar depres-sive disorders were not significantly different from the levels in a neurological control group. In this study, there was a positive cor-relation between the severity of the depression and CSF MHPG levels, but there was no meaningful correlation between CSF and urinary MHPG levels. In a small number of patients studied after recovery, there was a small but significant decrease in CSF MHPG levels and a significant increase in urinary MHPG levels.

Another group of investigators has reported that MHPG levels in the CSF were not different from control values in a small heterogeneous group of depressed patients; some manic patients showed markedly elevated levels of MHPG, but the mean level of CSF MHPG in the manic patients was not significantly higher than the control mean (47, 66). However, changes in the clinical state in some bipolar manic-depressive patients were associated with a change in CSF MHPG levels corresponding to the direction of the change in affective state. Similar changes in urinary MHPG in relation to changes in the clinical state have been observed in a number of longitudinal studies of manic-depressive patients, as described above.

In another small series of patients with recurrent (unipolar) depressions, manic-depressive depressions and manias, there were no differences in the mean levels of CSF MHPG between these various groups before treatment nor did any significant changes occur after treatment. However, the investigators noted that there was a wide scatter in the concentration of MHPG in the lumbar CSF of these patients. This study differs from others in that a spectrophotofluorometric rather than a gas chromatographic method was used to determine MHPG (67).

As noted above, measures of CSF MHPG may reflect changes in the rate of efflux of MHPG from the CSF, as well as in its rate of formation. In the absence of a technique to block the efflux of MHPG, these factors will remain confounded, and the interpretation of measurements of CSF MHPG will remain problematic.

D. HVA in Cerebrospinal Fluid

Homovanillic acid (HVA), a deaminated O-methylated metabolite of dopamine, can be determined in lumbar CSF and may provide information about the cerebral metabolism of dopamine (68). The interpretation of these findings is complicated by the fact that the concentration of HVA in lumbar CSF is considerably lower than in ventricular CSF, suggesting that there may be a transport system for the removal of HVA in the region of the fourth ventricle (68).

Moreover, as noted above, the rate of efflux of one or another metabolite from the CSF may vary over time and among subjects. Measurements of baseline levels of metabolites in lumbar CSF at an instant in time, therefore, do not necessarily reflect the rates of production of the metabolites during a given time interval. Information of this sort may be obtained for the acid metabolites of biogenic amines (e.g., HVA as well as 5-HIAA, a deaminated metabolite of serotonin) by blocking their efflux from the cerebrospinal fluid with probenecid, a drug which inhibits their transport (69). Several recent studies, therefore, have examined the accumulation of HVA in lumbar cerebrospinal fluid following the administration of probenecid in patients with affective disorders.

Baseline levels of HVA in the CSF* have been found to be lower in depressed patients than in control subjects in a number of studies (70-77), but not in all (78, 79). In one study, the baseline levels of HVA in lumbar CSF were significantly lower in unipolar depressions than in controls, but in bipolar depressions CSF HVA levels were within the normal range and significantly higher than in the unipolar group (80). However, other investigators have reported no differences in HVA levels between unipolar and bipolar depressions (72, 78).

Baseline levels of HVA in hypomanic and manic patients have been observed to be equal to, or lower than, control values in several studies (70, 72, 75, 76, 77, 80). However, in one study, increased baseline levels of HVA in CSF were observed in manic patients when compared with depressed patients or controls (78). In another study, patients with severe mania exhibiting a high degree of motor activity had elevated levels of HVA, whereas levels of HVA in hypomanic patients were slightly lower than control values; the increased levels of HVA in patients with severe mania were attributed to increased motor activity (81).

The accumulation of HVA following probenecid administration has been found to be decreased in at least certain subgroups of

---

* The term "baseline level of HVA (or 5-HIAA) in CSF" is used to distinguish this measurement from the accumulation of HVA (or 5-HIAA) in the CSF after administration of probenecid.

depressed patients when compared with controls (75, 77, 78, 79, 82, 83). However, levels of HVA following probenecid administration were higher in a diagnostically heterogeneous group of depressed patients than in a control population in one study (84). In two of these studies, no differences were observed in HVA accumulation after probenecid administration when depressed and hypomanic patients were compared (77, 78).

Several investigators have examined the probenecid-induced accumulation of HVA in depressed patients in relation to aspects of clinical phenomenology or diagnostic subtypes. Van Praag and his associates (79, 83) have reported that subnormal accumulation of HVA occurs in depressed patients with motor retardation. These investigators observed no difference in CSF levels of HVA after probenecid administration when patients with unipolar and bipolar depressions were compared (79). However, in another recent study, Goodwin et al. (77) found that patients diagnosed as bipolar I* had significantly higher CSF levels of HVA following probenecid administration than did patients diagnosed as bipolar II or as unipolar. In this study, depressed patients who had an antidepressant response to treatment with lithium had significantly lower levels of HVA in CSF after probenecid administration than did lithium nonresponders. Further studies will be required for clarification here, since these investigators have reported that an antidepressant response to treatment with lithium is observed more frequently in patients with bipolar depressive disorders than in patients with unipolar depressions (85).

In summary, a number of studies (though not all) have found that both the baseline levels of HVA in the CSF and the accumulation of HVA in the CSF after probenecid administration are reduced in at least some patients with depressive disorders. The

---

* The diagnosis of bipolar I was made by these investigators on the basis of a history of manic symptoms of sufficient severity to require hospitalization. The diagnosis of bipolar II was made on the basis of a history of periods of abnormally increased activity or euphoria, frequently at the termination of a depressive episode or during treatment with antidepressant drugs or ECT.

possibility that measures of HVA in the CSF may be of value in the clinical differentiation of various subtypes of depressive disorders is currently under investigation.

E. Levels of Serotonin or 5-HIAA in Human Brains After Suicide

Several studies have examined the levels of serotonin and 5-HIAA in the brains of depressed patients following suicide. In one study, the levels of serotonin in the hindbrain were lower in depressed patients after suicide than in a control group of subjects who had died from accidents or acute illnesses (86). However, in a subsequent study, this difference in serotonin levels was not replicated, but 5-HIAA was lower in depressed patients after suicide than in control subjects after death from natural causes. Statistically significant differences in the levels of norepinephrine were not observed (87).

In another study (88), serotonin levels were lower in the brain stem of patients after suicide than in control subjects; however, the major effect in this study was observed in patients with reactive depressions who had suicided rather than in patients with endogenous depressions. Moreover, in this study a positive correlation was found between age and serotonin concentration, and the authors noted that the decrease observed in patients after suicide was offset to some extent by the difference in age between the suicide and control groups. There were no significant differences in the concentrations of 5-HIAA in the brain stem, norepinephrine in the hypothalamus, or dopamine in the caudate nucleus when suicides and controls were compared (88).

Interpretation of these data is exceedingly difficult because of the many uncontrolled variables that may have influenced the results of these studies.

F. 5-HIAA in Cerebrospinal Fluid

Various findings suggest that measurements of 5-hydroxyindoleacetic acid (5-HIAA), a deaminated metabolite of serotonin, in the lumbar cerebrospinal fluid may yield information about the metabolism of serotonin in the brain (68), although some of the 5-HIAA in the lumbar CSF may come from the spinal cord (62, 89, 90). Since the initial report by Ashcroft and Sharman (91) that 5-hydroxyindole compounds were decreased in the cerebrospinal fluid of depressed patients, numerous investigators have reported that baseline levels of 5-HIAA in the CSF are lower in depressed patients than in controls. In a number of studies, statistically significant decreases (72, 92-99), or nonsignificant decreases (70, 74) in baseline levels of CSF 5-HIAA have been observed in depressed patients.

However, in several recent studies depressed patients have been found to have essentially normal baseline levels of 5-HIAA in the cerebrospinal fluid (73, 75-79). In several studies, the decrease in CSF 5-HIAA levels in depressed patients persisted after recovery (72, 80, 93) although a small rise to normal values upon recovery from depression was noted in one study of a small number of patients (94).

The variability observed in the studies of CSF 5-HIAA in depressions might be accounted for by a number of factors. These include the nature of the control group with which depressed patients were compared, the differences in age or sex of the various groups, the differences in the conditions under which the samples of cerebrospinal fluid were obtained, and the differences in techniques used for chemical determinations.

A number of investigators have studied baseline CSF 5-HIAA levels in depressed patients in relation to aspects of clinical phenomenology, diagnostic subtypes, or response to treatment. Depressed patients who were classified as psychotic (on the basis of the presence of delusions) had lower CSF levels of 5-HIAA than did nonpsychotic depressed patients in one study (72). In two other studies, patients with unipolar (recurrent) depressions had lower baseline levels of 5-HIAA in the CSF than did patients with bipolar (manic-depressive) depressions (72, 80). However, another study reported no differences in CSF 5-HIAA levels when patients with bipolar and unipolar depressions were compared (78).

In still another study, no differences in baseline CSF 5-HIAA levels were observed when patients with endogenous and neurotic depressions were compared (79). According to one recent investigation, the baseline levels of 5-HIAA in the CSF appeared to show a bimodal distribution in patients with endogenous depressions, but a unimodal distribution in patients with nonendogenous depressions. In this latter study, patients with relatively higher baseline levels of CSF 5-HIAA tended to show better antidepressant responses to treatment with nortriptyline than did patients with lower baseline levels of CSF 5-HIAA (100). In another recent study, depressions were classified into two types on the basis of differences in the baseline CSF 5-HIAA levels, clinical phenomenology and differential responses to treatment with 5-hydroxytryptophan or 1-dihydroxyphenylalanine (101).

In some studies, low baseline levels of CSF 5-HIAA have been observed in hypomanic or manic patients both before treatment and after recovery (70, 93, 94), but the lowering in pretreatment levels was not statistically significant in all of the studies. Other investigators, however, observed normal or increased CSF 5-HIAA levels in manic patients (75, 77, 78, 80, 92).

It should be pointed out in relation to these findings in patients with affective disorders that decreased baseline levels of 5-HIAA have been observed in other psychiatric conditions, including schizophrenic disorders (70, 92).

The accumulation of 5-HIAA in the CSF following administration of probenecid was found to be lower in depressed patients than in control subjects in a number of recent studies (77, 78, 82, 83, 97, 99, 102), but not in all (84). The possibility has been suggested that decreased 5-HIAA accumulation after probenecid administration may be characteristic of only a subgroup of patients with endogenous depressions who are not necessarily distinguishable on the basis of psychopathological features or of differences in motor activity (97, 99).

Van Praag and his associates reported that the accumulation of 5-HIAA in the CSF after probenecid administration was subnormal (i.e., lower than the lowest value found in the control group) in 12 of 28 patients with endogenous depressions, whereas the accumulation of 5-HIAA in the CSF in each of 10 patients with the diagnosis of neurotic depression fell within the range of the control group (79).

In a pilot study of the antidepressant effects of 5-hydroxytryptophan (5-HTP) in patients with vital (endogenous) depressions, these investigators observed that 3 of 5 patients improved after treatment with 5-HTP, whereas none of 5 subjects improved with a placebo. The 3 patients who improved during treatment with 5-HTP showed a low pretreatment accumulation of 5-HIAA in the CSF after probenecid, whereas the 2 patients who did not improve had a higher pretreatment accumulation of 5-HIAA (102).

In another recent study, Goodwin et al. (77) found no differences in the accumulation of 5-HIAA in the CSF after probenecid administration when these values were compared in patients with bipolar I, bipolar II, or unipolar depressive disorders. In this study, those depressed patients who had a favorable antidepressant response to treatment with lithium carbonate had a lower pretreatment accumulation of 5-HIAA in the CSF following probenecid administration than did lithium nonresponders (77).

Roos and Sjostrom have reported that 5-HIAA accumulation in the CSF after probenecid administration was significantly lower in manic patients than in control subjects (75, 78).

G. Enzymes Involved in Biogenic Amine Metabolism or Synthesis

A number of investigators have recently studied the enzymes which are involved in biogenic amine metabolism or synthesis in patients with affective disorders. In one study, the activities of tyrosine hydroxylase, dopamine-β-hydroxylase, monoamine oxidase, and catechol-O-methyl transferase were examined in various regions of brains obtained from depressive suicides, alcoholic suicides, and from persons who died of natural causes. No significant differences were found between enzyme activities in the brain regions of controls and suicides with the possible exception of tyrosine hydroxylase in the substantia nigra, where depressive (but not alcoholic) suicides showed greater activity (103).

In another recent study, Murphy and Weiss (104) found that platelet monoamine oxidase activity was significantly lower in bipolar depressed patients than in unipolar depressed patients or in normal controls of similar age and sex distribution. The levels of platelet monoamine oxidase activity in the unipolar depressed patients were slightly higher than those of controls, but this difference was not statistically significant. In a small number of bipolar patients studied longitudinally through both depressive and manic episodes, there was no consistent direction of change in platelet monoamine oxidase activity during either manic or depressed periods, suggesting that platelet monoamine oxidase activity does not vary with the phase of the illness in patients with manic-depressive disorders.

Murphy and Wyatt (105) have also reported that some schizophrenic patients have reduced platelet monoamine oxidase activity when compared with controls, and our recent findings suggest that the subgroup of schizophrenic patients with reduced platelet monoamine oxidase activity may be identified clinically by the presence of auditory hallucinations in conjunction with paranoid features (106). The occurrence of reduced platelet monoamine oxidase activity in paranoid schizophrenic disorders as well as in bipolar manic-depressive disorders suggests that there may be biochemical similarities between these groups of disorders.

Rosenblatt and Chanley found that after infusion with radioactive norepinephrine, patients with retarded depressions which were classified as manic-depressive had an elevated ratio of radioactive amines to deaminated metabolites in the urine when compared with normal controls and patients with agitated unipolar depressions (27, 28). Many factors could account for this finding, including an alteration in the disposition of the infused radioactive norepinephrine as well as a decrease in the deamination of norepinephrine or normetanephrine in the manic-depressive depressed group.

In contrast to the findings in bipolar manic-depressive disorders, platelet monoamine oxidase activity was found to be higher in a heterogeneous sample of depressed patients than in normal subjects matched for age (107). Plasma monoamine oxidase activity was reported to be significantly higher in premenopausal depressed women who did not require hospitalization than in control subjects (108).

It is difficult to compare the findings of these various studies since different methods and substrates were used in the assays of monoamine oxidase activity. Moreover, further investigation will be required to determine whether platelet (or plasma) monoamine oxidase activity provides an index of the monoamine oxidase activities in other tissues, particularly in the brain, which may have different isoenzymes.

In two studies of patients with primary affective disorders, the activity of catechol-O-methyl transferase in red blood cells was significantly reduced in depressed women but not in men (109, 110). However, another recent study found increased erythrocyte catechol-O-methyl transferase activity in patients with primary affective disorders (111). Further research will be required to resolve these apparent discrepancies.

In two recent studies, dopamine-β-hydroxylase activity was determined in serum or plasma in patients with affective disorders (112, 113). No differences in dopamine-β-hydroxylase activity were observed when values in manic or depressed patients were compared to control values. There also were no apparent differences in values in the different subtypes of depressive disorders examined in these two studies.

SUMMARY

Various clues to the underlying pathophysiology of depressive and manic disorders have emerged in recent years from studies of biogenic amine metabolism in patients with affective disorders.

A number of recent findings suggest that the urinary excretion of MHPG varies in relation to clinical state in patients with bipolar manic-depressive disorders. Moreover, the level of urinary MHPG, which is reduced in some types of depressive disorders, such as bipolar manic-depressive depressions, may provide a biochemical criterion for classifying the depressive disorders. Urinary MHPG levels may also help to predict differential responses to pharmaco-therapy with one or another of the tricyclic antidepressants.

Numerous studies have found that baseline levels of HVA in the CSF, and the accumulation of HVA in the CSF after its efflux is blocked by probenecid, are reduced in some patients with depressive disorders. This has not been an entirely consistent finding, however. The possible value of the level of CSF HVA as a criterion for differentiating subtypes of depressive disorders is currently under investigation.

A number of studies have also found reduced baseline levels of 5-HIAA in the CSF and reduced accumulation of CSF 5-HIAA after probenecid administration, in some patients with depressive disorders. It has been suggested that decreased 5-HIAA accumulation after probenecid administration may occur only in a subgroup of patients with depressive disorders who are not necessarily distinguishable on the basis of psychopathological features.

Several recent studies of patients with affective disorders have examined some of the enzymes involved in biogenic amine synthesis (e.g., tyrosine hydroxylase and dopamine-beta-hydroxylase), or metabolism (e.g., catechol-O-methyl transferase and monoamine oxidase). One of the most interesting findings to emerge from this research has been the observation that platelet monoamine oxidase activity was significantly reduced in depressed patients with bipolar manic-depressive disorders when compared with platelet MAO values observed in patients with unipolar depressive disorders and in normal controls.

The findings summarized in this review suggest that biochemical measures which relate to biogenic amine metabolism may be of value in classifying depressive disorders, and perhaps also in predicting differential responses to various antidepressant treatment modalities.

REFERENCES

1. SCHILDKRAUT, J. J.: *Neuropsychopharmacology and the Affective Disorders.* Boston: Little, Brown, 1970.
2. SCHILDKRAUT, J. J.: The catecholamine hypothesis of affective

disorders: A review of supporting evidence. *Am. J. Psychiat.*, 122:509-522, 1965.
3. STROM-OLSEN, R. and WEIL-MALHERBE, H.: Humoral changes in manic-depressive psychoses with particular reference to excretion of catecholamines in urine. *J. Ment. Sci.*, 104:696-704, 1958.
4. BUNNEY, W. E., JR., MURPHY, D. L. and GOODWIN, F. K.: The switch process from depression to mania: Relationship to drugs which alter brain amines. *Lancet*, 1:1022-1027, 1970.
5. GREENSPAN, K., SCHILDKRAUT, J. J., GORDON, E. K., LEVY, B. and DURELL, J.: Catecholamine metabolism in affective disorders II. Norepinephrine, normetanephrine, epinephrine, metanephrine and VMA excretion in hypomanic patients. *Arch. Gen. Psychiat.*, 21:710-716, 1969.
6. SHINFUKU, N., OMURA, M. and KAYANO, M.: Catecholamine excretion in manic-depressive psychosis. *Yonago Acta Medica*, 5:109-114, 1961.
7. SHINFUKU, N.: Clinical and biochemical studies with antidepressants. *Yonago Acta Medica*, 9:100-102, 1965.
8. SLOANE, R. B., HUGHES, W. and HAUST, H. L.: Catecholamine excretion in manic-depressive and schizophrenic psychosis and its relationship to symptomatology. *Canad. Psychiat. Assoc. J.*, 11:6-19, 1966.
9. TAKAHASHI, R., NAGAO, Y., TSUCHIYA, K., TAKAMIZAWA, M., KOBAYASHI, T., TORU, M., KOBAYASHI, K. and KARIYA, T.: Catecholamine metabolism of manic-depressive illness. *J. Psychiat. Res.*, 6:185-199, 1968.
10. MESSIHA, F. S., AGALLIANOS, D. and CLOWER, C.: Dopamine excretion in affective states and following Li_2CO_3 therapy. *Nature*, 225:868-869, 1970.
11. BERGSMAN, A.: Urinary excretion of adrenaline and noradrenaline in some mental diseases: Clinical and experimental study. *Acta Psychiatrica & Neurologica Scand.*, 54(Suppl. 133):5-107, 1959.
12. CURTIS, G. C., CLEGHORN, R. A. and SOURKES, T. L.: Relationship between affect and excretion of adrenaline, noradrenaline and 17-hydroxycorticosteroids. *J. Psychosom. Res.*, 4:176-184, 1960.
13. GREENSPAN, K., SCHILDKRAUT, J. J., GORDON, E. K., BAER, L., ARANOFF, M. S. and DURELL, J.: Catecholamine metabolism in affective disorders III: MHPG and other catecholamine metabolites in patients treated with lithium carbonate. *J. Psychiat. Res.*, 7:171-183, 1970.
14. WEIL-MALHERBE, H.: Biochemistry of functional psychoses. *Advances in Enzymology*, 29:479-553, 1967.
15. WYATT, R. J., PORTNOY, B., KUPFER, D. J., SNYDER, F. and ENGELMAN, K.: Resting plasma catecholamine concentrations in

patients with depression and anxiety. *Arch. Gen. Psychiat.*, 24: 65-70, 1971.

16. BUNNEY, W. E., JR., DAVIS, J. M., WEIL-MALHERBE, H. and SMITH, E. R. B.: Biochemical changes in psychotic depression: High norepinephrine levels in psychotic vs. neurotic depression. *Arch. Gen. Psychiat.*, 16:448-460, 1967.

17. SCHILDKRAUT, J. J., GORDON, E. K. and DURELL, J.: Catecholamine metabolism in affective disorders I. Normetanephrine and VMA excretion in depressed patients treated with imipramine. *J. Psychiat. Res.*, 3:213-228, 1965.

18. AXELROD, J.: Methylation reactions in the formation and metabolism of catecholamines and other biogenic amines. *Pharmacological Reviews*, 18:95-113, 1966.

19. KOPIN, I. J. and GORDON, E. K.: Metabolism of norepinephrine-H^3 released by tyramine and reserpine. *J. Pharm. Exper. Ther.*, 138:351-359, 1962.

20. KOPIN, I. J. and GORDON, E. K.: Metabolism of administered and drug-released norepinephrine-7-H^3 in rat. *J. Pharm. Exper. Ther.*, 140:207-216, 1963.

21. SCHILDKRAUT, J. J., GREEN, R., GORDON, E. K. and DURELL, J.: Normetanephrine excretion and affective state in depressed patients treated with imipramine. *Am. J. Psychiat.*, 123:690-700, 1966.

22. MAAS, J. W., FAWCETT, J. A. and DEKIRMENJIAN, H.: Catecholamine metabolism, depressive illness and drug response. *Arch. Gen. Psychiat.*, 26:252-262, 1972.

23. PRANGE, A. J., JR., WILSON, I. C., KNOX, A. E., McCLANE, T. K., BREESE, G. R., MARTIN, B. R., ALLTOP, L. B. and LIPTON, M. A.: Thyroid-imipramine clinical and chemical interaction: Evidence for a receptor deficit in depression. *J. Psychiat. Res.*, 9:187-206, 1972.

24. SCHILDKRAUT, J. J., KEELER, B. A., ROGERS, M. P. and DRASKOCZY, P. R.: Catecholamine metabolism in affective disorders: A longitudinal study of a patient treated with amitriptyline and ECT. *Psychosomatic Medicine*, 34:470, 1972; plus erratum *Psychosomatic Medicine*, 35:274, 1973.

25. KARKI, N. T.: Urinary excretion of noradrenaline and adrenaline in different age groups, its diurnal variation and effect of muscular work on it. *Act. Physiol. Scand.*, 39 (Suppl. 132): 5-96, 1956.

26. NELSON, G. N., MASUDA, M. and HOLMES, T. H.: Correlation of behavior and catecholamine metabolite excretion. *Psychosomatic Medicine*, 28:216-226, 1966.

27. ROSENBLATT, S. and CHANLEY, J. D.: Differences in metabolism of norepinephrine in depressions: Effects of various therapies. *Arch. Gen. Psychiat.*, 13:495-502, 1965.

28. ROSENBLATT, S., CHANLEY, J. D. and LEIGHTON, W. P.: The in-

vestigation of adrenergic metabolism with 7H³-norepinephrine in psychiatric disorders—II. Temporal changes in the distribution of tritiated metabolites in affective disorders. *J. Psychiat. Res.*, 6:321-323, 1969.

29. MANNARINO, E., KIRSCHNER, N. and NASHOLD, B. S., JR.: Metabolism of C¹⁴-noradrenaline by cat brain *in vivo. J. Neurochem.*, 10:373-379, 1963.

30. GLOWINSKI, J., KOPIN, I. J. and AXELROD, J.: Metabolism of H³-norepinephrine in rat brain. *J. Neurochem.*, 12:25-30, 1965.

31. RUTLEDGE, C. O. and JONASON, J.: Metabolic pathways of dopamine and norepinephrine in rabbit brain *in vitro. J. Pharmacol. Exper. Ther.*, 157:493-502, 1967.

32. MAAS, J. W. and LANDIS, D. H.: *In vivo* studies of metabolism of norepinephrine in central nervous system. *J. Pharmacol. Exper. Ther.*, 157:493-502, 1967.

33. MAAS, J. W., DEKIRMENJIAN, H., GARVER, D., REDMOND, D. E., JR. and LANDIS, D. H.: Catecholamine metabolite excretion following intraventricular injection of 6OH-dopamine. *Brain Res.*, 41:507-511, 1972.

34. SCHANBERG, S. M., SCHILDKRAUT, J. J., BREESE, G. R. and KOPIN, I. J.: Metabolism of normetanephrine-H³ in rat brain—identification of conjugated 3-methoxy-4-hydroxyphenylglycol as major metabolite. *Biochem. Pharmacol.*, 17:247-254, 1968.

35. SCHANBERG, S. M., BREESE, G. R., SCHILDKRAUT, J. J., GORDON, E. K. and KOPIN, I. J.: 3-Methoxy-4-hydroxyphenylglycol sulfate in brain and cerebrospinal fluid. *Biochem. Pharmacol.*, 17: 2006-2008, 1968.

36. WILK, S. and WATSON, E.: VMA in spinal fluid: Evaluation of the pathways of cerebral catecholamine metabolism in man. *In* E. Usdin and S. Snyder (Eds.), *Frontiers in Catecholamine Research.* New York: Pergamon, 1973, pp. 1067-1069.

37. AXELROD, J., KOPIN, I. J. and MANN, J. D.: 3-Methoxy-4-hydroxyphenylglycol sulfate, a new metabolite of epinephrine and norepinephrine. *Biochim. et Biophys. Acta.*, 36:576-577, 1959.

38. BREESE, G. R., PRANGE, A. J., JR., HOWARD, J. L., LIPTON, M. A., MCKINNEY, W. T., BOWMAN, R. E. and BUSHNELL, P.: 3-Methoxy-4-hydroxyphenylglycol excretion and behavioral changes in rat and monkey after central sympathectomy with 6-hydroxydopamine. *Nature New Biol.*, 240:286-287, 1972.

39. HOELDTKE, R. D., ROGAWSKI, M. and WURTMAN, R. J.: Effects of selective destruction of central and peripheral catecholamine containing neurons with 6-hydroxydopamine on catecholamine excretion in the rat. *Brit. J. Pharmacol.*, 50:265, 1974.

40. KAROUM, F., WYATT, R. and COSTA, E.: Estimation of the contribution of peripheral and central noradrenaline neurons to urinary 3-methoxy-4-hydroxyphenylglycol in the rat. *Neuropharmacology*, 13:165-176, 1974.

41. EBERT, M.: Personal communication.
42. SCHILDKRAUT, J. J., WATSON, R., DRASKOCZY, P. R. and HART-
    MANN, E.: Amphetamine withdrawal: Depression and MHPG
    excretion. *Lancet*, 2:485-486, 1971.
43. BOND, P. A., JENNER, F. A. and SAMPSON, G. A.: Daily varia-
    tions of the urine content of 3-methoxy-4-hydroxyphenylglycol
    in two manic-depressive patients. *Psychological Medicine*, 2:
    81-85, 1972.
44. JONES, F. D., MAAS, J. W., DEKIRMENJIAN, H. and FAWCETT,
    J. A.: Urinary catecholamine metabolites during behavioral
    changes in a patient with manic-depressive cycles. *Science*,
    179:300-302, 1973.
45. GOODWIN, F. K., BECKMANN, H. and POST, R. M.: Urinary 3-
    methoxy-4-hydroxyphenylglycol in subtypes of affective illness.
    *Scientific Proceedings in Summary Form, Annual Meeting of
    the American Psychiatric Association*, 1975, pp. 96-97.
46. BUNNEY, W. E., GOODWIN, F. K., MURPHY, D. L., HOUSE,
    K. M. and GORDON, E. K.: The "switch process" in manic-
    depressive illness. *Arch. Gen. Psychiat.*, 27:304-309, 1972.
47. SHOPSIN, B., WILK, S., GERSHON, S., ROFFMAN, M. and GOLD-
    STEIN, M.: Collaborative psychopharmacologic studies explor-
    ing catecholamine metabolism in psychiatric disorders. *In*
    E. Usdin and S. Snyder (Eds.), *Frontiers in Catecholamine
    Research*. New York: Pergamon, 1973, pp. 1173-1179.
48. MAAS, J. W., DEKIRMENJIAN, H. and FAWCETT, J.: Catechola-
    mine metabolism in depression and stress. *Nature*, 230:330-
    331, 1971.
49. RUBIN, R. T., MILLER, R. G., CLARK, B. R., POLAND, R. E. and
    ARTHUR, R. J.: The stress of aircraft carrier landings II.
    3-Methoxy-4-hydroxyphenylglycol excretion in naval aviators.
    Psychosomatic Medicine, 32:589-597, 1970.
50. EBERT, M. H., POST, R. M. and GOODWIN, F. K.: Effect of physi-
    cal activity on urinary MHPG excretion in depressed pa-
    tients. *Lancet*, 2:766, 1972.
51. MAAS, J. W., FAWCETT, J. A. and DEKIRMENJIAN, H.: 3-Me-
    thoxy-4-hydroxyphenylglycol (MHPG) excretion in depressive
    states: Pilot study. *Arch. Gen. Psychiat.*, 19:129-134, 1968.
52. SCHILDKRAUT, J. J., DRASKOCZY, P. R., GERSHON, E. S., REICH,
    P. and GRAB, E. L.: Effects of tricyclic antidepressants on
    norepinephrine metabolism: Basic and clinical studies. *In* B.
    T. Ho and W. M. McIsaac (Eds.), *Brain Chemistry and
    Mental Disease*. New York: Plenum, 1971, pp. 215-236.
53. SCHILDKRAUT, J. J., KEELER, B. A., PAPOUSEK, M. and HART-
    MANN, E.: MHPG excretion in depressive disorders: Relation
    to clinical subtypes and desynchronized sleep. *Science*, 181:
    762-764, 1973.
54. SCHILDKRAUT, J. J.: Catecholamine metabolism and affective

disorders: Studies of MHPG excretion. *In* E. Usdin and S. Snyder (Eds.), *Frontiers in Catecholamine Research.* New York: Pergamon, 1973, pp. 1165-1171.

55. SCHILDKRAUT, J. J., ORSULAK, P. J., GUDEMAN, J. E., ROHDE, W. A., CAHILL, J. F., SCHATZBERG, A. F., COLE, J. O. and FRAZIER, S. H.: Unpublished data.

56. MAAS, J. W., DEKIRMENJIAN, H. and JONES, F.: The identification of depressed patients who have a disorder of norepinephrine metabolism and/or disposition. *In* E. Usdin and S. Snyder (Eds.), *Frontiers in Catecholamine Research.* New York: Pergamon, 1973, pp. 1091-1096.

57. FEIGHNER, J. P., ROBINS, E., GUZE, S. B., WOODRUFF, R. A., JR., WINOKUR, G. and MUNOZ, R.: Diagnostic criteria for use in psychiatric research. *Arch. Gen. Psychiat.*, 26:57-63, 1972.

58. BECKMANN, H. and GOODWIN, F. K.: Antidepressant response to tricyclics and urinary MHPG in unipolar patients. *Arch. Gen. Psychiat.*, 32:17-21, 1975.

59. SCHILDKRAUT, J. J.: Norepinephrine metabolites as biochemical criteria for classifying depressive disorders and predicting responses to treatment—preliminary findings. *Am. J. Psychiat.*, 130:695-699, 1973.

60. GORDON, E. K. and OLIVER, J.: 3-Methoxy-4-hydroxyphenylethyleneglycol in human cerebrospinal fluid. *Clin. Chim. Acta.*, 35:145-150, 1971.

61. WILK, S., DAVIS, K. L. and THACKER, S. B.: Determination of 3-methoxy-4-hydroxyphenylethylene glycol (MHPG) in cerebrospinal fluid. *Anal. Biochem.*, 39:498-504, 1971.

62. POST, R. M., GOODWIN, F. K., GORDON, E. and WATKIN, D. M.: Amine metabolites in human cerebrospinal fluid: Effects of cord transection and spinal fluid block. *Science*, 179:897-899, 1973.

63. SHAW, D. M., O'KEEFE, R., MACSWEENEY, D. A., BROOKSBANK, B. W. L., NOGUERA, R. and COPPEN, A.: 3-Methoxy-4-hydroxyphenylglycol in depression. *Psychological Medicine*, 3:333-336, 1973.

64. SHOPSIN, B., WILK, S., SATHANANTHAN, G., GERSHON, S. and DAVIS, D.: Catecholamines and affective disorders revised: A critical assessment. *J. Nerv. Ment. Dis.*, 158:369-383, 1974.

65. POST, R. M., GORDON, E. K., GOODWIN, F. K. and BUNNEY, W. E., JR.: Central norepinephrine metabolism in affective illness: MHPG in the cerebrospinal fluid. *Science*, 179:1002-1003, 1973.

66. SHOPSIN, B., WILK, S., GERSHON, S., DAVIS, K. and SUHL, M.: Cerebrospinal fluid MHPG. *Arch. Gen. Psychiat.*, 28:230-233, 1973.

67. ASHCROFT, G. W., BROOKS, P. W., CUNDALL, R. L., ECCLESTON, D., MURRAY, L. G. and PULLAR, I. A.: Changes in the glycol metabolites of noradrenaline in affective illness. Presented at Fifth World Congress of Psychiatry, Mexico City, 1971.

68. MOIR, A. T. B., ASHCROFT, G. W., CRAWFORD, T. B. B., ECCLES-
    TON, D. and GULDBERG, H. S.: Cerebral metabolites in cere-
    brospinal fluid as a biochemical approach to the brain. *Brain*,
    93:357-368, 1970.
69. NEFF, N. H., TOZER, T. N. and BRODIE, B. B.: Application of
    steady-state kinetics to studies of the transfer of 5-hydroxy-
    indoleacetic acid from brain to plasma. *J. Pharmacol. Exper.
    Ther.*, 158:214-218, 1967.
70. BOWERS, M. B., JR., HENINGER, G. R. and GERBODE, F.: Cerebro-
    spinal fluid 5-hydroxyindoleacetic acid and homovanillic acid
    in psychiatric patients. *Int. J. Neuropharmacol.*, 8:255-262,
    1969.
71. BRODIE, H. K. H., SACK, R. and SIEVER, L.: Clinical studies of
    l-5-hydroxytryptophan in depression. *In* J. Barchas and E.
    Usdin (Eds.), *Serotonin and Behavior*. New York: Academic
    Press, 1973, pp. 549-559.
72. MENDELS, J., FRAZER, A., FITZGERALD, R. G., RAMSEY, T. A. and
    STOKES, J. W.: Biogenic amine metabolites in cerebrospinal
    fluid of depressed and manic patients. *Science*, 175:1380-1382,
    1972.
73. NORDIN, G., OTTOSON, J.-O. and ROOS, B.-E.: Influence of con-
    vulsive therapy on 5-hydroxyindoleacetic acid and homovanillic
    acid in cerebrospinal fluid in endogenous depression. *Psycho-
    pharmacologia* (Berl.), 20:315-320, 1971.
74. PAPESCHI, R. and MCCLURE, D. J.: Homovanillic and 5-hydroxy-
    indoleacetic acid in cerebrospinal fluid of depressed patients.
    Arch. Gen. Psychiat., 25:354-358, 1971.
75. ROOS, B.-E. and SJOSTROM, R.: 5-Hydroxyindoleacetic acid (and
    homovanillic acid) levels in the cerebrospinal fluid after pro-
    benecid application in patients with manic-depressive psy-
    chosis. *Pharmacologia Clinica*, 1:153-155, 1969.
76. WILK, S., SHOPSIN, B., GERSHON, S. and SUHL, M.: Cerebro-
    spinal fluid levels of MHPG in affective disorders. *Nature*,
    235:440-441, 1972.
77. GOODWIN, F. K., POST, R. M., DUNNER, D. L. and GORDON, E. K.:
    Cerebrospinal fluid amine metabolites in affective illness: The
    probenecid technique. *Am. J. Psychiat.*, 130:73-79, 1973.
78. SJOSTROM, R. and ROOS, B.-E.: 5-Hydroxyindoleacetic acid and
    homovanillic acid in cerebrospinal fluid in manic-depressive
    psychosis. *Eur. J. Clin. Pharmacol.*, 4:170-176, 1972.
79. VAN PRAAG, H. M., KORF, J. and SCHUT, D.: Cerebral mono-
    amines and depression—An investigation with the probenecid
    technique. *Arch. Gen. Psychiat.*, 28:827-831, 1973.
80. MEDICAL RESEARCH COUNCIL, BRAIN METABOLISM UNIT: Modified
    amine hypothesis for the etiology of affective illness. *Lancet*,
    2:537-577, 1972.
81. POST, R. M., KOTIN, J., GOODWIN, F. K. and GORDON, E. K.:

Psychomotor activity and cerebrospinal fluid amine metabolites in affective illness. *Am. J. Psychiat.*, 130:67-72, 1973.

82. SJOSTROM, R.: 5-Hydroxyindoleacetic acid in cerebrospinal fluid in manic-depressive psychosis and the effect of probenecid treatment. *Eur. J. Clin. Pharmacol.*, 6:75-80, 1973.

83. VAN PRAAG, H. M.: Towards a biochemical typology of depression? *Pharmakopsychiat.*, *Neuropsychopharmakol.*, 7:281-292, 1974.

84. BOWERS, M. B., JR.: Cerebrospinal fluid 5-hydroxyindoleacetic acid (5-HIAA) and homovanillic acid (HVA) following probenecid in unipolar depressives treated with amitriptyline. *Psychopharmacologia* (Berl.), 23:26-33, 1972.

85. GOODWIN, F. K., MURPHY, D. L., DUNNER, D. L. and BUNNEY, W. E., JR.: Lithium response in unipolar versus bipolar depression. *Am. J. Psychiat.*, 129:44-47, 1972.

86. SHAW, D. M., CAMPS, F. E., ECCLESTON, E. G.: 5-Hydroxytryptamine in hind-brain of depressive suicides. *Brit. J. Psychiat.*, 113:1407-1411, 1967.

87. BOURNE, H. R., BUNNEY, W. E., JR., COLBURN, R. W., DAVIS, J. M., DAVIS, J. N., SHAW, D. M. and COPPEN, A. J.: Noradrenaline, 5-hydroxytryptamine and 5-hydroxyindoleacetic acid in hindbrain of suicidal patients. *Lancet*, 2:805-808, 1968.

88. PARE, C. M. B., YEUNG, D. P. H., PRICE, K. and STACEY, R. S.: 5-Hydroxytryptamine in brainstem, hypothalamus and caudate nucleus of controls and of patients committing suicide by coalgas poisoning. *Lancet*, 2:133-135, 1969.

89. BULAT, M. and ZIVKOVIC, B.: Origin of 5-hydroxyindoleacetic acid in the spinal fluid. *Science*, 173:738-740, 1971.

90. WEIR, R. L., CHASE, T. N., NG, L. K. Y. and KOPIN, I. J.: 5-Hydroxyindoleacetic acid in spinal fluid. *Brain Res.*, 52:409-412, 1973.

91. ASHCROFT, G. W. and SHARMAN, D. F.: 5-Hydroxyindoles in human cerebrospinal fluids. *Nature*, 186:1050-1051, 1960.

92. ASHCROFT, G. W., CRAWFORD, T. B. B., ECCLESTON, D., SHARMAN, D. F., MACDOUGALL, E. J., STANTON, J. B. and BINNS, J. K.: 5-Hydroxyindole compounds in the cerebrospinal fluid of patients with psychiatric or neurological diseases. *Lancet*, 2:1049-1052, 1966.

93. COPPEN, A., PRANGE, A. J., JR., WHYBROW, P. C. and NOGUERA, R.: Abnormalities of indoleamines in affective disorders. *Arch. Gen. Psychiat.*, 26:474-478, 1972.

94. DENCKER, S. J., MALM, U., ROOS, B.-E. and WERDINIUS, B.: Acid monoamine metabolites of cerebrospinal fluid in mental depression and mania. *J. Neurochem.*, 13:1545-1548, 1966.

95. MCLEOD, W. R. and MCLEOD, M. S.: Serotonin and severe affective disorders. *Aust. N.Z. J. Psychiat.*, 5:289-295, 1971.

96. COPPEN, A.: Serotonin in the affective disorders. *In* N. S.

Kline (Ed.), *Factors in Depression*. New York, Raven Press, 1974, pp. 33-44.

97. VAN PRAAG, H. M. and KORF, J.: Endogenous depressions with and without disturbances in the 5-hydroxytryptamine metabolism: A biochemical classification? *Psychopharmacologia* (Berl.), 19:148-152, 1971.

98. VAN PRAAG, H. M. and KORF, J.: A pilot study of some kinetic aspects of the metabolism of 5-hydroxytryptamine in depressive patients. *Biol. Psychiat.*, 3:105-112, 1971.

99. VAN PRAAG, H. M., KORF, J. and PUITE, J.: 5-Hydroxyindoleacetic acid levels in the cerebrospinal fluid of depressive patients treated with probenecid. *Nature*, 225:1259-1260, 1970.

100. ASBERG, M., BERTILSSON, L., TUCK, D., CRONHOLM, B. and SJOQVIST, F.: Indoleamine metabolites in the cerebrospinal fluid of depressed patients before and during treatment with nortriptyline. *Clin. Pharm. Therapy*, 14:277-287, 1973.

101. FUJIWARA, J. and OTSUKI, S.: Subtype of affective psychoses classified by response on amine precursors and monoamine metabolism. *Folia Psychiat. et Neurologica Japonica*, 28:93-100, 1974.

102. VAN PRAAG, H. M., KORF, J., DOLS, L. C. W. and SCHUT, T.: A pilot study of the predictive value of the probenecid test in application of 5-hydroxytryptophan as antidepressant. *Psychopharmacologia* (Berl.), 25:14-21, 1972.

103. GROTE, S. S., MOSES, S. G., ROBINS, E., HUDGENS, R. W. and CRONINGER, A. B.: A study of selected catecholamine metabolizing enzymes: A comparison of depressive suicides and alcoholic suicides with controls. *J. Neurochem.*, 23:791-802, 1974.

104. MURPHY, D. L. and WEISS, R.: Reduced monoamine oxidase activity in blood platelets from bipolar depressed patients. *Am. J. Psychiat.*, 128:1351-1357, 1972.

105. MURPHY, D. L. and WYATT, R. J.: Reduced monoamine oxidase activity in blood platelets from schizophrenic patients. *Nature*, 238:225-226, 1972.

106. SCHILDKRAUT, J. J., HERZOG, J. M., ORSULAK, P. J., EDELMAN, S. E., SHEIN, H. M. and FRAZIER, S. H.: Reduced platelet monoamine oxidase activity in a subgroup of schizophrenic patients. *Am. J. Psychiat.*, 133:438-440, 1976.

107. NIES, A., ROBINSON, D. S., RAVARIS, C. L. and DAVIS, J. M.: Amines and monoamine oxidase in relation to aging and depression in man. *Psychosomatic medicine*, 33:470, 1971.

108. KLAIBER, E. L., BROVERMAN, D. M., VOGEL, W., KOBAYASHI, Y. and MORIARTY, D.: Effects of estrogen therapy on plasma MAO activities and EEG driving responses of depressed women. *Am. J. Psychiat.*, 128:1492-1498, 1972.

109. COHN, C. K., DUNNER, D. L. and AXELROD, J.: Reduced catechol-

O-methyl transferase activity in red blood cells of women with primary affective disorders. *Science*, 170:1323-1324, 1970.

110. DUNNER, D. L., COHN, C. K., GERSHON, E. S. and GOODWIN, F. K.: Differential catechol-O-methyl transferase activity in unipolar and bipolar affective illness. *Arch. Gen. Psychiat.*, 25: 348:353, 1971.

111. GERSHON, E. S. and JONAS, W. Z.: Erythrocyte soluble catechol-O-methyl transferase activity in primary affective disorders. *Arch. Gen. Psychiat.*, 32:1351-1356, 1975.

112. SHOPSIN, B., FREEDMAN, L. S., GOLDSTEIN, M. and GERSHON, S.: Serum dopamine-β-hydroxylase (DBH) activity and affective states. *Psychopharmacologia* (Berl.), 27:11-16, 1972.

113. WETTERBERG, L., ABERG, H., ROSS, S. B. and FRODEN, O.: Plasma dopamine-β-hydroxylase activity in hypertension and various neuropsychiatric disorders. *Scand. J. Clin. Lab. Invest.*, 30: 283-289, 1972.

9

Depression and Sleep Research: Basic Science and Clinical Perspectives

David R. Hawkins, M.D.

A great amount of research effort has been devoted to the study of the sleep of patients with depression; this is the disease or syndrome in which disturbances of sleep are the most usual and the most profound. Most of this paper will be devoted to research into sleep in depression, a field which remains complex and uncertain in spite of all of the investigations that have been carried out.

The paper will begin with the presentation of a patient with unipolar psychotic depression (1) which was successfully treated by electroconvulsive therapy and studied longitudinally in the sleep laboratory throughout his hospitalization, and again for two nights three weeks after his discharge from the hospital. This case exemplifies the conduct of a longitudinal sleep study, demonstrates typical findings, and raises questions about the possible presence of certain anatomical and physiological mechanisms in depression. Following the case presentation and discussion, there will be a review of the anatomy and physiology of depression, with the exclusion of those aspects of these subjects covered by other authors in this volume. Some information about the state of the art in sleep research will be given, followed by a more comprehensive consideration of sleep research as it relates to the affective disorders.

CASE HISTORY

A white 51-year-old married dairy farmer was brought to the hospital by his son. He stated that he was "all mixed up," felt "blue," had lost his appetite, and had trouble sleeping.

He related his difficulties to having been severely gored by a bull about three months earlier; he had suffered multiple fractures of the left ribcage and fractures of the right superior and inferior pubic rami. For several days before the attack by the bull, the patient had suffered from what he described as an influenza-like illness. As he began to improve from this, he noticed that his bull was restless and needed to be taken out into the field. At the time he saw this as too dangerous a task for his sons, but in retrospect he felt he had shown poor judgment in trying to do it himself while in a weakened condition. He spoke of the bull anthropomorphically, saying that it had sensed his anxiety and lack of confidence, and attacked him for that reason. It was clear that the patient saw this as a struggle with a personified adversary, a struggle in which his manhood was in question. He had had two previous accidents with bulls, one about six years earlier, and one as a youngster. The content of his depressive rumination and delusion was that his own inadequacies and errors of judgment had placed his whole family in a situation where financial disaster was imminent.

Initially, in his hometown hospital, he had a brief hypomanic type of episode that was diagnosed as an anxiety reaction. His depression began shortly before he left the hospital, not quite two months before this admission. It was characterized by feelings of impending disaster. For about two weeks before admission he was markedly withdrawn and uncommunicative, slept poorly, ate little, and lost a considerable amount of weight. No drugs were being used.

The patient was the youngest of five siblings. His father, described as a quiet, hard-working man, died at the age of 54, when the patient was nine. He left many debts, and things were extremely difficult for his family. The mother died when the patient was 17. She was an extremely strict, hard-working woman who kept her children close to her. After her husband's death, she worked in the fields. As the youngest child, the patient was very close to her and regularly accompanied her to church. He described himself as having been a very shy, quiet youngster, afraid of his elders. He had to work hard after his father died, and he left school at age 14 because of financial problems. Feeling it important that he make money to pay off the family's debts, he worked on the farm thereafter.

He married at age 20 and had three sons, all of whom remained close to home. He was disappointed that he did not have more education. Until about six years before admission, an older brother had worked with him on the farm, handling all of the paperwork connected with the business; since his brother's departure the patient felt a continuing sense of inadequacy and anxiety about the business aspects of the farm, and this undoubtedly contributed to his sense of loss of power and manhood in his encounter with the bull.

He appeared shy, obviously depressed, and retarded, and looked somewhat older than his stated age. He was restless; his speech was slow; he had a poverty of ideas, and was vague, indirect, and repetitive. There was no evidence of hallucinations. He was negativistic, and cooperated poorly. Physical examination was unremarkable except for the finding of mild emphysema. The degree of retardation and impoverishment of ideation was such as to raise seriously the question of organic brain disease. A routine electroencephalogram, skull films, and brain scan were interpreted as normal. He was successfully treated by nine electroconvulsive treatments (ECT) and was discharged on day 37 of hospitalization, markedly improved. The only drugs that were used were sodium thiopental and succinylcholine to modify the ECT. The patient was studied in the sleep laboratory for 31 out of 36 hospital nights, and then again on two consecutive nights three weeks after discharge from the hospital. The usual measurements were made; eye movements were monitored by means of a ceramic strain gauge. The methodology and results have been presented in more detail elsewhere (1).

Figure 1 indicates the patient's overall sleep pattern. Total sleep for the five nights not spent in the laboratory was estimated by his nurses. With the exception of nights 5 and 9 (which followed the first ECT), his sleep was markedly impoverished, with frequent long periods of wakefulness. On night 17, following his sixth ECT, the total sleep time rose abruptly to normal values, and continued so throughout the rest of the study. There was some slight decrease in the amount of sleep during the last two nights before discharge. This has been a relatively consistent finding in our longitudinal sleep studies, and we assume it represents anxiety related to impending discharge. The Hamilton score began to change as the total sleep improved; it was entirely normal on discharge. Appetite was estimated on a 4-point scale. A change from marked anorexia to normal eating accompanied the sleep change. Weight was measured weekly, and some time during the week of sleep change a continuing and rapid weight loss was reversed; the patient gained 24 pounds in from two-and-a-half to three weeks and a marked constipation was relieved. Other aspects of the case in Figure 1 will be discussed at appropriate points later in this paper.

During the first part of his hospitalization the patient was withdrawn, severely retarded, and negativistic, and had a depressed affect. The striking sudden improvement in sleep was not noted at the time and was appreciated only after sleep records were analyzed. The observations of professional personnel indicated that it was not until day 19, or two days after the marked sleep improvement, that the patient appeared to take an interest in his surroundings and to be more actively participant in ward activities. His depressive mood gradually lifted, and except for mild anxiety about returning home he seemed quite normal at the time of discharge. He had initially been most uncooperative when electrodes were applied in the laboratory, but the lab log book indicated that starting with day 17 he was much less so. During the recovery phase he frequently started drifting off to sleep in the daytime. Although he was not

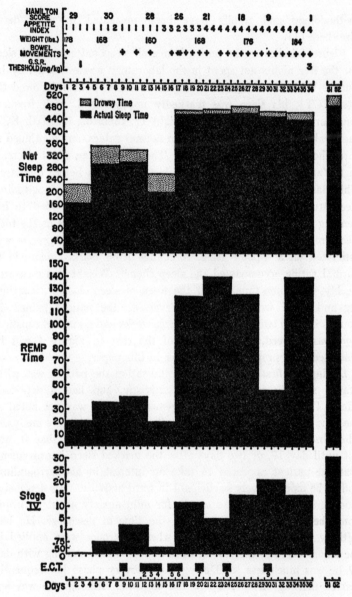

Reprinted by courtesy of American Journal of Psychiatry

allowed to nap because of his participation in the sleep study, the pressure for sleep was obvious.

The abrupt normalization of most sleep dimensions and other somatic manifestations has not been as striking in other patients we have studied longitudinally. Following an ECT treatment, there is some improvement in overall sleep, with some return in the direction of the disease pattern on subsequent nights, and then again improvement after a succeeding treatment. In the case of treatment with tricyclic medication, there is a slower but more consistent trend toward normal.

This case raises a number of interesting issues and questions:

1. The abrupt normalization suggests a mechanism for the control of depression, which, under certain conditions, can be promptly switched off. Those patients who rapidly and regularly cycle from depression to mania and back suggest a similar concept. This raises the question as to whether there is a discrete anatomical center that is responsible for control and switching, in one or more anatomical locations, or whether there is a functional system in control of the depressive mechanism.

2. This notion of a controlling or switching system fits with the observation of our clinical predecessors that severe depressions, once under way, have a life of their own. Our predecessors, of course, had no specific treatment for depression available.

3. This case strongly suggests—and other experience generally confirms—that the biological phenomena tend toward normality somewhat in advance of the behavioral changes and subjective mood improvement. This raises the question as to whether or not sleep abnormalities and/or sleep deprivation play any role in the development of depressive illness.

4. This case may have some relevance to the reactive-endogenous dichotomy in depression. There seems little doubt that this patient's depressive illness was related to a life event that was specifically stressful for him, but it had all the signs of what would ordinarily be classified as an endogenous depression. The use of the term

"reactive-endogenous dichotomy" may not be the most felicitous expression; rather we should probably ask the question in a depressive illness whether or not the biological mechanisms are involved. Klein (2) addresses this issue when he speaks of "endogenomorphic depression." Obviously, if one takes this point of view and assumes a genetic predisposition, the degree of vulnerability will be variable, and the contribution of external events variable also.

Having set the stage with this case presentation, let us return to a general discussion of the anatomy and psychophysiology of depression.

ANATOMY

The only substantial proposal for a special anatomy of depression is that proposed by Kraines (3), to be discussed shortly. The name *affective disorders* immediately suggests that we should ask what we know about brain control of affects. Papez (4) pointed out that emotion is "a physiological process which depends on an anatomic mechanism." He suggested that the structure known as the limbic lobe deals with "the various phases of emotional dynamics, consciousness and related functions. The various structures in the limbic system form a part of a circuit by which impulses are transferred from the hypothalamus to the cortex, and return by the cortex to the hypothalamus." MacLean (5) investigated this area extensively, termed it the limbic system, and suggested that this system, also known as the visceral brain, is composed of several structures: the subcallosal, cingulate, and parahippocampal gyri; and the hippocampus proper. Included are associated subcortical nuclei such as the amygdaloid complex, septal nuclei, hypothalamus, epithalamus, anterior thalamic nuclei, and parts of the basal ganglion. None of the experimental manipulations, whether stimulation or extirpation, has demonstrated depressive syndrome, but it has been shown that portions of the septal region act as a pleasure center. Olds (6) and, subsequently, Heath (7) have shown that mammals, including some humans studied, will strive to get self-stimulatory shocks through electrodes implanted in this area. These studies suggest a major relationship to mania, but obviously only to some of its dimensions. Lilly (8) demonstrated centers in the monkey brain the stimulation of which led to withdrawal and debility; these may be similar to the punishment centers found by Olds. These findings do suggest anatomical bases for some of the aspects of depression. Brain (9) indicates that rage, fear, and depression may be present in uncinate fits.

Lobotomy has, of course, been used to treat depressive illness. Kelly et al. (10) performed limbic leucotomy, which interrupts the connections between the frontal cortex and the limbic system, on 40 patients with a variety of disorders, and saw the greatest improvement (80 percent) among those who were depressed. This finding implicates the frontal lobe in depression in some way, but it does not appear to be the whole answer.

Many—if not most—of the somatic systems involved in depression are somehow controlled by the hypothalamus, which is clearly linked to all emotional expression. Stimulation of the hypothalamus during neurosurgery is said to have induced manic-like behavior. Drawing on existent knowledge of the central nervous system and the natural history of manic-depressive illness without specific therapy, Kraines (3), in a most provocative paper, developed the thesis that manic-depressive illness is physiologic in origin. He hypothesized that pathology of the emotional circuit of Papez (4) can explain the symptoms and the course of this illness. He implicated the hypothalamus as the primary site for the mechanism of the manic-depressive syndrome. Certainly, however, everything we know indicates the hypothalamus to be a final way-station; its various control functions are in turn controlled by hormonal and neural mechanisms at higher levels; there is nothing to indicate that affective illness is in any way related to anatomical abnormalities of the hypothalamus.

PSYCHOPHYSIOLOGY

Zung et al. (11) demonstrated that depressed patients have a lower auditory threshold for awakening in every stage of sleep than do normal controls, but that it returns to normal when depression has been overcome. Thus, the lowered threshold must be seen as a function of depressive illness rather than idiosyncratic among the patients studied. Evidence suggests an increase in the activity of the reticular activating system during depression. The depressed presumably have a higher level of arousal than normals. Hill (12), among others, has discussed the combination of heightened arousal and general inhibition as an important manifestation of depression, although heightened arousal related to RAS activation is but one dimension of this disorder.

There is some evidence that alpha rhythm is more persistently suppressed in response to stimuli in depressed patients than in controls. Shagass (13) has noted a prolongation of the recovery phase of the cortical evoked potential in psychotically depressed patients. These are other evidences of an apparently increased activity of the reticular activating system in psychotic depressives. Satterfield (14) studied the auditory evoked cortical response in depressed patients and found two patterns of abnormality—hyperrecovery and hyporecovery. Patients with the former have increased central nervous system excitability, whereas in the latter it may be decreased. Preliminary evidence suggests that these two patterns of recovery are associated with what the family history is in respect to affective disorders.

Perez-Reyes (15) followed up Shagass's earlier studies of the sedation threshold, investigating the inhibition threshold of the galvanic skin response (GSR) and the sleep threshold. He found that it took significantly more sodium thiopental to reach the GSR inhibition threshold or the sleep threshold in neurotic depressives than in normal controls, and significantly less to reach the same thresholds in psychotically depressed patients. The patient described here had a very low GSR inhibition threshold at the time of admission, but it was quite normal at the time of discharge.

In explaining these differences, Perez-Reyes suggested that neurotic depressives have an increased central excitatory state, a decreased central inhibitory state, or a combination of both. He postulated that psychotically depressed patients have an increased central inhibitory state and/or a decreased central excitatory state. The findings in the psychotically depressed patients seem paradoxical in the light of the well-known fact that they have greater difficulty maintaining sleep than normals, and are much more easily aroused. Another way of viewing this, and one more consonant with my view, is that depressives in general maintain a chronic state of high arousal, with overactivity of the reticular activating systems and perhaps other activating systems as well. The explanation of the low GSR inhibition and sleep threshold of psychotic depressed patients would be that the centers responsible for sleep are in a higher state of activation leading toward sleep because of a relative sleep deprivation, so it would take less sodium thiopental to inhibit the arousal system enough for sleep "pressure" to take over. The confirmation of this is that while less sodium thiopental is required, psychotically depressed patients awake sooner. Data on our patient clearly suggest this. Although when he was admitted he desperately wanted to sleep, he could get only three or four hours a night. His sleep deprivation was marked. It took a relatively small amount of sodium thiopental to eliminate the spontaneous GSR and to induce sleep. When he recovered and slept normally except for some limitations of delta sleep, and with satisfaction to himself, the usual dose of sodium thiopental was needed to inhibit GSR and induce sleep. The interpretation of the Perez-Reyes studies must be regarded as preliminary. Improved methodology for working out the details of the multiple central nervous system mechanisms involved will be necessary before a clear understanding of these phenomena is achieved.

PSYCHOPHYSIOLOGY OF SLEEP

Although we have considerable psychophysiological knowledge about sleep, the mechanisms involved are still obscure. The rest of this paper will be devoted to a discussion of the investigation of sleep in affective illness. Before taking a comprehensive look at what has been learned in recent years about the relationship of sleep to depression, it may be useful to review briefly what the present state of our knowledge of sleep is and how it is studied in the sleep laboratory.

Our current scientific sleep studies would be impossible without the electroencephalograph; the electromyograph and other polygraphic measures are helpful also. We are able to divide sleep by laboratory criteria into a number of different stages and two different states, although we are only dimly aware of the functional significance of the classification. Standard terms and directions for scoring sleep studies have been prepared by Rechtschaffen and Kales (16). A more comprehensive summary that includes basic norms of sleep and extensive references is available in a book by Williams et al. (17).

As the subject becomes drowsy, there is immediately some decrease in muscle potential (EMG) as measured by the electromyogram, and an increase in the amplitude of alpha, with some slowing. Shortly thereafter the EEG activity changes to low amplitude and irregularity, often accompanied by some slow, rolling movements of the eyes. This is known as Stage 1 sleep; it normally occupies 5 percent or less of a night's sleep, although in depression it is often considerably increased. In the normal sleeper Stage 1 is rapidly followed by Stage 2, which is characterized by the appearance of so-called sleep spindles—bursts of 14 cycles/second activity in the EEG. Stage 2 normally occupies about 50 percent of total sleep time. Stage 3 is heralded by the appearance of delta waves, which are much greater in voltage—75-100 microvolts—and of a slow rate of 1-2 cps. Any given epoch (usually 30 or 60 seconds) occupied by more than 50 percent delta waves is classified as Stage 4. It is during Stage 4 that most activity of the body, the brain, and, presumably, the mind, is at its lowest level. During this stage there is the highest threshold for being awakened by external stimuli. This is the stage that recovers at the expense of all others after a number of nights of total sleep deprivation. Figure 2 illustrates the EEG patterns found in waking and the different stages of sleep.

These four stages of sleep were identified early by electroencephalograms, although they were classified in a slightly different way. In 1953 Aserinsky and Kleitman identified what has come to be recog-

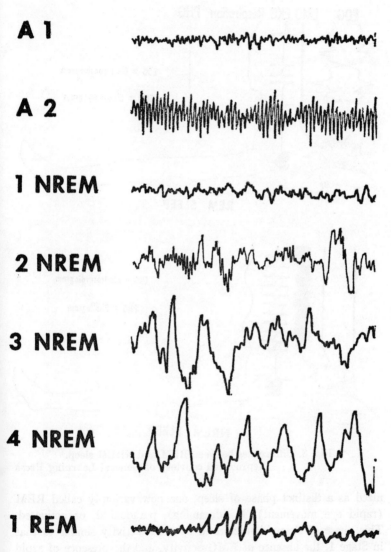

A 1

A 2

1 NREM

2 NREM

3 NREM

4 NREM

1 REM

Fig. 2. Classification of wakefulness and sleep by EEG.

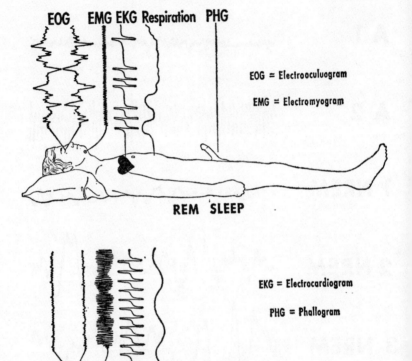

Fig. 3. Differences between REM and NREM sleep.
Reproduced courtesy of General Learning Press

nized as a distinct phase of sleep, one now variously called REM (rapid eye movement), D (dreaming), paradoxical, or activated. This phase of sleep, characterized by EEG activity similar to that in Stage 1, the absence of EMG activity, and the presence of rapid eye movements, is thought to be the phase of sleep during which dreaming takes place. It occupies between 20 and 25 percent of a normal night's sleep, and is clearly a neurophysiologically distinct type of sleep. Most vital functions such as respiration and heart rate are increased and are often irregular. Penile erection occurs regularly in men. This is a phase of activation with CNS metabolism and activity as great as that in waking, or greater. CNS inhibition of motor activity keeps the sleeper from actually moving, however. Figure 3 graphically illustrates the differences between NREM and REM sleep. The control center for REM sleep appears to be in the rostral part of the pons.

These stages of sleep follow one another in regular cyclical patterns throughout the night; there are from four to six cycles in a normal night of sleep. Stages 1 to 4 follow in sequence, with Stage 4 occupying most of the first cycle of approximately 90 minutes. Toward the end of a cycle, muscle tension decreases and there is a slight shift from Stage 4 to 3 to 2, and then Stage 1 REM. The first REM period is typically quite brief; it is soon followed by Stage 2, and the cycle repeats itself. Most delta sleep generally occurs in the first cycle of the night. As the night progresses, REM periods are longer. There seems to be a greater necessity for REM and Stage 4 sleep than for the other stages. Figure 4 shows a normal night's sleep.

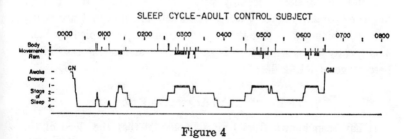

Figure 4

To summarize, sleep is now known to be an active process rather than a simple absence of activation—from the reticular activating system, for example. It consists of two distinct neurophysiological states and a number of different stages as indicated by the EEG which follow each other sequentially in a series of from four to five cycles during a normal night's sleep. Probably because of its association with dreaming and because of the unexpectedness of such great activation, investigative attention has tended to focus on REM sleep, which Snyder (18) called the third organismic state.

Selective REM deprivation studies show that a "pressure" for REM builds up. Evidence for this is that it becomes increasingly difficult to awaken the subject from this phase of sleep and that he returns directly to REM sleep after being awakened, a behavior that would not normally occur. After several nights of selective REM deprivation, the normal subject, allowed to sleep freely, will have more than usual REM sleep, in what has been termed a rebound effect.

These findings suggest that there is some special function of this phase of sleep that is especially needed. However, the hypothesis that originally stimulated studies of REM—that the prevention of dreaming would lead to psychological disturbances—has not been borne out. There is accumulating evidence as more attention is paid to all dimensions of sleep that Stage 4 is the one most compellingly needed. After several nights of total sleep deprivation, this stage "rebounds" on the first recovery night. If normal subjects are allowed to sleep for only three to five hours a night for a number of nights, Stage 4 sleep returns to amounts that are nearly normal, which means that the percentage of sleep occupied by Stage 4 is greatly increased. There is only a very modest increase in the percentage of REM sleep.

SLEEP RESEARCH IN AFFECTIVE DISORDERS

It has been known from time immemorial that the sleep of the mentally ill, worried, or guilty is disturbed. A German saying, "Ein gutes Gewissen ist ein sanftes Ruhkissen," means "a good conscience is a soft pillow." Coleridge's Ancient Mariner, who suffered a long period of guilty depression after killing the albatross, said of the sleep he was finally able to obtain when his depression lifted:

> *... Oh sleep, it is a gentle thing,*
> *Beloved from pole to pole;*
> *To Mary Queen the praise be given—*
> *She sent the gentle sleep from heaven*
> *That crept into my soul.*

Shakespeare recognized the restorative nature of a good night's sleep when he called sleep the "balm of hurt minds" (Macbeth, Act III, Scene 4). In the Winter's Tale (Act II, Scene 3) there is an excellent description of the onset of depression:

> *He straight declin'd, droop'd, took it deeply,*
> *Fasten'd and fix'd the shame on't in himself,*
> *Threw off his spirit, his appetite, his sleep*
> *And downright languish'd.*

All clinicians are well aware of the troubled sleep of psychiatric patients, particularly those who are depressed. These patients complain of shortened, broken sleep, difficulty in falling asleep, and a tendency to awaken early in the morning. Moreover, they awake feeling unrefreshed. The development of the electroencephalogram and other polygraphic methods has enabled us to study objectively in the sleep laboratory the sleep of patients with affective illness, and objective evidence of sleep abnormalities has been found. It often becomes evident that the patient's sleep is not as greatly reduced quantitatively as he had supposed, but qualitative changes are present and may account for the sleeper's feeling that it has been insufficient.

The first laboratory studies of the sleep of depressed patients were performed in 1946 by Diaz-Guerrero and his colleagues (19) before REM or paradoxical sleep was known. They studied six patients classified as manic-depressives and found that they had difficulty falling asleep and awakened frequently during the night; the subjects tended to awaken early in the morning, had more fluctuations from one level of sleep to another than control subjects, and lighter sleep in general.

It was almost 20 years after the Diaz-Guerrero study that the sleep of depressives was studied again in the laboratory, but during the past decade many such studies have been undertaken (1, 11, 20-35). Initially, large numbers of depressive patients selected with little precision as to the type and severity of illness were studied for a few nights in the laboratory. Some generally similar findings emerged, as will be noted, but it became apparent that longitudinal studies and more precise diagnostic classification would be necessary.

There is general documentation that the sleep of depressive patients is fragmented by many periods of awakening and a tendency toward early-morning awakening. The laboratory findings seldom match the subjective account given by the subject, especially in regard to distinctive very early morning waking, perhaps because the controlled environment of the sleep laboratory is more conducive to continuous sleep than the average bedroom. The sleeper in the laboratory is not bothered by light, temperature changes, or noise. It is likely that the depressed patient is easily awakened by external stimuli, and he probably does awaken in the early morning more often at home than in the laboratory in which the environment is so closely controlled. The sleep of depressed patients is generally quite light during the later hours of sleep; probably some of his sleep at this time is experienced by the patient as partial awakening. The time depressed patients take to fall asleep, while more than normal persons require, is not as long as it is with some patients having other types of mental disorder. Neurotic patients or those in waxing or waning stages of acute schizophrenia often have considerable difficulty in falling asleep.

It is extremely difficult to score sleep records of many depressed patients, there being an admixture of wave forms which would not be seen in juxtaposition in the sleep of the normal individual. For example, sleep spindles may briefly appear during an epoch of REM sleep. Periods of delta waves briefly interposed on a background of slow alpha are often seen, in so-called alpha-delta sleep (36). This fragmentation or uneven transition from one stage of sleep to another may indeed reflect interference with usual sleep mechanisms by a high state of arousal; resultant sleep deficit; and competition, not only among the stages of sleep, but between the pressure of sleep and the pressure to wake. The most pervasive and persistent abnormality is a decrease or even absence of Stages 3 and 4 (delta wave sleep).

Among the original reasons for our decision to study the sleep of patients with depression were several hypotheses about REM sleep. This was when modern sleep research was in its infancy, but it was known that the greater part of REM sleep occurs during the latter third of the night. We wondered if depressives might be suffering from REM deprivation as a result of their early morning awakening; or, we speculated, it might be that early morning awakening was related to excessive waking from REM sleep that occurred because the psychological conflicts coming to expression in the depressive's dreams might be stronger than the sleeping state could contain. Neither of these hypotheses was borne out, however.

Cross-sectional Studies

In the original series of 21 patients we studied cross-sectionally, we found the mean amount of REM sleep lower than in the controls. The difference was not striking, however, and it was certainly less significant than the decrease in delta sleep, but when one looked at the values for individual patients it was apparent that there was a great deal of variation in the amount of REM sleep, some subjects clearly having higher than normal REM values, and others considerably lower. Longitudinal studies subsequently indicated that there is often a considerable variation in the amount of REM sleep from night to night in the same patient.

The finding of wide variation in the amount of REM sleep raised a number of questions. Since our original series contained patients with differing types and degrees of depression, as well as differences in age, we considered these as possibly accountable. It was also possible that the variation was idiosyncratic, related to the constitution of the individual patient. However, what seemed most plausible was that an initial period of REM deprivation was followed from time to time by REM rebound. This conclusion resembled the ideas being developed independently at that time by Snyder (37). Consideration of the latter possibility was among the major reasons, but by no means the only one, for shifting to longitudinal studies in the sleep of depressed patients. Our early longitudinal studies tended to bear out the low amount of REM in psychotic patients and some other severely depressed persons. We also found reduced REM onset latency in some patients on some nights.

Snyder and his colleagues (37) were also studying depressed patients at the Clinical Research Center at NIH. In some instances they were able to study over a considerable period of time depressed patients who received no ECT or pharmacotherapy, and were impressed with the variability of the amount of REM and with decrease in REM onset latency. They also noted in some of their subjects a frequent transition from REM to waking, and vice versa; subjects often returned directly to REM sleep after periods of wakefulness. This group also pointed out that during REM periods frequent intense bursts of actual REM activity took place, and periods of the relative absence of any actual eye movements were recorded. Snyder postulated that a deficit in REM sleep, which was thought to be a period of sleep much more susceptible to change because of stresses, was greater than overall sleep loss early in the course of developing depression, and that when recovery began there was a rebound of REM sleep that would account for the increase of REM sleep and the reduction of REM latency. Studies of a larger series of patients in a variety of laboratories have begun to suggest that REM is usually not reduced in depression but is, in fact, often more than in normal individuals.

Mendels and Chernik (38) emphasize their new findings about REM sleep and discuss this matter at some length. They suggest that the decrease in REM sleep often found in early studies may have been due to recent drug use. This was, however, not the case with the patient presented at the beginning of this paper; he had a clearly marked reduction of REM sleep and considerable rebound after successful treatment with ECT, as was the case with some other patients who were carefully studied in longitudinal fashion.

Kupfer (39) in particular expresses the conviction that one of the hallmarks of sleep in patients with depression is lowered REM latency. Short REM latency in depression has been seen in other

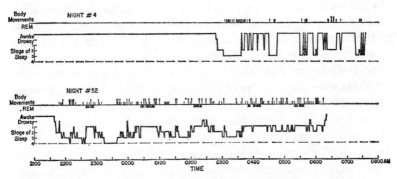

Fig. 5. Sleep during psychotic depression (Night 4) and recovery (Night 52—three weeks after hospital discharge). (Note increase in total sleep, REM and Stage 4 sleep.)

laboratories but by no means consistently. There are evidences that variations in the course of the illness or in the psychopathology are related to the amount of REM sleep (37, 39-43).

Hauri and Hawkins (41), in a study of a series of depressed patients, developed a measure called *percentage of phasic REM*. We divided the entire period of REM sleep into 30-second epochs and counted the number of epochs that contained at least one eye movement. This number was expressed as a percentage of the total number of 30-second segments of REM sleep. We found an inverse correlation between the percentage of phasic REM and the severity of the depression as measured by the Beck Depression Inventory. The more percentage phasic REM a patient showed during a given night, the lower was his score on the Beck Depression Inventory on the night before and the night after the sleep. This study should be replicated, particularly in view of the fact that a significant proportion of the patients were receiving drugs known to affect REM sleep.

It may be that Snyder's (37) original notion of REM deprivation early in the course of the illness has some validity. It may also be the case that a number of the later studies not showing lowered REM amounts involved patients less severely depressed than those in the earlier ones, or patients further along in the development of their depression. In a follow-up study in which previously depressed patients were studied at quarterly intervals, Mendels (38) found significant change in the sleep of four out of ten. Three of the four had a clinical relapse shortly thereafter. In the sleep of the three subjects who relapsed a prior reduction in REM sleep ranged from 15 to 30 percent. The investigator also found a change in delta wave sleep. Two of the three former patients had a marked reduction in delta wave sleep, and a third had a threefold increase. This would lend credence to the notion of REM deprivation early in the course of depression and also to the notion that sleep difficulties might, in fact, play a role in the evolution of the depressive illness.

Severity of Depression

In general, observation tends to confirm reports in the literature that sleep fragmentation and other abnormalities are usually most severe among the most severely depressed patients. The case presented here exhibited both severe depression and major sleep abnormalities. Figure 5 shows graphically his sleep pattern at the height of his depression, and after clinical recovery on night 52 of the study, three weeks after discharge from the hospital. When we used the Beck Depression Inventory in our original studies of depressed patients and related the scores to changes in their sleep patterns, we found no significant correlation, although there was a trend for the more severely depressed patients to be more wakeful and to have less delta and REM sleep (28). Such evaluation should be used with a larger series. It seems clear that most severely depressed persons do have major sleep difficulties (24, 42).

Psychotic vs. Neurotic Depressives

In the same series (28) we contrasted the sleep of patients who were delusional and hence classified as psychotic with the sleep of neurotic depressives. The psychotic depressives had much less delta or Stage 4 sleep, averaging less than a minute per night; less REM sleep; more wakefulness; and longer periods of Stage 1. Snyder

(32) and his co-investigators also found that the sleep of psychotically depressed patients tended to be more severely disrupted.

Aging and Depression

Comparison of the sleep of depressed patients 50 years old or older with that of those under 50 (28) showed a striking difference in wakefulness and Stage 4 sleep. The older depressives were more wakeful, and had almost no delta or Stage 4 activity. REM sleep seemed unaffected by age. Stage 4 sleep has been shown to decrease with age; the decrement begins to be significant in the late 40's (17, 44). The older depressives in our series had much less Stage 4 sleep than matched controls. There seems to be a definite age-illness interaction.

The sleep of elderly normals has not yet been studied in sufficiently comprehensive or detailed a manner as to demonstrate whether the falloff in Stage 4 is linear, or whether it comes in increments; nor is it clear whether this is a regular feature of aging, or an accompaniment of clear deficits in the central nervous system. Since depression is more prevalent in the elderly as Stage 4 decreases, and since Stage 4 deficit is such a constant feature of sleep in depression, one wonders if the fall-off in Stage 4 sleep plays a role in the development of depression in the aged.

Sleep in Young Depressives

Clinically, one gets the impression that when young people become depressed they sleep more and longer than they do normally. Prior to the study to be described, no study of the sleep of young depressed patients under controlled and measured laboratory conditions has been reported. In our sleep laboratory we have to date studied 13 depressives under the age of 26, all of whom were selected on the basis of their suffering from a primary depression and scoring above normal on a self-rated Beck Depression Inventory and a Hamilton Inventory administered by an observer (45). One of the most striking findings of this study is the small number of patients who fit our criteria, in spite of our access to a university

TABLE 1

Young Depressives' Mean Sleep Measures

N=13 9♀ 4♂	$\bar{X}$	RANGE	AGE RANGE: 17-24 EXTENDED NIGHT	RANGE
TOTAL SLEEP	445	142-528	623	528-757
SLEEP LATENCY	35	2-116		
REM LATENCY	111	8-264		
% STAGE 0	3	0-11		
% STAGE 4	8	0-26		
% STAGE REM	21	11-33		

population of close to 15,000 and to young people from the community at large. Depression seems to be the most common clinical diagnosis made in this age group, but there seems to be something unique about depression seen at this time of life. Among the young subjects in our study there is considerable fluctuation in the clinical picture, with variations from day to day in the depth of depression. Table 1 (45) shows preliminary results. There is little wakefulness, and no shortening of the sleep period. Most sleep measures do not appear abnormal although occasional nights of fragmented sleep appear. There is a definite decrease in Stage 4 sleep. Preliminary evidence on the basis of a sample too small to be statistically evaluated suggests a positive correlation between the depth of depression and the reduction of Stage 4. After several nights of regular measurement the subjects were allowed to sleep as long as they liked. In each instance the depressed subjects slept more than nine hours; to date the study bears out the clinical impression that depression does not curtail sleep in the young, but that they may indeed be hypersomniac by way of defending themselves from unpleasant affect they experience while awake. Such a defensive use of sleep does not seem to be available to their elders.

These preliminary findings raise the question whether the depression of young people is a different disorder (or combination of disorders) from depression as it appears among older people, or whether the physiologic and/or ego flexibility of the young allows an adaptation not later available. Can this age-disease interaction account in some way for the fact that depression in later life is more fixed and severe than among the young?

Bipolar versus Unipolar Depression

A problem which plagues many, if not most, of the studies of the biology of depression concerns the lack of specificity in defining the types and/or degree of depression from which the subjects suffer. A not inconsiderable reason for this is a lack of clear understanding of how to classify depressive patients. At the present time many investigators feel that the most useful distinction is that between bipolar and unipolar depressions, although now the bipolar group has been subclassified, and subgroups within the unipolar classification seem likely. Bipolar I refers to patients who were hospitalized for mania some time before becoming subjects in a depression study. Bipolar II includes those depressed patients whose history suggests previous hypomania or mania not clear-cut enough to have required hospitalization (46). The unipolar group includes those with no psychiatric history other than that of recurrent depression. The early studies of sleep in depression are particularly troublesome in respect to imprecise diagnostic classification. We have noted the variations in the sleep patterns in depression, and the influence of age, severity of the depression, and psychosis. Hartmann (22, 47), studying the sleep of bipolar patients in the depressed phase, found their total sleep time to be approximately normal, with an increase in REM time and percent, and a decrease in mean REM onset latency. Stage 4 sleep was not greatly changed. These findings are somewhat different from those of other sleep studies, possibly because although the subjects were clearly depressed they may not have been as severely depressed as the subjects of other studies. Kupfer et al. (48) found that bipolar patients in their depressive phase have more than the usual amount of sleep. Jovanovic et al. (43) conversely found that sleep in bipolar patients in the depressed state, when studied longitudinally in both mania and depression, showed much awakening, and reduction of REM and Stage 4. Their claim that the sleep records of bipolar depressives are variable according to the severity and the stage of the depressive illness is well founded.

There are two studies which compare the sleep characteristics of bipolar and unipolar patients. Mendels and Clernik (38) compared bipolar I, bipolar II, and unipolar patients, finding that the bipolar patients had less sleep disturbance than the others, and slightly more delta-wave sleep. They cautioned, however, that the values based on individual differences overlapped considerably. Gillin et al. (49) found that the only statistically significant difference between bipolars and unipolars was a shortened REM latency. They reported on bipolar I patients only. They did find that depressed patients as a group in each category had less total sleep, less delta sleep, shorter REM latencies, and more periods of wakefulness either intermittently or in the early morning, but there were no significant differences in REM. It therefore seems premature to draw any major inferences about differences in sleep between unipolar and bipolar depressives. A rather large series of longitudinal sleep studies of bipolar patients, that continues, through both the depressive and manic stages, is needed, but, unfortunately for research, it seems unlikely that such studies could be accomplished in the absence of the confounding effects of the specific therapy used. It would be unethical to withhold therapeutic intervention for the sake of uncontaminated research except, perhaps, briefly in the case of a rapidly cycling manic depressive.

Manic Patients

Relatively few manic or hypomanic patients have been studied in the sleep laboratory (38, 50). Some manic patients have very little actual sleep, others have relatively normal amounts. In general, their REM percent time has tended to remain normal, or even increase somewhat, and their delta sleep is ordinarily reduced. Bunney et al., in studying rapidly cycling manic-depressive patients, found that total hours of sleep and REM time decreased before and during manic episodes. They did find one patient, however, who showed an increase of REM sleep during the manic period. They, too, emphasized the inconsistencies in reported changes in REM sleep of depressed patients and suggested that it may have to do with the clinical characteristics of the patient population, noting that the population they studied was moderately retarded rather than being agitated. It should be pointed out that sleep abnormalities are quite similar in mania and depression. Indeed, it would be impossible to tell from a sleep record alone whether the subject was manic or depressive. This likeness is but one of a number of features that both states share; thus the usual notion of their being at

polar extremes is an oversimplification, and probably an obfuscating
concept. Although they have some opposite characteristics, it seems
likely that they have more that are similar (51, 52, 53).

Sleep in Depressed Patients during Remission

A follow-up study of the original series of depressed patients
we had studied in the sleep laboratory (26) indicated that with
improvement in the clinical condition, sleep tended to return toward
normal, although at the time of discharge some residual indications
of less than normal sleep were likely. We noted particularly that
Stage 4 sleep was often not back to normal levels; this finding is
borne out by the patient presented early in this paper, who showed
distinctly low Stage 4 values three weeks after discharge—at a
time when he was symptomatically improved and his other sleep
measures were normal. We decided to investigate whether or not
sleep tended to return entirely to normal with remission. Since depression is often a recurring disorder, we also thought that we
might learn something about the long-range illness by looking at
the dimension of sleep during remission.

We studied 14 patients who had been previously hospitalized for
at least one depressive episode but who had been symptom-free and
drug-free for at least six months, and had no history of mania (63).
When contacted, many of the patients we found by searching the
hospital charts refused to sleep in the sleep laboratory. It seemed
to us that this reluctance was often related to some insecurity
about their sleep patterns, and perhaps a fear of not being able to
sleep well in a strange environment. The 14 who finally agreed to
come to the sleep laboratory were studied for five consecutive nights
and compared with controls individually matched for age, sex, and
education. A first and superficial look at the sleep data we gathered
disclosed little out of the ordinary, but when they were compared
with data from the controls definite evidence of continuing sleep
disturbance became apparent. The formerly depressed patients had
more difficulty falling asleep, more Stage 1, and less delta sleep;
there was greater night-to-night variability in practically all sleep

parameters. Curiously, REM sleep periods seemed to be longer and less subject to interruptions among the remitted patients than among the controls. The former scored statistically significantly higher than the controls on the Beck and Zung Inventory, although their scores were not outside the normal range.

This study clearly indicates that there are continuing abnormalities in the sleep patterns of previously depressed patients, even in the absence of clinical signs of disease. This raises a number of interesting questions. Does the sleep abnormality arise from some genetic difference in these subjects? If so, is this simply one of many genetic differences from the norm? Or is it the case that the experience of having a depressive illness severe enough to require hospitalization leaves the individual with permanent functional central nervous system abnormalities that affect sleep regulation?

The Effect on Sleep of Therapeutic Agents

Accepted therapeutic means for the treatment of depression include electroconvulsive therapy, monoamine oxidase inhibitors, tricyclics, and, in some selected cases, lithium. Two novel experimental techniques have been described. The first (54) involves total sleep deprivation for one night or more, which seems to have an energizing therapeutic effect that lasts for several days. The second (55) invokes selective REM deprivation over three weeks' time, and is reported to have the same degree of efficacy in endogenous depressed patients as imipramine, and no effect in reactive depression.

ECT

The case presented in this paper illustrates the effect of ECT on the sleep of a severely depressed patient. The changes in this case are more abrupt than we usually find, but are otherwise typical. Whether ECT directly affects the sleep mechanism or whether the results are an indirect outcome of changes in the basic depressive mechanism is unknown. Obviously, no one has been able to study effects of ECT on the sleep pattern of normal human beings. Early studies of ECT effects on cats (56, 57) indicated that ECT suppressed REM sleep, and raised speculation that REM suppression was the means by which ECT works. Zarcone et al. (58) published a study of ECT effects on the sleep of several schizophrenic and depressed patients; this seemed to confirm the cat studies. However, close examination of their data makes their conclusions seem tenuous, and subsequent studies (59) confirm the initial finding of improved sleep with ECT and an increase in REM sleep where it had been low. The basic action of ECT on sleep remains a mystery, as does its action in the alleviation of depression.

Tricyclics and MAO Inhibitors

The role of tricyclics and MAO inhibitors in the treatment of depression has been written on extensively. Their effects on the sleep of depressives are complex and still somewhat controversial. It can be said, however, that successful treatment of depression tends to improve the patient's overall sleep.

The relation of tricyclics and MAO inhibitors to REM sleep is of special interest. Both drugs repress REM sleep. Wyatt and his colleagues (60) showed that improvement in 6 anxious-depressed subjects treated with phenelzine was temporally related to the suppression of REM characteristics, which was total. Marked REM rebound followed the cessation of therapy and the reappearance of symptoms. Dunleavy et al. (61) found that mood improvement followed closely the degree of REM suppression in 22 patients treated with phenelzine. They associated the improvement with a profound neurophysiological change that takes up to three weeks to be accomplished, and point out that REM suppression is not inevitably accompanied by mood improvement. Both groups of investigators are careful to emphasize that it would be premature to assume that the improvement was due to REM suppression. It could well be that the suppression was but a byproduct of other changes that were directly responsible for the alleviation of depression.

The tricyclic antidepressants have been studied with respect to their effect on the sleep of normal as well as depressed subjects.

For a more thorough discussion and a more comprehensive list of references, the reader is referred to papers by Mendels and Chernik (38) and Vogel et al. (55). These antidepressants produce significant but by no means total suppression of REM sleep in normals as well as depressed patients. Unlike the MAO inhibitors, they have a tendency to permit a return of REM sleep as therapy continues. Some investigators have found an increase in delta sleep, but others report a decrease. Some have noted increased intrasleep restlessness in patients given tricyclics.

Lithium

Lithium, which is now being used in the treatment of selected depressive as well as manic patients, and for prophylactic effect in remitted manic depressives, is the only treatment that seems truly to normalize sleep patterns. Of all the antidepressive medications it seems the only one that leads to an increase in delta sleep. When increased REM is present, it tends to lower it, but no lower than the normal range. Whether or not it acts directly on the sleep mechanism is unknown. However, individuals on prophylactic lithium who are free of symptoms show no detectable abnormalities of sleep.

Sleep Deprivation as Therapy

A unique approach to the treatment of depression, and one that is as yet experimental, has been used by Vogel (55). Reasoning as follows, he hypothesized that depression might be treatable by REM deprivation: 1) the major antidepressant drugs (tricyclics and monoamine oxidase (MAO inhibitors) produced substantial, persistent suppression of REM sleep, much more so than non-antidepressant drugs; 2) electroshock therapy (ECT), an efficacious antidepressant, was reported to decrease REM sleep; 3) reserpine, which induced depression, substantially increased REM sleep; and 4) prolonged REM sleep deprivation of animals was reported to produce behavioral changes opposite to the behavioral changes of human depression.

His first point certainly seems true. As we have pointed out, ECT does not seem to decrease the REM sleep of depressed human beings although it does so with animals. A close reading of the relevant literature, and a review of films showing the behavior of animals deprived of REM sleep for long periods, do not appear to this observer to bear out the notion that they are manifesting the reverse of depressed behavior.

Vogel and his colleagues have by now studied 34 endogenous and 18 reactive depressive patients who were treated over three weeks' time by being awakened from REM sleep. These investigators used a double-blind crossover technique, and controlled by comparing wakings from NREM sleep to wakings from REM. The patients' depression was evaluated by the Hamilton Depression Rating Scale, a global disability scale, the Zung Self-Rating Depression Scale, and tests of psychomotor slowness. By the end of this study 17 of the 34 endogenous depressives improved enough with REM deprivation as the only treatment to be discharged from the hospital. This treatment was, however, without efficacy in the case of the reactive depressives. Reviewing the literature about imipramine therapy, the authors concluded that they had obtained approximately equivalent results with REM deprivation. Some of the patients not improved by REM deprivation were successfully treated by ECT. They claim that REM deprivation relieves the symptoms of endogenous depression in about 50 percent of the cases, and hypothesize that the improvement is related to increased pressure for REM sleep, which may be the mechanism for the action of antidepressant drugs. These carefully performed and complex studies are hard to evaluate. It is to be hoped that other investigators will see fit to replicate these experiments, but with the present efficacy of drug therapy it may be some time before another investigator feels sufficiently motivated to replicate Vogel's study.

Pflug and his associates (62) have attempted to treat depression by one night of total sleep deprivation. The abatement of symptoms often occurs between 2 and 4 A.M. Apparently, improvement depends on total continuing wakefulness, so no napping is permitted during the following day. The improvement, which lasts for only one to two days, is accompanied by an increase in systolic blood pressure. Normal subjects and neurotic depressives react quite differently from those with endogenous depression, generally feeling worse after a night of sleep deprivation. Normal subjects have a very slight increase in blood pressure; the neurotics have a decrease. The authors suggest using a night of deprivation at the start of treatment coincident with the initiation of tricyclic medication; they indicate that a subsequent night of deprivation may be helpful. One is hard pressed to account for these findings. The polarity of the endogenous and neurotic depressives in respect to blood pressure, and the central position of normals, is reminiscent of Perez-Reyes's (16) polar findings with the GSR inhibition threshold test. The authors suggest that the mechanism may be a shift in neurohumoral transmitter balance as a result of the sleep deprivation.

SUMMARY

Depression is a complex, multifaceted group of disorders probably consisting of differing genetically determined predispositions for different patterns of disorder, with final common pathways that lead to generally similar clinical manifestations. There is no anatomical lesion or specific abnormality implicated, although a number of functional systems must play a role. Included among these are almost certainly the frontal lobe, limbic system, and reticular activating system. With the major cognitive aspects of the syndrome in human beings, the associated network of the cortex must certainly play a role.

Numerous psychophysiological functions seem to be involved, but no very clear-cut abnormalities have been defined. Certainly there is some curious combination of arousal and inhibition. While there are striking differences between mania and depression, the similarities of disturbance are probably greater.

The longstanding clinical impression of sleep abnormalities as a major manifestation of most depressive disorders has been clearly established through many studies in many sleep laboratories. There is generally some difficulty getting to sleep, but frequent and long periods of waking constitute the most characteristic picture. The most consistent and pervasive abnormality is the diminution or absence of delta sleep.

The findings with regard to REM sleep are inconsistent, and there is generally no real abnormality. Variation is the rule. Hints of other disturbances are found in the frequent shortening of REM onset latency and in changes in percentage phasic REM sleep manifestations. One careful investigator finds that REM deprivation seems to be effective in some cases of depression; although this is an intriguing finding it is poorly understood.

Of interest and concern is the finding that remitted patients, although clinically normal, continue to have slight but definite sleep abnormalities. Whether abnormal or insufficient sleep plays any role in the development of depressive illness remains a major question. While not discussed in this paper, the fact that biogenic amines serving as neurohumoral transmitters seem to play a role in the mechanism of depression, as well as a role in the mechanisms that control sleep, suggests that better understanding of their metabolism and function will clarify our understanding of both sleep and affective illness.

Finally, the relationship of both sleep and affective illness to the aging process needs further study. Both the clinical manifestations of depression and the sleep pattern of depressives change as the organism ages. Young depressives, for example, seem to be able to oversleep, but sleep is often difficult to achieve in later life.

REFERENCES

1. HAWKINS, D. R., MENDELS, J., SCOTT, J., BENSCH, G. and TEACHEY, W.: The psychophysiology of sleep in psychotic depression: A longitudinal study. *Psychosom. Med.*, 29(4):329-344, 1967.
2. KLEIN, D. F.: Endogenomorphic depression: A conceptual and terminological revision. *Arch. Gen. Psychiat.*, 31:447-454, 1974.
3. KRAINES, S. H.: Manic-depressive syndrome: A physiologic disease. *Dis. Nerv. Syst.*, 27:573-582, 670-676, 1966.
4. PAPEZ, J. W.: A proposed mechanism of emotion. *Arch. Neurol. Psychiat.*, 38:725, 1937.

5. MacLean, P. D.: Some psychiatric implications of physiological studies on frontotemporal portion of limbic system (visceral brain). *Electroenceph. Clin. Neurophysiol.*, 4:407, 1952.

6. Olds, J.: Differentiation of reward systems in the brain by self-stimulation techniques. *In* S. R. Ramey and D. S. O'Doherty (Eds.), *Electrical Studies on the Unanesthetized Brain.* New York: Hoeber, 1960, p. 17.

7. Heath, R. G.: Pleasure and brain activity in man: Deep and surface electroencephalograms during orgasm. *J. Nerv. Ment. Dis.*, 154:3, 1972.

8. Lilly, J. C.: Learning motivated by subcortical stimulation: The "start" and "stop" patterns of behavior. *In* S. R. Ramey and D. S. O'Doherty (Eds.), *Electrical Studies on the Unanesthetized Brain.* New York: Hoeber, 1960.

9. Brain, W. R.: The physiological basis of consciousness: A critical review. *Brain*, 81:426, 1958.

10. Kelly, D., Richardson, A., Mitchell-Heggs, N., Greenup, J., Chen, C. and Hafner, R. J.: Stereotactic limbic leucotomy: A preliminary report on forty patients. *Brit. J. Psychiat.*, 123: 141, 1973.

11. Zung, W. W. K., Wilson, W. P. and Dodson, W. E.: Effect of depressive disorders on sleep EEG responses. *Arch. Gen. Psychiat.*, 10:439-445, 1964.

12. Hill, D.: Depression: Disease, reaction, or posture? *Amer. J. Psychiat.*, 125:445-457, 1968.

13. Shagass, C.: *Evoked Brain Potential in Psychiatry.* New York: Plenum Press, 1972.

14. Satterfield, J. H.: Auditory evoked cortical response studies in depressed patients and normal control subjects. *In* T. A. Williams, M. M. Katz and J. A. Shields (Eds.), *Recent Advances in the Psychobiology of the Depressive Illnesses.* Washington: U.S. Government Printing Office, 1972, pp. 87-98.

15. Perez-Reyes, M.: Differences in sedative susceptibility between types of depression: Clinical and neurophysiological significance. *In* T. A. Williams, M. M. Katz and J. A. Shields (Eds.), *Recent Advances in the Psychobiology of the Depressive Illnesses.* Washington: U.S. Government Printing Office, 1972, pp. 119-130.

16. Rechtschaffen, A. and Kales, A. (Eds.): *A Manual of Standardized Terminology, Techniques and Scoring System for Sleep Stages of Human Subjects.* NIH Publication #204. Public Health Service, U.S. Government Printing Office, 1968.

17. Williams, R. L., Karacan, I. and Hursch, C. J.: *EEG of Human Sleep: Clinical Applications.* New York: John Wiley & Sons, 1974.

18. Snyder, F.: The new biology of dreaming. *Arch. Gen. Psychiat.*, 8:381-391, 1963.

19. DIAZ-GUERRERO, R., GOTTLIEB, J. S. and KNOTT, J. R.: The sleep of patients with manic-depressive psychosis, depressive type. *Psychosom. Med.*, 8:399, 1946.
20. GREEN, W. J. and STAJDUHAR, P. P.: The effect of ECT on the sleep-dream cycle in a psychotic depression. *J. Nerv. Ment. Dis.*, 143:123-134, 1966.
21. GRESHAM, S., AGNEW, H. and WILLIAMS, R.: The sleep of depressed patients: An EEG and eye movement study. *Arch. Gen. Psychiat.*, 12:503-507, 1965.
22. HARTMANN, E.: Longitudinal studies of sleep and dream patterns in manic-depressive patients. *Arch. Gen. Psychiat.*, 19: 312-329, 1968.
23. HAWKINS, D. R. and MENDELS, J.: Sleep disturbance in depressive syndromes. *Am. J. Psychiat.*, 123:682-690, 1966.
24. LOWRY, F. H., CLEGHORN, J. M. and MCCLURE, D. J.: Sleep patterns in depression: Longitudinal study of six patients and brief review of literature. *J. Nerv. Ment. Dis.*, 153:10-26, 1971.
25. MENDELS, J. and HAWKINS, D. R.: Sleep and depression: A controlled EEG study. *Arch. Gen. Psychiat.*, 16:344-354, 1967.
26. MENDELS, J. and HAWKINS, D. R.: Sleep and depression: A follow-up study. *Arch. Gen. Psychiat.*, 16:536-540, 1967.
27. MENDELS, J. and HAWKINS, D. R.: Studies of psychophysiology of sleep in depression. *Ment. Hyg.*, 51:501-510, 1967.
28. MENDELS, J. and HAWKINS, D. R.: Sleep and depression: Further considerations. *Arch. Gen. Psychiat.*, 19:445-452, 1968.
29. MENDELS, J. and HAWKINS, D. R.: Sleep and depression: IV. Longitudinal studies. *J. Nerv. Ment. Dis.*, 153:251-272, 1971.
30. MENDELS, J. and HAWKINS, D. R.: Sleep studies in depression. *In* T. A. Williams, M. M. Katz and J. A. Shields (Eds.), *Recent Advances in the Psychobiology of the Depressive Illnesses.* Washington: U.S. Government Printing Office, 1972, pp. 147-170.
31. OSWALD, I., BERGER, R. J., JARMILLO, R. A., et al.: Melancholia and barbiturates: Controlled EEG, body and eye movement study of sleep. *Brit. J. Psychiat.*, 109:66-78, 1963.
32. SNYDER, F.: Sleep disturbance in relation to acute psychosis. *In* A. Kales (Ed.), *Sleep: Physiology and Pathology.* Philadelphia: Lippincott, 1969, pp. 170-182.
33. SNYDER, F.: Electrographic studies of sleep in depression. *In* N. S. Kline and E. Laske (Eds.), *Computers and Electronic Devices in Psychiatry.* New York: Grune & Stratton, 1968, pp. 272-303.
34. MENDELS, J. and CHERNIK, D. A.: REM sleep and depression. *In* M. H. Chase, W. C. Stern and P. L. Walter (Eds.), *Sleep Research*, Vol. 1. Los Angeles: Brain Information Service, Brain Research Institute, 1972, p. 141 (Abstract).
35. MURATORIO, A., MAGGINI, C. D. and MURRI, L.: Il sonno notturno

nelle sindromi depressive studio poligrafico di 33 casi. *Estratto da Neopsichiatria*, 33 (196), pp. 1-28.

36. HAURI, P. and HAWKINS, D. R.: Alpha-delta sleep. *Electroencephalography and Clinical Neurophysiology*, 34:233-237, 1973.

37. SNYDER, F.: NIH studies of sleep in affective illness. *In* T. A. Williams, M. M. Katz and J. A. Shields (Eds.), *Recent Advances in the Psychobiology of the Depressive Illnesses*. Washington: U.S. Government Printing Office, 1972, pp. 171-192.

38. MENDELS, J. and CHERNIK, D. A.: Sleep changes and affective illness. *In* F. F. Flack and S. C. Draghi (Eds.), *The Nature and Treatment of Depression*. New York: John Wiley & Sons, 1975, pp. 309-333.

39. KUPFER, D. J. and FOSTER, F. G.: Interval between onset of sleep and rapid eye movement sleep as an indicator of depression. *Lancet*, 2:684-686, 1972.

40. BUNNEY, W. E., JR., GOODWIN, F. K. and MURPHY, D. I.: The "switch process" in manic-depressive illness: II. Relationship to catecholamines, REM sleep and drugs. *Arch. Gen. Psychiat.*, 27:304-309, 1972.

41. HAURI, P. and HAWKINS, D. R.: Phasic REM, depression, and the relationship between sleeping and waking. *Arch. Gen. Psychiat.*, 25:56-63, 1971.

42. HAURI, P. and HAWKINS, D. R.: Individual differences in the sleep of depression. *In* U. J. Jovanovic (Ed.), *The Nature of Sleep*. Stuttgart: Gustav Fischer Verlag, 1973, pp. 193-197.

43. JOVANOVIC, U. J., DOGAN, S., DURRIGL, V., GUVAREV, N., HAJNSEK, F., GUBAREV, N., ROGINA, V. and STOJANOVIC, V.: Changes of sleep in manic-depressive patients dependent on the clinical state. *In* U. J. Jovanovic (Ed.), *The Nature of Sleep*. Stuttgart: Gustav Fischer Verlag, 1973, pp. 208-211.

44. FEINBERG, I.: The ontogenesis of human sleep and the relationship of sleep variables to intellectual function in the aged. *Comprehensive Psychiatry*, 9(2):138-147, 1968.

45. HAWKINS, D. R., VAN DE CASTLE, R., TEJA, J. S., TRINDER, J. GREYSON, B. and BARTELS, S.: Sleep patterns among young depressed patients. Second International Sleep Research Congress, 15th Annual Meeting of APSS, at Edinburgh, Scotland, June 30-July 4, 1975, p. 203 in *Proceedings* (abstract).

46. DUNNER, D. L., GOODWIN, F. K., GERSON, E. S. et al.: Excretion of 17-OHCS in unipolar and bipolar depressed patients. *Arch. Gen. Psychiat.*, 26:360-363, 1972.

47. HARTMANN, E.: Mania, depression and sleep. In A. Kales (Ed.), *Sleep Physiology and Pathology: A Symposium*. Philadelphia: Lippincott, 1969, pp. 183-191.

48. KUPFER, D. J., IMMELBHOCK, J. M., SWARTZBURG, M., ANDERSON, C., BYCK, R. and DETRI, T. P.: Hypersomnia in manic-depressive disease. *Dis. Nerv. Syst.*, 73:720-724, 1972.

49. GILLIN, J. C., BUNNEY, W. E., BUCHBINDER, R. and SNYDER, F.:
    Sleep changes in unipolar and bipolar depressed patients as
    compared with normals. Second International Sleep Research
    Congress, 15th Annual Meeting of APSS, at Edinburgh, Scot-
    land, June 30-July 4, 1975, p. 204 in *Proceedings*.
50. MENDELS, J. and HAWKINS, D. R.: Longitudinal sleep study in
    hypomania. *Arch. Gen. Psychiat.*, 25:274-277, 1971.
51. WHYBROW, P. C. and MENDELS, J.: Toward a biology of depres-
    sion: Some suggestions from neurophysiology. *Am. J. Psychiat.*,
    125:1491-1500, 1969.
52. MENDELS, J.: *Concepts of Depression*. New York: Wiley, 1970.
53. MENDELS, J.: Biological aspects of affective illness. *In* S. Arieti
    (Ed.), *American Handbook of Psychiatry*. New York: Basic
    Books, 1974, pp. 448-479.
54. PFLUG, B. and TOLLE, R.: Disturbance of the 24-hour rhythm in
    endogenous depression and the treatment of endogenous de-
    pression by sleep deprivation. *Int. Pharmacopsychiat.*, 6:187-
    196, 1971.
55. VOGEL, G. W., THURMOND, A., GIBBONS, P., SLOAN, K., BOYD, M.
    and WALKER, M.: REM sleep reduction effects on depression
    syndromes. *Arch. Gen. Psychiat.*, 32:765-777, 1975.
56. KAELBLING, R.: REM sleep suppression and rebound after anti-
    depressant therapy. *In* H. Goldman (Ed.), *Research in Com-
    prehensive Psychiatry*. Columbus, Ohio: Columbus State Uni-
    versity, 1972, pp. 61-75.
57. COHEN, H. B. and DEMENT, W. C.: Sleep: Suppression of rapid
    eye movement phase in the act after shock. *Science*, 154:396-
    398, 1966.
58. ZARCONE, V., GULEVICH, G. and DEMENT, W.: Sleep and electro-
    convulsive therapy. *Arch. Gen. Psychiat.*, 16:567-573, 1967.
59. MENDELS, J., VAN DE CASTLE, R. and HAWKINS, D. R.: Electro-
    convulsive therapy and sleep. *In* M. Fink, S. Kety, J. McGaugh
    and T. A. Williams (Eds.), *Psychology of Convulsive Therapy*.
    New York: Halstead Press, 1974, pp. 41-46.
60. WYATT, R. J., FRAM, D. H., KUPFER, D. J. and SNYDER, F.: Total
    prolonged drug-induced REM sleep suppression in anxious-
    depressed patients. *Arch. Gen. Psychiat.*, 24:145-155, 1971.
61. DUNLEAVY, D. L. F. and OSWALD, I.: Phenelzine, mood response,
    and sleep. *Arch. Gen. Psychiat.*, 28:353-356.
62. PFLUG, B. and TOLLE, R.: The influence of sleep deprivation on
    the symptoms of endogenous depression. *In* U. J. Jovanovic
    (Ed.), *The Nature of Sleep*. Stuttgart: Gustav Fischer Verlag,
    1971, pp. 177-180.
63. HAURI, P., CHERNIK, D., HAWKINS, D. R. and MENDELS, J.: Sleep
    of depressed patients in remission. *Arch. Gen. Psychiat.*, 31:
    386-391, 1974.

10

Depression: Somatic Treatment Methods, Complications, Failures

Heinz E. Lehmann, M.D.

DIAGNOSIS AND THE DIFFERENT TREATMENT OPTIONS OF DEPRESSION

One recognizes depression by one or all of the following three methods:

1. Observation
2. History
3. Empathy

The first two are basic for the diagnosis of any pathology and are thus shared by all of medicine. The third—empathy—is a diagnostic approach that is specific for the psychiatrist and has to substitute for the important third diagnostic method that is available to most physicians, but not to psychiatrists, that is, objective instrumental and laboratory findings. A nosological survey of current diagnostic concepts of depression is presented in Figure 1.

Once he has recognized that his patient is depressed, the psychia-

FIGURE 1: NOSOLOGICAL SCHEME OF AFFECTIVE DISORDERS

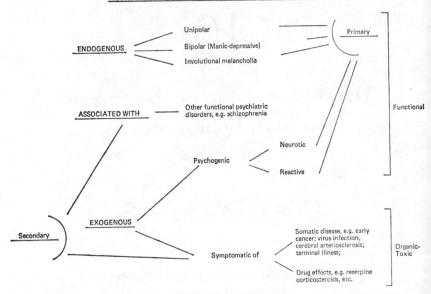

trist has to ask himself the following strategic questions, approximately in the given order:

1. Is the depression pathological or is it a grief reaction or plain unhappiness?
2. Does the patient require treatment?
3. Does he require hospitalization?
4. Is the depression primary or secondary?
5. Is he suffering from an endogenous or a psychogenic depression?
6. What treatment should the patient receive?
7. Will he require maintenance treatment?

Answers to questions 1, 2 and 3 will be based on the patient's history or on the intensity of his symptoms. Questions 4 and 5 will have to be answered partly on the basis of the history, i.e., the presence or absence of a time-related traumatic event (loss), or of a previous non-affective psychiatric disorder, and partly on the basis of existing symptoms, e.g., diurnal variation, early morning insomnia, or the presence of symptoms characteristic of a non-affective psychiatric disorder.

Finally, the answers to questions 6 and 7 depend to considerable extent on the answers to the other questions. The different options for use of somatic antidepressant therapy are discussed in this paper.

The psychiatric treatment of depression may be divided into three historic phases. During the first phase, psychotherapy alone was probably sometimes helpful, but all somatic treatments were hardly any more than ineffective nostrums.

Many of the old physical treatments of depression would be considered today as cruel, aversive procedures: painful cold showers, unexpectedly being plunged into deep water, being whirled around while strapped into a machine until severe vomiting and weakness set in (1, 2, 3). The second phase began in the late 1930's when metrazol, electroconvulsive therapy, and, to some extent, psychosurgery, provided the first effective physical treatments of depressions. The third phase—that of modern pharmacotherapy of depression—began about 20 years later.

TABLE 1

Somatic Treatment Modalities for the
Management of Depression

1. Pharmacotherapy
2. Sleep Deprivation
3. Electroconvulsive Treatment (ECT)
4. Psychosurgery

Table 1 gives the repertoire of somatic treatment modalities that is available today for the management of depressive syndromes. Although pharmacotherapy is currently the treatment of first choice of the experts, and by far the most widely used form of antidepressant treatment (4), its discussion will be left to the end, and the other somatic treatments will be dealt with first.

ELECTROCONVULSIVE THERAPY (ECT)

ECT is the physical treatment in psychiatry that has survived for almost 40 years, although we do not yet have any plausible theory of its action mechanism (5). It is the most effective treatment for depression. Curiously, it is also an excellent treatment for manic states and is helpful in many schizophrenic conditions. It is contraindicated in anxiety and hysterical states, as well as in brain-damaged patients. One of its drawbacks is the susceptibility to frequent relapses of patients treated with convulsive therapy.

The other main disadvantage of ECT is the memory impairment that invariably occurs after a few treatments. ECT produces a short-lasting acute brain syndrome with confusion, memory disturbances, disinhibition of affect, and slowing of the EEG. These symptoms are reversible and usually disappear completely within two to four weeks after the last treatment. However, in older people some permanent memory impairment may be observed. A more subtle, persistent memory disorder, that may not appear on tests but may be disturbing to patients who depend much on their intellectual organization, can also be observed occasionally in younger persons. Unilateral ECT, administered over the non-dominant hemisphere, causes less memory impairment, but is possibly somewhat less effective (6).

ECT may be the treatment of choice in very severe and suicidal depressions, when it might be dangerous and intolerable for the patient to have to wait one or two weeks for the effects of antidepressant drugs to occur. It is also indicated in depressed patients who are not responding to antidepressant drugs within a month or two.

A recent survey in Massachusetts has shown clearly that in private hospitals ECT is administered much more frequently than in state hospitals (7). This may be due to the fact that in private hospitals more nursing staff and anesthetists are available, in contrast to the more restricted economics prevailing in state hospitals. It may also be a question of fees for service available in private but not in state hospitals; or it may reflect a greater need in private hospitals to see quick, dramatic and gratifying results. For with ECT, the first signs of improvement appear rapidly and are subjective: The patient feels well and immediately acknowledges this gratefully, even while his objective test performance is still impaired. With antidepressant drug treatment, the improvement is slower and first noticeable objectively in the patient's behavior. The patient himself may not acknowledge that he feels any better and does so, often somewhat grudgingly, only later.

To some clinicians it is a drawback of ECT that the patient recovers so rapidly and with such complete amnesia that he has virtually no recollection of becoming sick or getting well. He accepts good-humoredly that he must have been sick since he has received the treatment, but the experiences of becoming ill and becoming well again, for what they are worth, are not available to him, and he will not be able to draw on what he may have learned from them should he ever be threatened with a recurrence of his illness at some later time.

SLEEP DEPRIVATION

Sleep deprivation is a new antidepressant treatment modality that has been developed during the last three years in Germany (8). It consists in keeping the depressed patient awake continuously for 36 hours. The procedure may be carried out once or twice a week and, if the first two treatments have been successful, may be repeated six or seven times. At our hospital we have had amazing success with sleep deprivation in 9 of 15 severely depressed, hospitalized patients who had not responded to antidepressant drug therapy (9). In certain cases the results were as dramatic as with ECT.

The action mechanism of this unspecific procedure is not well understood. It is the converse of continuous sleep, which was one of the first successful somatic treatments used in psychiatry (10). Stress-induced stimulation of the adrenergic system may be involved in sleep deprivation, with the resulting metabolic and endocrine changes. It has also been demonstrated recently that REM sleep

deprivation has a favorable influence on depression, a factor that
may enter into the picture of sleep deprivation. Total sleep deprivation, like REM sleep deprivation, is effective mainly in endogenous,
particularly unipolar, depressions and not in reactive or neurotic
depressions (11).

PSYCHOSURGERY

Psychosurgery has today become the target of attacks by activists
who advocate its outlawing, protesting that psychosurgery constitutes
"murder of the soul," that it may be used as a weapon against
helpless minorities, and that it reduces its "victims" to "vegetables."
Without wishing to enter into the controversy, this writer must
state that a thorough review of the literature and his personal clinical experience have convinced him that modern psychosurgery can
be a valuable therapeutic weapon and, in certain desperate cases,
may constitute the only effective relief available. In the 1930's and
1940's, when its technique was still rather primitive and its use
often indiscriminate, there were indeed many therapeutic failures
and disastrous complications. Today, with stereotactic techniques,
and used only for its restricted indications, one should expect 60-70
percent therapeutic successes, with very few physical complications
and virtually no gross psychological deterioration following psychosurgery. The only indications for the use of psychosurgery are, in
the writer's opinion, severe depression, anxiety, or obsessive-compulsive symptoms that have persisted for at least two years and
have not been relieved by adequate treatment with any other available therapeutic methods, i.e., psychotherapy, pharmacotherapy and
ECT. In other words, psychosurgery should be used only as a last
resort and for some specific symptomatology in the relatively few
cases where these qualifications apply (12). While it is true that
there is a dearth of controlled trials of psychosurgery, some retrospective studies with matched controls and even one placebo-
controlled experiment—only skin incisions under anesthesia—have
been reported and have clearly shown the therapeutic value of psychosurgery when performed under the right conditions (13, 14).

PHARMACOTHERAPY

Many drugs had been used in treating depressed patients before modern antidepressant substances were introduced. Drugs used in past centuries include hellebore and opium, and more recently hematoporphyrin (15), dinitrile succinate (16) and nicotinic acid (17). Of these, only the treatment with tincture opii found general acceptance and probably did give severely depressed patients some modest relief. However, reliably effective pharmacotherapy of depression became available only with the almost simultaneous discovery of the monoamine oxidase inhibitors and the tricyclic antidepressants in the late 1950's.

Monoamine Oxidase Inhibitors (MAOI's)

Since Kline (18) introduced iproniazid into antidepressant therapy, a great deal of research has been centered on the MAOI's and their effects of increasing the biogenic indoleamines and catecholamines and their metabolites in the brain, since this increase seems to be associated with an antidepressive action.

The pharmaceutical industry has developed two classes of MAOI's: those with and those without a hydrazide complex in their structure. The first MAOI—iproniazide (Marsilid)—was a hydrazide compound and proved to be hepatotoxic. Because of several fatal complications which occurred with its use, iproniazide was eventually withdrawn from the market in the U.S. This has been regretted by many psychiatrists who claim that iproniazide was probably the most effective of the MAOI antidepressants. Other, less toxic MAOI's, possessing hydrazide groups in their structure, include isocarboxazide (Marplan), nialamide (Niamide) and phenelzine (Nardil). Tranylcypromine (Parnate) is an MAO without a hydrazide group, which is characterized by a biphasic action: an immediate stimulating and mood-lifting, amphetamine-like effect and a delayed, more gradual and sustained antidepressant action which appears after the typical 8-10 days that are required for most antidepressant drugs to take effect (see Figure 2 for the chemical structure of some MAOI's).

MAO - INHIBITORS

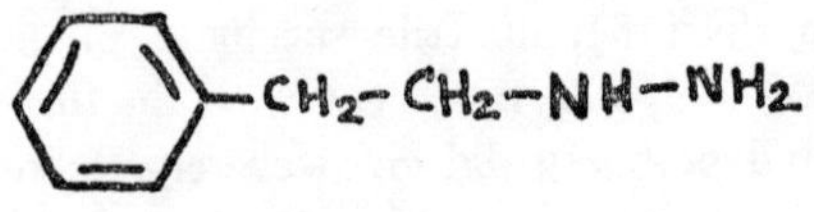

PHENELZINE

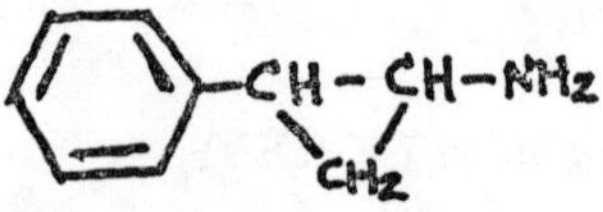

TRANYLCYPROMINE

Figure 2

The therapeutic efficacy of MAOI's is probably about the same as that of other (tricyclic) antidepressants, i.e., from 60-70 percent improvement in unselected cases of depression. However, it has been frequently claimed that the MAOI's are specifically indicated in the more atypical depressions when hysterical, impulsive, obsessive, anhedonic, and phobic symptoms prevail (19-23). This clinical impression has not been confirmed in some controlled studies (24, 25), and many clinicians have seen the same type of depression also respond well to antidepressants other than MAOI's.

One serious inconvenience of all MAOI's is their incompatibility —and often intensely adverse interaction, in the form of paroxysmal hypertension—with adrenaline, noradrenaline, and practically all adrenergic drugs, such as the amphetamines, methylphenidate, etc., as well as alcohol, thyroxin, meperidine, tricyclic antidepressants, and many food items which contain tyramine, a noradrenaline-releaser. Unfortunately, such food items comprise a great variety of the common diet, e.g., aged cheeses, pickles, chicken liver, beer, Chianti wine, etc. A sudden surgical emergency in a patient who is on MAOI treatment, may present problems to the anesthetist because of the many interactions and the long sustained actions of MAOI's with other drugs; even a local anesthetic for dental procedures would be contraindicated if it would be used together with epinephrine.

As a general rule, one should prescribe MAOI's only to patients who are sufficiently intelligent and reliable to adhere to all the warnings and instructions, which must necessarily be made very explicit to all patients for whom this type of drug is prescribed. Special caution is indicated with young persons who might be suspected of being multiple-drug abusers.

If a patient has been started on an MAOI and it has been decided to change to tricyclic antidepressants, 8 to 10 days must be allowed to elapse before the new medication can be prescribed, since the drug's inhibition of MAO is complete and it takes about a week after its discontinuation before a sufficient amount of new MAO has been produced by the organism.

Daily doses of MAOI antidepressants marketed in the U.S. are listed in Table 2.

Tricyclic Antidepressants

The prototype of the tricyclic antidepressants is imipramine (Tofranil) whose antidepressant properties were first discovered and reported by Kuhn (26). Chemically, the tricyclic antidepressants are iminodibenzyl derivatives which resemble phenothiazines in their chemical structure. They are referred to as tricyclic, because their nucleus is represented by three benzol rings (Figure 3). Other widely used drugs of the same type are amitriptyline (Elavil) which produces more sedation and drowsiness than imipramine, and the demethylated derivatives of imipramine: desipramine (Pertofrane; Norpramin), and of imitriptyline: nortriptyline (Aventyl). The last named drugs produce less sedation and, as some reports indicate, fewer other side-effects; however, they may be slightly less effective in their specific antidepressant action (27, 28).

TABLE 2

Usual Doses of Antidepressant Drugs in mg.

MAO Inhibitors

Isocarboxazide (Marplan):	20- 80
Nialamide (Niamide):	100-200
Phenelzine (Nardil):	45- 75
Tranylcypromine (Parnate):	20- 30

Tricyclics

Imipramine (Tofranil):	50-300
Amitriptyline (Elavil):	50-300
Desipramine (Norpramin; Pertofrane):	50-300
Nortriptyline (Aventyl):	30-200
Protriptyline (Vivactil; Triptil):	10- 80
Doxepin (Sinequan):	50-250

Lithium

For maintenance treatment aimed at preventing depressive or manic episodes:	Serum level between 0.6 and 1.1 meq/1.
For treatment of acute manic syndrome:	Serum level between 1.0 and 1.4 meq/1.

There has been a neck-and-neck race between the antidepressant efficacy of imipramine (Tofranil) and amitriptyline (Elavil) for some years. One recent review reports that amitriptyline (Elavil) was superior to imipramine (Tofranil) in four of seven comparative studies and inferior to it only once (29). Another review states that of six such studies amitriptyline (Elavil) was found to be superior to imipramine in two and inferior to it in one study (30). Furthermore, a follow-up of the most extensive study that had shown the superiority of amitriptyline (Elavil) over a six-month period revealed that twelve months after the study had been completed there were more relapses among patients on amitriptyline (Elavil) than among those on imipramine (Tofranil) (31).

TRICYLIC ANTIDEPRESSANTS

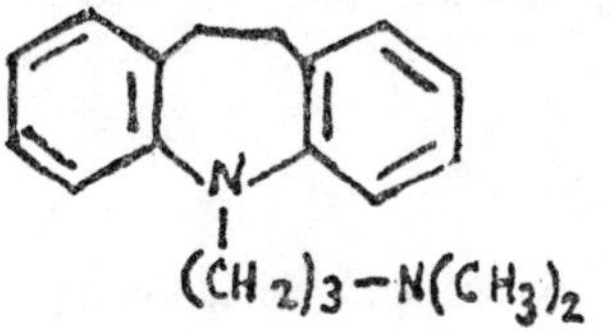

IMIPRAMINE 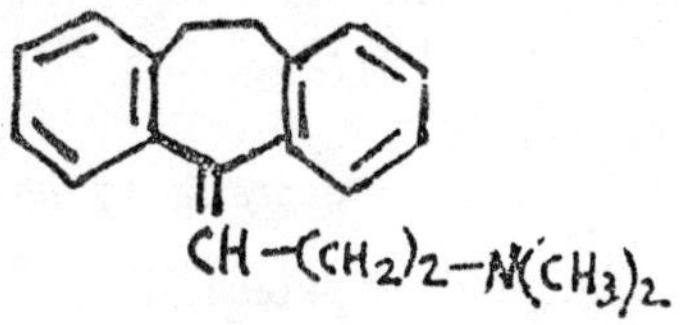   AMITRIPTYLINE

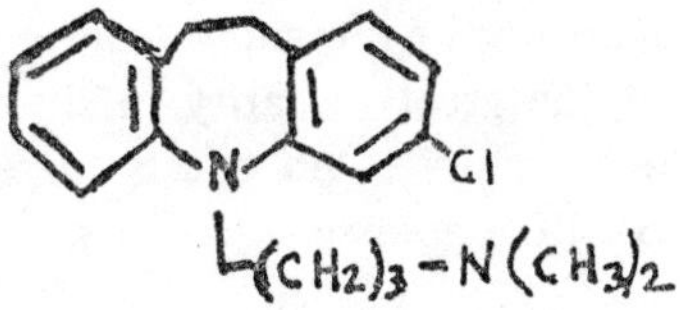

CHLORIMIPRAMINE

Figure 3

Another tricyclic antidepressant whose chemical structure is somewhat different, because of changes in its side chain, is protriptyline (Vivactil, Triptil). The latest compound to join the family of tricyclic antidepressants is doxepin (Sinequan) which, like amitriptyline, has a primary anxiolytic-sedative effect in addition to its antidepressant action and, unlike most other tricyclics, is claimed not to interact with antihypertension drugs (32, 33) and to produce fewer cardiotoxic effects when given in therapeutic doses.

Daily doses of tricyclic antidepressants, marketed in the U.S., are listed in Table 2.

Clomipramine (Anafranil), a tricyclic, and maprotiline (Ludiomil), a compound with four rings (tetracyclic), and viloxazine hydrochloride (Vivalan), a new antidepressant compound that differs from the tricyclics in chemical structure and side-effects, are three other antidepressants for which much pharmacological and clinical data are now available. Most of the work with these compounds has been done in Europe, and the drugs are not yet marketed in the U.S. (34-37).

Efficacy of Antidepressant Pharmacotherapy

Hundreds of published reports on antidepressant pharmacotherapy have established the fact that tricyclic antidepressants are definitely —and MAOI's almost certainly—more effective than placebo. It has been pointed out that negative results with MAOI's in controlled studies might have been due to the administration of inadequate doses. Direct comparisons of the many reported results is extremely difficult because of the great disparity in the type of patients admitted to the different studies. All efforts to reliably isolate homogeneous subgroups of depressed patients have so far proved unsuccessful.

Nevertheless, most results converge toward 60-70 percent efficacy of MAOI's or tricyclic drugs in the treatment of unselected depressions (38, 39). It is instructive to view these results within the perspective of the whole range of possible physical interventions in depressive illness. Figure 4 represents the probability of favorable therapeutic outcomes with various methods of treatment, as well as with placebo or without any specific treatment.

It is probably justified at this time to conclude that significant spontaneous improvement of depression within a month occurs in about 20 percent of patients (40). Placebos may increase the depressed patient's chances of improvement by another 20-30 percent (39, 41). Effective antidepressant drugs which are available today give the patient an additional 20-30 percent chance of improvement. Finally, electroconvulsive treatment (ECT) may be counted on to produce reliable improvement in another 10-15 percent of those patients who have resisted all other treatments.

However, even if the actual therapeutic contribution of antidepressive pharmacotherapy is only from 20-30 percent over and above spontaneous recovery or placebo effects, this is nevertheless

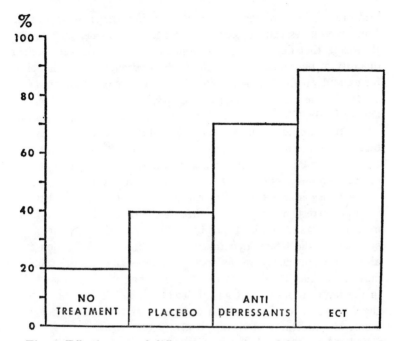

Fig. 4. Effectiveness of different treatment modalities in depressed patients (percent of patients much improved after three weeks).

an important therapeutic gain, and every attempt to exploit it should be made by the clinician. ECT—even though it has been shown to be the most effective antidepressive therapy (42, 43)—is more difficult to administer than drugs, causes special, disturbing side-effects, and does not lend itself easily to maintenance treatment.

Mechanisms of Action

Two major hypotheses about the somatic substrate of psychiatric depressions are competing at present: One explains depression as the result of deficient catecholamines—more specifically, norepinephrine—at crucial receptor sites in the brain; the other assumes that a deficiency of indoleamines—more specifically, serotonin—at brain receptors is responsible for the manifestations of depression. Both hypotheses can be brought under a common denominator by theorizing that depression is the result of a disturbed ratio and/or quantity of biogenic amines in the CNS, as Prange's group is doing, for example, with their permission theory of affective disorders (44).

Monoamine inhibitors increase the available amounts of biogenic amines in the CNS by interfering with their metabolic degradation, while tricyclic antidepressants achieve the required increase of biogenic amines by inhibiting the re-uptake of these substances from the synaptic cleft into the neuron. Both classes of antidepressant drugs, therefore, counteract a reduction of either catecholamines or indoleamines in the CNS. Experimental work has shown that the rewarding (response-excitatory) effect of electrical stimulation of the medial forebrain bundle depends on the activation of adrenergic synapses in the lateral hypothalamus and that this activation may also be brought about by the action of amphetamine and, probably, norepinephrine. Thus, an increase of catecholamines at these sites in the brain would correct any deficient adrenergic transmission at the synapse—a condition which may serve as a neuro-physiological model of antidepressant therapy (45).

It has been reported that the secondary amines, e.g., desipramine and protriptyline, inhibit more selectively the uptake of noradrenaline, and the tertiary amines, e.g., imipramine and amitriptyline, the uptake of serotonin (46). An interesting parallel appears in the clinical observation that the secondary amines, which affect mainly the noradrenergic neurons, are producing more pronounced motor activation and increased drive, while the tertiary amines, which act predominantly on serotonin-sensitive neurons, are more effective in improving the mood of depressed patients (47).

Side-effects and Drug Interactions

The interactions of MAOI's with other drugs and various food substances have already been discussed. The most disturbing side-effect of MAOI's is orthostatic hypotension. Other side-effects which are not uncommon are weight gain and effects on the CNS, e.g., restlessness and insomnia, impairment of sexual functioning in the form of delayed ejaculation and orgasm, loss of erection, and reduced libido.

The most important side-effect of the tricyclics is their potential cardiotoxic action (48), which is probably of clinical importance only in pre-existing cardiovascular disorder (but the presence of the latter may not always be known). Arrhythmias and a widening of the QRS complex in the ECG are the manifestations of this cardiotoxic effect, which is always reversible when the drug is discontinued. In elderly patients and in those with known cardiovascular disease, a pre-treatment ECG and subsequent ECG monitoring may be indicated.

Other side-effects of tricyclic antidepressants are: drowsiness, particularly during the first week of administration, dryness of mouth, tremor, sweating, dizziness, constipation, difficulty with voiding, hypotension, delayed ejaculation, headache, and—particularly in the elderly—confusional states. None of these symptoms is, as a rule, important enough to interfere seriously with the administration of the antidepressant, except for severely neurotic patients who seem to be specially sensitive to side-effects, and for alcoholics who find it impossible to take adequate doses of tricyclic antidepressants if they continue to drink heavily at the same time.

Because all tricyclic antidepressants have anti-cholinergic properties, caution is indicated when prescribing these drugs for patients suffering from untreated closed angle glaucoma (49) or symptoms of disturbed micturition. For the same reason, it is unwise to prescribe tricyclic antidepressants in a triple combination with a neuroleptic drug, e.g., a phenothiazine, and an antiparkinson drug, since most neuroleptics—and practically all antiparkinson drugs—have anticholinergic properties of their own, which have an additive or potentiating effect on the anticholinergic activity of the tricyclic antidepressant and may produce dangerous, even fatal complications, e.g., adynamic ileus (50). The combination of a tricyclic antidepressant with a neuroleptic (major tranquilizer) alone is usually well tolerated, as long as no antiparkinson drug is added to it. Tricyclic antidepressants may also be administered together

TABLE 3

Tricyclic Antidepressants: Interactions with Other
Drugs (Several not definitely established)

INTERACTING DRUGS	PROBABLE EFFECTS
Barbiturates	Reduced Plasma Level
Methylphenidate	Increased Plasma Level
Thyroid (Tri-iodothyronine)	Enhanced Antidepressant Effect in Female Patients
MAO Inhibitors	Enhanced Antidepressant Effect and Toxicity
Guanethidine	Decreased Hypotensive Effect
Phenothiazines	Enhanced Sedation and Increased Plasma Level
Anticholinergics	Enhanced Side-Effects
Physostigmine	Reduction of Anticholinergic Effects
Minor Tranquilizer	Enhanced Sedation
Alcohol	Enhanced Sedation
Cigarettes	Reduced Plasma Level
Estrogens (oral contraceptives?)	Increased Plasma Level
Reserpine	Enhanced Antidepressant Effects and Toxicity

with most anxiolytic sedatives (minor tranquilizers), except barbiturates, without adverse effects, although confusional states have
occasionally been observed following the simultaneous administration of tricyclics with benzodiazepines (51). Some of the interactions
of antidepressant drugs with other drugs are listed in Table 3 and
relative contraindications to the different treatment modalities in
depression in Table 4.

Barbiturates—probably by means of enzyme induction—lower
the plasma level of tricyclic antidepressants and thus their thera-

TABLE 4

Relative Contraindications to Different Treatment
Modalities in Depression

ECT	Age over 60. (Persistent memory defect) Organic Brain Lesion. Decompensated Circulatory Disease. Fever. States of high anxiety.
Tricyclic *Antidepressants*	Glaucoma, particularly of the untreated closed angle type. Prostatic Hypertrophy. Myocardial Disease. Cardiac Arrhythmias. Age over 60. (Monitor ECG for cardiac toxicity)
MAO-Inhibitors	Hypotension. Alcoholism. Low Intelligence. Low Reliability. Patients on thyroid, adrenergic or tricyclic anti- depressant drugs.
Lithium	Age over 60. (Unstable renal clearance; difficult control of serum level; lower threshold of toxicity) Kidney, Liver, Circulatory Disease. Patients on Diuretics.

peutic efficacy (52, 53). Methylphenidate (Ritalin), on the other
hand, inhibits the metabolism of imipramine and causes an increase
in serum levels of imipramine and desipramine; this may have a
potentiating effect on the therapeutic action of these antidepressants.
A similar interaction has been observed with some phenothiazines,
also resulting in an increase of tricyclic plasma levels (54-57).
Inhibition of the metabolism of imipramine has also been observed
when high doses of oestrogen are taken (58, 59). Furthermore, an
antagonism has been observed between the hypotensive action of
guanethidine and imipramine, possibly because the tricyclics com-
pete successfully with guanethidine, bethanidine and bretyllium for

the adrenergic receptor sites and thus prevent their full hypotensive action. An interaction with methyldopa (Aldomet) has not been definitely demonstrated but is suspected (60, 61, 62).

Sleep studies have shown that imipramine, desipramine, amytriptyline, and doxepin produce an immediate reduction of REM sleep. Some tricyclic antidepressants increase intrasleep restlessness, e.g., imipramine and desipramine, while others seem to decrease restlessness during sleep, e.g., doxepin (63, 64).

Finally, lithium, which is frequently used in the maintenance treatment of recurrent depressions, interacts with most diuretics to the effect that its clearance is impaired and its serum level increased; under these conditions there is a greater risk of toxicity.

Methodological Problems

The pathophysiology of depression has not yet been definitively established. One is tempted to accept the existing theory involving a disturbed balance of biogenic amines in the brain, but because it is based on circumstantial evidence only, the theory lacks experimental proof and furnishes us with little detail.

Since there is as yet *no real animal model* for emotional depression, pharmacologists have circumvented the problem by adopting certain pharmacologically or physiologically produced experimental states in animals as some approximation to, or models of, depression, e.g., the reserpine-induced state of altered behavior and metabolism. In a provocative review of the existing data, McKinney and Bunney (65) have proposed research strategies which could be used to create animal models of depression which etiologically and phenomenologically represent better approximations of depressive disorders in humans.

Another problem arises from the fact that it is impossible to know what proportion of metabolites of catecholamines or indoleamines measured in various body fluids, e.g., urine, blood or cerebrospinal fluid, reflects processes in the CNS, and *how much it results from peripheral processes.*

Still another unsolved problem faces the clinical investigator whose controlled clinical trials with antidepressant drugs require *homogeneous groups* of depressed patients. Until now, no clear criteria are known that would enable a researcher to screen depressed patients, in order to form such homogeneous samples. However, much experimental, genetic, epidemiological, and statistical work is going on in this area, and there is reason to hope that the identification of homogeneous groups of depressed patients will be achieved with greater precision in the not too distant future.

Predictors of Treatment Outcome and Choice of Drugs

Unlike ECT, pharmacotherapy of depression, even if effective, does not produce dramatic improvement within a few days. As a rule, it takes from one to three weeks before it becomes evident whether or not a patient is responding to treatment. Because of this long waiting period, it would be helpful if there were methods to predict the patient's eventual response to chemotherapy and the specific drugs before embarking upon the treatment. No generally applicable predictors of this kind exist today.

However, there are methods of predicting therapeutic outcome which are effective in certain special situations. Applying pharmacogenetic principles, Pare et al. (66) and Angst (67) have observed that a depressed patient will often respond to the same antidepressant treatment that has been effective in other members of his family. For instance, if a relative of a depressed patient has previously responded well to a MAOI, the patient himself is likely to improve with the same type of treatment. Similarly, therapeutic responsiveness to tricyclic antidepressants also seems to run in families.

The probenecid test is a procedure which prevents the excretion of biogenic amines and metabolites from the CNS, so that their accumulation in the cerebro-spinal fluid may be measured (68). Van Praag and his coworkers (69) have reasoned that those depressed patients in whom it could be demonstrated that serotonin metabolism was specifically disturbed would show a therapeutic response to treatment with the serotonin precursor 5-hydroxytryptophan. Having selected those patients in whom the probenecid test revealed a relative decrease of serotonin turnover, they reported encouraging results of this type of biochemically selected treatment in depressed patients who had previously been therapy-resistant.

A biochemical predictor of therapeutic response in depressed patients whose catecholamine metabolism is specifically affected, may be 3-methoxy-4-hydroxyphenylglycol (MHPG) which has been claimed to reflect more central than peripheral catecholamine turnover. Schildkraut (70) reported tentative findings that imipramine seems to be most effective in those depressed patients whose MHPG excretion is lowest, and that amitriptyline seems to produce the best therapeutic response in depressed patients with relatively higher levels of MHPG.

An interesting predictor for phenelzine-responsive depressed patients has been studied by Johnstone and Marsh (71). These investigators measured the genetically determined speed of metabolic acetylation in depressed outpatients and related it to the therapeutic response to phenelzine. The results suggested that phenelzine was effective for slow acetylators. The variable results that have been observed with phenelzine may be explained by the fact that this drug may be indicated only in depressed patients who are slow acetylators.

The possibility of using measurements of the monoamine oxidase content of blood platelets as indicators and predictors of the efficacy of antidepressant therapy has also been discussed (72).

Attempts to relate the plasma level of tricyclic antidepressants directly to the clinical response have so far been unsuccessful. Burrows et al. (73) found that in patients receiving 150 mg. nortriptyline per day, there was considerable inter-individual variability of plasma levels, but no prediction of the therapeutic response could be made on the basis of these differences. Others have shown that side-effects may be related to the plasma level of a tricyclic drug and that best clinical results are observed in a middle range of plasma levels which may be related, in non-linear fashion, to tricyclic plasma levels (53, 74, 75, 76).

Wittenborn (77) has studied possible correlations of premorbid personality factors with antidepressant treatment outcome and observed that depressed patients with a history of manic-depressive illness, involutional melancholia, or paranoid personality features reacted poorly, while the reactive diagnostic group responded favorably to imipramine. This is in contrast to most other published findings which report a better therapeutic response of endogenous depressions to tricyclic antidepressants (38, 41).

Exploring the influence of socioeconomic factors on the therapeutic response of depressed patients to amitriptyline and chlordiazepoxide (Librium), alone and in combination, Rickels et al. (78) observed that in the treatment of mildly to moderately depressed outpatients the type of drug is of much less importance in patients belonging to the lower socioeconomic classes than in the middle social class patients, who also responded less frequently to placebo than the lower class patients.

Perhaps the most reliable predictors of therapeutic responses to antidepressant drugs are still the clinical symptoms. It has already been mentioned that some clinicians feel MAOI's are more specifically indicated in neurotic depressions with hysterical and anxiety symptoms. Nevertheless, a recent controlled comparative study established that the tricyclic amitriptyline, given to depressed outpatients, produced not only somewhat faster relief from their depressive symptoms than the MAOI phenelzine, but also greater improvement in the neurotic features (79). For the treatment of episodic panic attacks, Klein (80) found imipramine and MAOI's equally effective.

Hollister and Overall (81) reported that imipramine was particularly effective in the treatment of retarded depressions, while hostile and anxious depressions responded better to the neuroleptic thioridazine (Mellaril). However, a recent study with imipramine in neurotic, depressed patients proved the effectiveness of this tricyclic in the anxious as well as the retarded patients (81). A fairly consistent finding in various studies was a tendency for female depressed patients to show a poor response to imipramine if they had a history of suicide attempt or paranoid features (21, 83, 84).

Finally, in two controlled comparative studies on the effects of various psychotropic drugs on depressed patients, it was observed that imipramine, chlorpromazine (Thorazine) and diazepam (Valium) were equally effective for sleep disturbances, imipramine was best for depressive and anergic symptoms, and diazepam was most suited for the treatment of anxiety symptoms (41).

Maintenance Treatment

Until recently, the prophylactic maintenance treatment of patients suffering from recurring depressions was much less reliable than that of schizophrenic patients. Relatively few controlled studies of this problem are available. Imlah et al. (85) could show that patients who had recovered from a depressive episode and were maintained on imipramine had a significantly lower relapse rate in the following six months than patients who were given placebo. In a recent double-blind, controlled study, Mindham et al. (86) could show that the relapse rate of patients who had recovered from a depressive episode and were continued on tricyclic antidepressants at lower than treatment doses for the following six months had a relapse rate of 22 percent, while patients continued on placebo had a 50 percent incidence of relapse.

A controlled, large-scale study, undertaken by the U.S. Veterans Administration (87), has recently demonstrated convincingly that the maintenance of depressed patients—that is, prevention of recurring depressive episodes—is equally effective with imipramine or lithium carbonate in unipolar depressions, but is significantly more effective with lithium than with imipramine in bipolar depressions. This finding allows the clinician a rational choice of the chemical agent he wants to administer to patients with recurrent depressions, if he has decided to keep the patient on continued pharmacotherapy for some time once he has recovered from his depressive episode. In most cases, this is a wise precaution to adopt (28).

How long such maintenance treatment should be continued is a question which at this time only clinical judgment can decide. Lithium maintenance treatment often does not become fully effective for a year, and once it has been embarked upon it should not be given up—except for severe side-effects or toxicity—before at least one year has elapsed. In some cases maintenance treatment must be continued for several years, sometimes for the lifetime of the patient.

Whether, for a patient suffering from unipolar depressions, one should choose a tricyclic, e.g., imipramine, or lithium, as the maintenance drug would depend on several considerations. How well does the patient tolerate imipramine or lithium? Can he be trusted to come regularly for the periodic determinations of lithium plasma levels? How long are the phases when the patient is well? Has he had more than one affective episode during the last three years? Answers to these questions enter into the making of the final clinical decision.

Since the significance of apparent interactions of lithium with the plasma levels of tricyclic antidepressants has not yet been clarified, it would, at the present time, seem advisable to interrupt any lithium maintenance treatment for the duration of an acute depressive episode that may require tricyclic antidepressant therapy.

Other Treatments

Although it is known that the combination of MAOI's with tricyclic antidepressants may result in dangerous hypertensive reactions, states of hyperpyrexia, agitation, confusion, convulsion, coma and death (88, 89, 90), some clinicians—particularly in Britain—recommend this combined chemotherapy as being often successful in depressed patients who have failed to respond to all other available treatments (91, 92). Apparently, complications of such combined treatment can be minimized if the doses of the MAOI and tricyclic antidepressant are built up very slowly and simultaneously over a period of two to three weeks (92), and if amitriptyline is chosen as the tricyclic drug, because it is a weaker potentiator of noradrenaline than imipramine (93).

The addition of the thyroid hormone triiodothyronine to imipramine enhances the therapeutic action of imipramine in depressed patients, as Prange et al. (94) first reported. The authors explained this by postulating an interaction of triiodothyronine and imipramine to produce an elevation of adrenergic activity, a hypothesis which later could be experimentally confirmed (95).

The intravenous instead of the traditional oral route of administration of tricyclic antidepressants has been employed by some clinicians. The drug most frequently chosen for intravenous infusion is clomipramine (available in Canada, but not yet in the U.S.), and this kind of therapy has been claimed to be effective not only in depressions but also for the relief of obsessive-compulsive and phobic symptomatology (96-99). However, because side-effects and complications may be more frequent with this kind of administration, Rigby et al. (100) suggest that the use of the intravenous route be reserved for those who have failed to respond to oral medication.

Because it is currently assumed that intracerebral catecholamines play a significant role in the etiology of depressive conditions, treatment of depressed patients with L-dopa, alone or in combination with other antidepressants, has been tried by a number of investigators with varying success (101, 102). Bunney et al. (103) reported that the use of L-dopa as an antidepressant was clearly ineffective in most of their patients, and that the drug almost regularly evoked manic symptoms in those patients who suffered from a bipolar depression.

Tryptophan, a precursor of serotonin, has been introduced as an antidepressant by those investigators who consider a deficient serotonin turnover as the principal etiological factor of the depressive state (104, 105). L-Tryptophan, by itself and in combination with an MAOI antidepressant, has been reported to give good clinical results (106). A dose of 9 mg. of L-tryptophan per day proved to be as effective as 150 mg. of imipramine per day in its antidepressant action. The addition of triiodothyronine enhanced the antidepressant action of imipramine, but not that of tryptophan (107).

Thyrotropin Releasing Hormone (TRH) is one of the latest antidepressant agents. Prange and Wilson (108) had observed that TRH will potentiate L-dopa-induced behavioral activation in mice and then tested the hormone for possible antidepressant activity. They found that single doses of TRH, given intravenously, produced a distinct improvement of depressive symptoms. Onset of this improvement was observed after two hours, and the antidepressant effect lasted from six to thirty hours. A replication of the clinical trial with TRH confirmed the earlier observations (109). The antidepressant action of TRH is probably not mediated through the pituitary, but seems to be a central effect, since potentiation of L-dopa-induced activation of behavior by TRH occurs also in hypothysectomized animals (110). Whether or not this interesting observation will acquire clinical significance and eventually produce more lasting improvement, only the future will show. Several studies conducted in Europe have thrown doubt on the antidepressant effectiveness of TRH (111).

A therapeutic approach to the treatment of depression, which differs in several aspects from most other antidepressant chemotherapies, has been tried by Lehmann et al. (112). They treated a group of depressed patients—including some geropsychiatric patients—with injections of 50 mg. of meperidine (Demerol) and the simultaneous oral administration of 10 mg. of dextro-amphetamine (Dexedrine) on alternate days, repeated five times. Their results, as measured by clinical findings and ratings on the Hamilton Depression Rating Scale, were encouraging: In most cases considerable improvement occurred and was maintained for long periods. The mechanism of action of this therapy may be partly based on shifts in the central turnover of biogenic amines, e.g., a meperidine-induced increase of noradrenaline, and partly on a reconditioning of affective and mood-related processes occurring after the repeated experience of pharmacologically-induced states of well-being. However, these findings have not been confirmed by others or by double-blind controlled observations.

Lithium, which has proved so successful in the treatment of manic episodes and in the prevention of relapses of manic or depressive episodes in patients with bipolar affective disorders, has also been tried in the treatment of depressive episodes. Although good results in the treatment of both unipolar and bipolar depressions have been reported by some (113), others have observed favorable therapeutic results mainly with bipolar depressions. Himmelhoch et al.

TABLE 5

Effectiveness of Established and Experimental Antidepressants on Different Dimensions of Psychopathology

	Depressive Symptoms	Anxiety Symptoms	Psychotic Symptoms
Antidepressants (Tricyclics or MAOI's)	++	+	-
Anxiolytics.	+	++	0
Neuroleptics	(+)	+	++
Amphetamine-like drugs	(+)	-	-
Lithium	(+)	(+)	0
L-dopa	(+)	0	(-)
Tryptophane	(+)	0	(-)(+)
Peptides, e.g. TRH: MIF, etc.	(+)	0	(+)

```
++ or +:    effective
   (+):     sometimes effective
    0 :     ineffective
   (-):     antitherapeutic
   (-):     sometimes antitherapeutic
```

(114) were successful with the combination of lithium and an MAOI in a group of 9 bipolar depressed patients who had resisted previous treatment with tricyclics, and Goodwin et al. (115) observed some improvement with lithium—as the only antidepressant—in 80 percent of bipolar, but in only 33 percent of unipolar depressions.

Table 5 gives an overview of the effectiveness of various established and experimental antidepressants on different dimensions of psychopathology.

Treatment-resistant Depressions

Every clinician has probably had the bad fortune to encounter depressed patients who did not improve, in spite of all his efforts. Although, in general, depression is a disease with a good prognosis, and most depressions would eventually terminate by self-recovery, there are certain depressive syndromes where all therapeutic efforts are doomed to failure. One or more of the following eight factors are usually involved in these cases:

1. inappropriate mode of treatment, inappropriate drug or inadequate dosage and duration of therapy;
2. association of the depression with organic brain damage or alcoholism;
3. ongoing life situations and existential contingencies which are inevitable and intolerable, e.g., severe, permanent disability, advanced age, and loneliness;
4. a life history with uniquely traumatizing situations, e.g., concentration camp experiences;
5. a lifelong depressive character structure with a specific, antitherapeutic psychodynamic constellation;
6. hypochondriasis or schizophrenic admixture;
7. over 45 years of age;
8. duration of depression longer than 1 year.

Fortunately, the first factor, i.e., inappropriate or inadequate treatment, accounts for most cases of treatment-resistant depressions; it is also the factor that can most easily be changed in the patient's favor. The other factors are difficult or sometimes impossible to modify. However, psychotherapy, continued interest, support and encouragement on the part of the psychiatrist, combined with his sustained medical efforts to provide at least some measure of relief for the patient, can in some of these patients improve their prognosis.

SUMMARY AND CONCLUSIONS

Chemotherapy of depression is today well established as the treatment of choice for all pathological, persistent, depressive states. Sleep deprivation is an easily administered treatment that, in endogenous depressions, may enhance the effects of antidepressant drugs. Whenever the state of depression is extremely acute and life-threatening, because of unmanageable agitation or suicidal impulses, or when chemotherapy has proved unsuccessful for more than 4 weeks, ECT is indicated. Psychosurgery may, in refractory cases, be considered as a last resort. Psychotherapy is often required, particularly in reactive depressions after the acute symptoms have subsided.

There are two principal types of antidepressant drugs: the MAOI's and the tricyclics. The choice of the particular drug to be used is today still best determined by clinical symptoms, but may soon be based on biochemical factors.

Maintenance treatment of patients after the termination of their depressive episode is recommended, at least for some months, but often for years. In patients who have suffered from a bipolar depression, lithium is the most effective maintenance treatment; in unipolar patients, imipramine is equally effective.

Active research into the physico-chemical substrate of depression is rapidly progressing, and although the ideal antidepressant has not yet been found, many original, provocative, and promising leads are being offered to the perceptive and knowledgeable clinician.

REFERENCES

1. PINEL, P.: Ellébore. In: Encyclopédie méthodique, Série Médecine, Bd. 5, 2. Paris: Teil, 1972.

2. REIL, J. C.: Rhapsodien über die Anwendung der psychischen Curmethode auf Geistes-zerrüttungen, 2. Aufl., Halle 1818 (1. Aufl. 1803).
3. COX, J. M.: Practical Observations on Insanity. London, 1804.
4. KLEIN, D. F.: Indications for specific treatments of depressions. Psychopharmacol. Bull., 11/3:3-13, July 1975.
5. HURWITZ, T. D.: Electroconvulsive therapy: A review. Comprehens. Psychiat., 15/4:303-314, 1974.
6. LEVY, R.: The clinical evaluation of unilateral ECT. Brit. J. Psychiat., 114:459-463, 1968.
7. DIEPZ, J.: ECT study reveals disparity between public, private units. Psychiatric News, 10/5:1, August 6, 1975.
8. PFLUG, B.: Über den Schlafentzug in der ambulanten Therapie endogener Depression, Der Nervenazt, 43:614-622, 1972.
9. COLE, M. G. and MULLER, H. F.: The treatment of endogenous depression by 36-hour sleep deprivation. Paper presented at the Canadian Psychiatry Association Annual Meeting in Banff, Alberta, September 1975.
10. KLAESI, J.: Dauernarkose mittels Somnifen bei Schizophrenen. Ztschr. Ges. Neurol. Psychiat., 74:557-592, 1922.
11. BHANJI, S. and ROY, G. A.: The treatment of psychotic depression: A replication study. Brit. J. Psychiat., 127:222-226, 1975.
12. OSTROW, D. E. and LEHMANN, H. E.: Quizzing the expert: Clinical criteria for psychosurgery. Hospital Physician, 2:24-31, 1973.
13. LIVINGSTON, K. E.: Cingulate cortex isolation for the treatment of psychoses and psychoneuroses. Res. Publs. Ass. Res. Nerv. Ment. Dis., 31:374-378, 1953.
14. TAN, E., MARKS, I. M. and MARSET, P.: Bimedial leucotomy in obsessive-compulsive neurosis: A controlled serial enquiry. Brit. J. Psychiat., 118:155-164, 1971.
15. STEINBERG, D. L.: Hematoporphyrin treatment of severe depressions. Am. J. Psychiat., 92:901-913, January 1936.
16. GILLIS, A. and SALFIELD, D. J.: Treatment of depressive states with dinitrile succinate. J. Ment. Sci., 99:542-546, July, 1953.
17. WASHBURNE, A. C.: Nicotinic acid in depressed states: Preliminary report. Ann. Int. Med., 32:261-269, February, 1950.
18. KLINE, N. S.: Clinical experience and iproniazid (Marsilid). J. Clin. Exp. Psychopath., 19/2 (Suppl. 1):72, 1958.
19. ALEXANDER, L. and BERKELEY, A. W.: The inert psychasthenic reaction (anhedonia) as differentiated from classic depression and its response to iproniazid. J. N.Y. Acad. Sci., 80:669, 1959.
20. CRISP, A. H., HAYS, P. and CARTER, A.: Three amine oxidase inhibitor drugs in the treatment of depression. Lancet, 1:17, 1961.

21. KILOH, L. G., BALL, J. R. B. and GARSIDE, R. F.: Prognostic factors in treatment of depressed states with imipramine. *Brit. Med. J.*, 1:1225-1227, 1962.

22. SARGANT, W.: Treatment of anxiety states and atypical depressions by the monoamine oxidase inhibitor drugs. *J. Neuropsychiat.* 3 (Suppl.) :S96-102, 1962.

23. WEST, E. M. and DALLY, P. J.: Effects of iproniazid in depressive syndrome. *Brit. Med. J.*, 1:1491-1494, 1959.

24. SPEAR, F. G., HALL, P. and STIRLAND, P.: A comparison of subjective responses to imipramine and tranylcypromine. *Brit. J. Psychiat.*, 110:53-55, 1964.

25. LEITCH, A. and SEAGER, C. P.: A trial of four antidepressant drugs. *Psychopharmacologia*, 4:72-77, 1963.

26. KUHN, R.: Über die Behandlung depressiver Zustände mit einem Iminodibenzylderivat (G 22355). *Schw. Med. Wchnschr.* 35/36: 1135-1140, Aug. 31, 1957.

27. HOLLISTER, L. E., OVERALL, J. E., JOHNSON, M., KATZ, G., KIMBELL, I. and HONIGFELD, G.: Evaluation of desipramine in depressive states. *J. New Drugs*, 3:166-171, 1963.

28. LEHMANN, H. E.: Problems of differential diagnosis and choice of therapy in depressive states. *Psychosomatics*, VI:266-272, Sept.-Oct. 1965.

29. MORRIS, J. B. and BECK, A. T.: The efficacy of antidepressant drugs: A review of research 1958-1972. *Arch. Gen. Psychiat.*, 30:667-674, 1974.

30. BAN, T. A.: *Depression and the Tricyclic Antidepressants.* Montreal: Ronalds Federated Graphic Limited, 1974.

31. KESSELL, A. and HOLD, N. F.: Depression—an analysis of followup study. *Brit. J. Psychiat.*, 3:1143-1153, 1965.

32. CASTROGIOVANNI, P., PLACIDI, G. F., MAGGINI, C., GHETTI, B. and CASSANO, G. B.: Clinical investigation of doxepin in depressed patients. Pilot open study, controlled double-blind trial versus imipramine and all-night polygraphic study. *Pharmacopsychiatrie Neuropsychopharmacologie*, 4:170-181, 1971.

33. WHITING, B., GOLBERT, A. and WALDIE, P.: The drug disc warning to drug interaction. *Lancet*, 1(7811) :1037-1038, 1973.

34. ANAFRANIL SYMPOSIUM: MURPHY, J. (Ed.) : *The Journal of International Medical Research*, 1/5:271-488, 1973.

35. BALESTRIERI, A., BENASSI, G. B., CASTROGIOVANNI, P., CATALANO, A., COLOMBI, A., CONFORTO, C., DEL SOLDATA, G., GILBERTI, F. and SARTESCHI, P.: Clinical comparative evaluation of maprotiline, a new antidepressant drug. *Int. Pharmacopsychiat.*, 6:236-248, 1971.

36. EDITORIAL: New drug shows promise in depressive patients. *J. Am. Med. Assn.*, 220/5:661-662, 1972.

37. MURPHY, J. E.: Vivalan: Drug profile. *J. Int. Med. Res.*, 3 (Suppl.), 3/122:122-124, 1975.
38. KLERMAN, G. L. and COLE, J. O.: Clinical pharmacology of imipramine and related antidepressant compounds. *Pharmacological Reviews*, 17/2:101-141, 1965.
39. LEHMANN, H. E.: Non-MAO inhibitor antidepressants in clinical perspective. Antidepressant drugs of Non-MAO inhibitor type—Proceedings of a Workshop. National Institute of Mental Health, U.S. Department of Health, Education and Welfare, Public Health Service, 1966.
40. BURT, C. G., GORDON, W. F. and HORDERN, A.: Amitriptyline in depressive states: A controlled trial. *J. Ment. Sci.*, 108:711, 1962.
41. RASKIN, A.: Drugs and depression subtypes. *In: Depression in the 70's.* Excerpta Medica, 1971.
42. GREENBLATT, M., GROSSER, G. H. and WECHSLER, H.: A comparative study of selected antidepressant medications and EST. *Amer. J. Psychiat.*, 119:144-153, 1962.
43. *British Medical Journal*, 1:881, 1965: Clinical trial of the treatment of depressive illness. Report to the Medical Research Council by its Clinical Psychiatry Committee.
44. PRANGE, A. J., LIPTON, M. A. and WILSON, I. C.: Clinical intimations of amine balance and permission. *Psychopharmacol. Bull.*, 10/3:53-55, July 1974.
45. STEIN, L.: Psychopharmacological substrates of mental depression. Proceedings of the First International Symposium on Antidepressant Drugs, Milan, April 1966. *Excerpta Medica, International Congress Series No. 122*, 130-140.
46. MODIGH, K.: Effects of clomipramine (Anafranil) on neurotransmission in brain monoamine neurones. *J. Int. Med. Res.*, 1:274-280, 1973.
47. KIELHOLZ, P.: Die Behandlung endogener Depressionen mit Psychopharmaka. *Deutsche Chirurg. Mediz. Wochenschrift*, 93: 701, 1968.
48. MOIR, D. C., CROOKS, J., SAWYAR, P., TURNBULL, M. J. and WEIR, R. D.: Cardiotoxicity of tricyclic antidepressants. *Brit. J. Pharmacol.*, 44:371, 1972.
49. *Drug Therapy Bulletin*, 13/2:7-8, 1975: Tricyclic antidepressives and glaucoma: What's the risk?
50. WARNES, H., LEHMANN, H. E. and BAN, T. A.: Adynamic ileus during psychoactive medication: A report of three fatal and five severe cases. *Canad. Med. Assn. J.*, 92:1112-1113, 1967.
51. MARTIN, E. W.: *Hazards of Medication.* Philadelphia: J. B. Lippincott, 1971.
52. NAKAZAWA, K.: Studies on the demethylation, hydroxylation and N-oxidation of imipramine in rat liver. *Biochem. Pharmacol.*, 19:1363-1369, 1970.

53. SJOQVIST, F. W., HAMMER, W., IDESTROM, C. M., LIND, M., TUCK, D. and ASBERG, M.: Plasma level of monomethylated tricyclic antidepressants and side effects in man. Proceedings of the European Society for Study of Drug Toxicity, Paris 1967, *Excerpta Medica*, International Congress Series Number 145, Amsterdam, 246-253, 1968.

54. PEREL, J. M., BLACK, N., WHARTON, R. N., and MALITZ, S.: Inhibition of imipramine metabolism by methylphenidate. *Federal Proceedings*, 28:418, 1969.

55. GARRETTSON, L. K., PEREL, J. M. and DAYTON, P. G.: Methylphenidate interaction with both anticonvulsants and ethyl biscoumacetate. *J. Am. Med. Assn.*, 207/11:2053-2056, 1969.

56. WHARTON, R. N., PEREL, J. M., DAYTON, P. G. and MALITZ, S.: A potential clinical use for methylphenidate with tricyclic antidepressants. *Am. J. Psychiat.*, 127:12, 1971.

57. RAFAELSEN, O. J. and GRAM, L. F.: Interaction between antidepressants and other groups of psychopharmaca. *In* Symposia Medica Hoechst (8) (Eds.), *Classification and Prediction of Outcome of Depression.* Stuttgart, Germany: F. K. Schattauer Verlag GmbH., 1974, pp. 253-256.

58. PRANGE, A. J.: Therapeutic and theoretical implications of imipramine-hormone interactions in depressive disorders in psychiatry. Proceedings of the V World Congress of Psychiatry. *In* R. de la Fuente and M. N. Weisman (Eds.), *Excerpta Medica*, Amsterdam, 1973, 1023-1031.

59. KHURANA, R. C.: Estrogen imipramine interaction, *J. Amer. Med. Assn.*, 222/6:702-703, 1972.

60. LEISHMANN, A. W. D., MATTHEWS, H. L. and SMITH, A. J.: Antagonism of guanethidine by imipramine. *Lancet*, 1:112, 1963.

61. MITCHELL, J. R., CAVANAUGH, J. H., ARIAS, L. and OATES, J. A.: Guanethidine and related agents. III. Antagonism by drugs which inhibit the norepinephrine pump in man. *Journal of Criminal Investigation*, 39:1596, 1970.

62. STOCKLEY, I. H.: Drug interactions: 5 tricyclic antidepressants. Pt. 1. Interactions with drugs affecting adrenergic neurones. *Pharmaceutical Journal*, 208:559-562, 1972.

63. FRAM, D. H., WYATT, R. J. and SNYDER, F.: Longitudinal sleep patterns in depressed patients treated with amitriptyline. *Psychophysiology*, 7/2:317, 1970.

64. DUNLEAVY, D. L. F., BREZINOVA, V., OSWALD, I., MACLEAN, A. W. and TINKER, M.: Changes during weeks in effects of tricyclic drugs on the human sleeping brain. *Brit. J. Psychiat.*, 120:663-672, June, 1972.

65. MCKINNEY, W. T., JR. and BUNNEY, W. E., JR.: Animal model of depression—I. Review of evidence: Implications for research. *Arch. Gen. Psychiat.*, 21:240-248, August, 1969.

66. PARE, C. M. B., REES, L. and SAINSBURY, M. J.: Differentiation of two genetically specific types of depression by response to antidepressant drugs. *Lancet*, 11:1340, 1962.
67. ANGST, J.: Antidepressiver Effekt und genetische Faktoren. *Arzneimittel-Forsch*, 14:496, 1964.
68. GOODWIN, F. K. and GORDON, E. K.: Cerebrospinal fluid amine metabolites in affective illness: The probenecid technique. *Amer. J. Psychiat.*, 130/1:73-79, 1973.
69. VAN PRAAG, H. M., KORF, J., DOLS, L. C. W. and SCHUT, T.: A pilot study of the predictive value of the probenecid test in application of 5 hydroxytryptophan as antidepressant. *Psychopharmacologia* (Berl.), 25/1:14-21, 1972.
70. SCHILDKRAUT, J.: Norepinephrine metabolites as biochemical criteria for classifying depressive disorders and predicting responses to treatment: Preliminary findings. *Am. J. Psychiat.*, 130/6:695-698, 1973.
71. JOHNSTONE, E. C. and MARSH, W.: Acetylator status and response to phenelzine in depressed patients. *Lancet*, 1:567-570, March 17, 1973.
72. ROBINSON, D. S., NIES, A., RAVARIS, C. L., IVES, J. O. and LAMBORN, K. R.: Treatment response to MAO inhibitors: Relation to depressive typology and blood platelet MAO inhibition. *In* Symposia Medica Hoechst (8) (Eds.), *Classification and Prediction of Outcome of Depression.* Stuttgart, Germany: F. K. Schattauer Verlag GmbH., 1974, 259-267.
73. BURROWS, G. D., DAVIES, B. and SCOGGINS, B. A.: Plasma concentration of nortriptyline and clinical response in depressive illness. *Lancet*, 2:619-623, 1972.
74. ASBERG, M., KRAGH-SORENSEN, P., BERTILSSON, L., CRONHOLM, B., EGGERT-HANSEN, CH., SJOQVIST, F. and TUCK, J. R.: Studies of relationship between plasma level and clinical effects of nortriptyline—Methodological problems. *In* Symposia Medica Hoechst (8) (Eds.), *Classification and Prediction of Outcome of Depression.* Stuttgart, Germany: F. K. Schattauer Verlag GmbH, 1974, pp. 181-192.
75. BRAITHWAITE, R. A., GOULDING, R., THEANO, GINETTE, BAILEY, J. and COPPEN, A.: Plasma concentration of amitriptyline and clinical response. *Lancet*, 1:1297-1300, June 17, 1972.
76. KRAGH-SORENSEN, P., ASBERG, M. and EGGERT-HANSEN, C.: Plasma-nortriptyline levels in endogenous depression. *Lancet*, 1:113, 1973.
77. WITTENBORN, J. R.: Diagnostic classification and response to imipramine. Unpublished manuscript, 1967.
78. RICKELS, K., GORDON, P. E., JENKINS, B. W., PERLOFF, M., SACHS, T. and STEPANSKY, W.: Drug treatment in depressive illness (amitriptyline and chlordiazepoxide in two neurotic populations). *Dis. Nerv. Syst.*, 31:30-42, Jan., 1970.

79. KAY, D. W. K., GARSIDE, R. F. and FAHY, T. J.: A double-blind trial of phenelzine and amitriptyline in depressed out-patients. A possible differential effect of the drugs on symptoms. *Brit. J. Psychiat.*, 123:63-67, 1973.

80. KLEIN, D. F.: Delineation of two drug-responsive anxiety syndromes. *Psychopharmacologia*, 5:397-403, 1964.

81. HOLLISTER, L. E. and OVERALL, J. E.: Reflections on the specificity of action of antidepressants. *Psychosomatics*, 6:361-365, 1965.

82. COVI, L., LIPMAN, R., DEROGATIS, L. R., SMITH, J. E. and PATTISON, J. H.: Drugs and group psychotherapy in neurotic depression. *Am. J. Psychiat.*, 13: February 2, 1974.

83. ROBIN, A. A. and LANGLEY, G. E.: A controlled trial of imipramine. *Brit. J. Psychiat.*, 110:419-422, 1964.

84. WITTENBORN, J. R.: Factors which qualify the response to iproniazid and imipramine. *In* J. R. Wittenborn and P. R. A. May (Eds.), *Prediction of Response to Pharmacotherapy.* Springfield, Ill.: Charles C Thomas, 1966.

85. IMLAH, N. W., RYAN, E. and HARRINGTON, J. A.: The influence of antidepressant drugs on the response to ECT and subsequent relapse rates. Presented at the Fourth Annual Meeting of the Collegium Internationale Neuropsychopharmacologicum: Birmingham, 1964, 438-442. Excerpta Medica Foundation, Amsterdam.

86. MINDHAM, R. H. S., HOWLAND, C. and SHEPHARD, M.: Continuation therapy with tricyclic antidepressants in depressive illness. *Lancet,* 2/7782-854-855, 1972.

87. PRIEN, R. F., KLETT, C. J. and CAFFEY, E. M., JR.: Lithium carbonate and imipramine in prevention of affective disorders. *Arch. Gen. Psychiat.*, 29:420-425, 1973.

88. BOWEN, L. W.: Fatal hyperpyrexia with antidepressant drugs. *Brit. Med. J.*, 2:1465, 1964.

89. LOCKETT, M. F. and MILNER, G.: Combining the antidepressant drugs. *Brit. Med. J.*, 1:921, 1965.

90. BEAUMONT, G.: Drug interactions with clomipramine (Anafranil). *J. Int. Med. Res.*, 1:480-484, 1973.

91. GANDER, D. R.: The clinical value of monoamine oxidase inhibitors and tricyclic antidepressants in combination. *In* S. Garattini and M. N. G. Dukes (Eds.), *Antidepressant Drugs.* Excerpta Medica Foundation, 1967.

92. PARE, C. M. B.: Recent advances in the treatment of depression. *In* A. Coppen and A. Walk (Eds.), *Recent Developments in Affective Disorders.* Ashford, Kent: Headley Brothers Ltd., 1968, pp. 137-150.

93. SETHNA, E. R.: A study of refractory cases of depressive illnesses and their response to combined antidepressant treatment. *Brit. J. Psychiat.*, 124:265-272, 1974.

94. PRANGE, JR., A. J., WILSON, I. C., LIPTON, M. A., et al.: Use of a thyroid hormone to accelerate the action of imipramine. *Psychosomatics*, 11/5:442-444, 1970.

95. BREESE, G. R., TRAYLOR, T. D. and PRANGE, A. J., JR.: The effect of triiodothyronine on the disposition and actions of imipramine. *Psychopharmacologia* (Berl.), 25/2:101-111, 1972.

96. CORDOBA, F. E. and LOPEZ-IBOR, J. J.: Monochlorimipramine in psychiatric patients resistant to other forms of treatment. *Acta Luso-Espanolas de Neurologia y Psiquiatrica*, 26:119, 1967.

97. CAPSTICK, N.: Clomipramine (Anafranil) in the treatment of obsessional states. Paper read at the 7th Congress of the Collegium Internationale Neuro-Psychopharmacologicum, Prague, 1970.

98. MARSHALL, W. K. and MICEV, V.: Clomipramine (Anafranil) in the treatment of obsessional illnesses and phobic anxiety states. *J. Int. Med. Res.*, 1:403-412, 1973.

99. RACK, P. H.: Clomipramine (Anafranil) in the treatment of obsessional states with special reference to the Leyton obsessional inventory. *J. Int. Med. Res.*, 1:397-402, 1973.

100. RIGBY, B., CLARREN, S. and KELLY, D.: A psychological and physiological evaluation of the effects of intravenous clomipramine (Anafranil). *J. Int. Med. Res.*, 1:308-316, 1973.

101. KLERMAN, G. L., SCHILDKRAUT, J. J., HASENBUSH, L. L., GREENBLATT, M. and FRIEND, D. G.: Clinical experience with dihydroxyphenylalanine (Dopa) in depression. *J. Psychiat. Res.*, 1:289-297, 1963.

102. FRACASSO, G. L., FRISONE, L. and PARMIGIANI, P.: Clinical effect of combined administration of levodopa and tricyclic antidepressive agents in the treatment of depressive syndromes. *Rass. Stud. Psychiat.*, 61/2:176-185, 1972.

103. BUNNEY, W. E., JR., GERSHON, E. S., MURPHY, D. L. and GOODWIN, F. K.: Psychobiological and pharmacological studies of manic depressive illness. *J. Psychiat. Res.*, 9/3:207-226, 1972.

104. COPPEN, A., SHAW, D. M., HERZBERG, B. and MAGGS, R.: Tryptophan in the treatment of depression. *Lancet*, 1178-1180, December 2, 1967.

105. SANO, I.: L-5-hydroxytryptophan ((L-5-HTP) treatment in endogenous depression. *Munch. Med. Wschr.*, 114/40:1713-1716, 1972.

106. AYUSO GUTIERREZ, J. L. and LOPEX IBOR ALINO, J. J.: Tryptophan and an MAOI (nialamide) in the treatment of depression. A double blind study. *Int. Pharmacopsychiat.* (Basel), 6/2:92-97, 1971.

107. COPPEN, A., WHYBROW, P. C., NOGUERA, R., MAGGS, R. and PRANGE, A. J., JR.: The comparative antidepressant value of L-tryptophan and imipramine with and without attempted

potentiation by liothyronine. *Arch. Gen. Psychiat.*, 26:234-240, March 1972.

108. PRANGE, A. J. and WILSON, I. C.: Thyrotropin releasing hormone (TRH) for the immediate relief of depression: A preliminary report. *Psychopharmacologia* 26 (Suppl.):82, August 1972.

109. KASTIN, A. J., ELWENSING, R. H., SCHALCH, D. S. and ANDERSON, M. S.: Improvement in mental depression with decreased thyrotropin response after administration of thyrotropin-releasing hormone. *Lancet*, 2:740-742, 1972.

110. PRANGE, A. J., JR., LARA, P. P., WILSON, I. C., ALLTOP, L. B. and BREESE, G. R.: Effects of thyrotropin-releasing hormone in depression. *Lancet*, 999-1002, November 11, 1972.

111. BENKERT, O., MARTSCHEK, I. and GORDON, A.: Comparison of T. R. H., L.H.-R.H., and placebo in depression. *Lancet*, 2:1146, November, 1974.

112. LEHMANN, H. E., ANANTH, J. V., GEAGEA, K. C. and BAN, T. A.: Treatment of depression with dexedrine and demerol. *Current Therapeutic Research*, 13/1:42-49, January 1971.

113. RYBAKOWSKI, J.: Lithium carbonate in endogenous depression. *Psychiat. Pol.*, 6/5:547-550, 1972.

114. HIMMELHOCH, J. M., DETRE, T., KUPFER, D. J., et al.: Treatment of previously intractable depressions with tranylcypromine and lithium. *J. Nerv. Ment. Dis.*, 155/3:216-220, 1972.

115. GOODWIN, K., MURPHY, L., DUNNER, L. and BUNNEY, W. E.: Lithium response in unipolar versus bipolar depression. *Amer. J. Psychiat.*, 129/1:76-79, July, 1972.

11

Clinical Toxicology of Psychotropic Medications

Bruce H. Bailey, M.D. and
James R. Guidy, Pharm.D.

I. INTRODUCTION

Suicide is an unfortunate but frequent outcome for the person suffering a depressive mood disorder and/or a state of hopelessness. It has reached a high level of incidence as a cause of death in all age groups and in all socioeconomic levels in our own culture, as well as others (1). Although well recognized, it is worth repeating that every depressed person has some suicidal risk which must be assessed initially and monitored through the course of treatment, especially in early phases when the patient may be improving but still have "bad days." The frequency, distribution, method used, and prevention of suicide are the subjects of a major area of specialization having a sizable literature of its own (2, 3). This chapter will address a particular aspect: the use of medication in a suicidal attempt; its prevention, recognition and assessment; and its treatment.

It is perhaps ironic that an increasingly frequent phenomenon is the choice of a prescribed antidepressant medication as the instrument of a suicidal attempt. This has certainly been our experience, as well as that of others (4). In a recent Medical Grand Rounds, where the authors had presented material related to the assessment, physiologic effects, and treatment of a person who had overdosed with a tricyclic antidepressant, one medical staff member queried, "If these damn drugs are so dangerous, why don't we get them off our formulary?" This was evaluated as a positive reflection of continuing education effort, such that a proposal was made and accepted that the topic "Assessment and Management of Depression" be soon placed on the schedule.

The most effective treatment of suicide is prevention. After the clinician has reached a degree of assessment to warrant treatment of a mood disorder, he will not only titrate the dosage of medication to establish a therapeutic level, but will also titrate the *amount* of medication made available to the patient depending on the clinician's own index of suicidal potential. This raises the issue of what we have called the "loaded-gun syndrome." In treating a patient with a mood disorder, we might ask the patient, or a member of his family, to eliminate guns from the house. We might also ask that the medicine cabinet be emptied. It is equally important that we carefully monitor the amount of medication available to the patient so that he does not have a lethal stockpile available, should he reach such a degree of hopelessness that suicide is his alternative.

Faced with this issue, in instances of some patients who are under care at the Phoenix VA Hospital, we have recently, with the full understanding and consent of the patient, written letters to community emergency facilities asking that they not prescribe more than one day's supply of medication for the patient, specifically indicating that this is a patient who has repeatedly made suicide attempts by stockpiling of medication. It should be understood that this was not an attempt to deprive the patient of treatment, but to clarify that his treatment was under the responsibility of one agency.

The physician is now in an arena of proliferation of pharmaco-therapeutic agents. It behooves the clinical psychiatrist to be knowledgeable about the direct effects, side effects, and synergism or antagonism of drug interactions. After taking a family history of the patient, a family *drug* history as well as a drug history of the patient may be useful both in diagnostic assessment and in choice of appropriate therapeutic agent. In addition, the clinician should review the *current drug profile* of the patient before prescribing potent medications (particularly the tricyclic antidepressants because of their potent anticholinergic activity). An effective technique is to ask the patient to bring in all of the bottles of medication he is taking. It is frequently useful to consult with the patient's primary physician. This will assist the clinician in monitoring and altering the overall treatment progress of the patient, and in adequately informing the patient as to potential drug effects. The patient should always be cautioned as to the synergistic effects of alcohol.

II. SPECIFIC ANTAGONISTS

It would normally be appropriate to next discuss in detail the diagnostic evaluation of the patient and the general supportive measures important to his critical care and recovery. However, we should like to put information about drug-specific antagonists at the forefront because of our awareness that this information is not widely known.

A. *Physostigmine salicylate (Antilerium)*

Physostigmine salicylate is a cholinergic agent which has the ability to reverse the entire spectrum of anticholinergic toxicity. We will be discussing the triad of peripheral, cardiac and central nervous system toxicity with tricyclic antidepressant overdose later in this paper. However, we must recognize the potential for anticholinergic toxicity in other therapeutic agents. Table 1 represents a partial list of such agents.

It is not uncommon to find patients taking several therapeutic agents for their various medical problems, many of which, as side effects, possess anticholinergic activity.

EXAMPLE: A patient with neuropsychiatric disorder receiving a phenothiazine and an antiparkinson agent. He may also be receiving medical treatment for peptic ulcer disease, resulting in the addition of an antispasmodic, such as dicyclomine (Bentyl). For colds, flu, chronic rhinitis or sinusitis he may be prescribed an antihistamine, or choose one for himself from the shelf of any drug store or supermarket. In all, this patient is receiving at least four separate therapeutic classes of drugs having potent anticholinergic side effects. The result: potential anticholinergic toxicity.

El-Yousef et al. (5) have demonstrated that a significant number of patients on combination psychotropic agents experience a toxic psychosis, referred to often as the "central anticholinergic syndrome," and recommend the use of physostigmine diagnostically when this is suspected.

As mentioned earlier, anticholinergic drugs may cause peripheral, cardiac, and central nervous system toxicity. While most of these agents are capable of eliciting some peripheral and cardiac activity, only the tertiary ammonium compounds are capable of crossing the blood-brain barrier and producing a central anticholinergic syndrome (Table 1). Those anticholinergics not producing central effects are quaternary ammonium compounds, which do not cross the blood-brain barrier.

Physostigmine salicylate (Antilerium), neostigmine (Prostigmin) and pyridostigmine (Mestinon, Regonol) are all cholinergic agents. They act by inhibiting the enzyme cholinesterase, resulting in an increase in the activity of the endogenous parasympathetic neurotransmitter, acetylcholine, at parasympathetic, or cholinergic, receptor sites. Neostigmine and pyridostigmine are *quaternary ammonium* compounds. Like the quaternary ammonium anticholinergic agents, they are unable to cross the blood-brain barrier. Therefore, they cannot elicit a central nervous system cholinergic response, and are incapable of reversing the "central anticholinergistic syndrome" (5, 8, 9, 10-18). Physostigmine salicylate, the remaining cholinesterase inhibitor, is a *tertiary ammonium* compound, can cross the blood-brain barrier, and is therefore the only one of the three anticholinesterases capable of reversing central anticholinergic toxicity (19).

TABLE 1

A Representative List of Agents Producing "Central Anticholinergic Syndrome" (6, 7)

Antipsychotics

Chlorpromazine (Thorazine)　　　Thiothixene (Navene)
Thioridazine (Mellaril)　　　　　Chlorprothixene (Taractan)

Antihistamines

Chlorpheniramine (Chlor-trimeton, Teldrin, Ornade)
Brompheniramine (Disomer, Dimetapp)
Diphenhydramine (Benadryl)
Promethazine (Phenergan)
Tripelennamine (Pyribenzamine)

Antispasmodics

Atropine and Scopolamine　　　Belladonna alkaloids (Donnatal)
Dicyclomine (Bentyl)　　　　　Oxyphencylimine (Daricon)

Antiparkinson agents

Trihexyphenidyl (Artane)　　　Benztropine (Cogentin)
Ethopropazine (Parsidol,　　　Chlorphenoxamine (Phenoxene)
　(also phenothiazine))　　　　Procyclidine (Kemadrin)

Muscle relaxant

Orphenadrine (Norflex, Norgesic)

Proprietary drugs (sedative-hypnotic)

Compoz (scopolamine and antihistamine)
Sleep-eze (scopolamine and antihistamine)
Sominex (scopolamine and antihistamine)
Nytol (antihistamine)
Excedrin-PM (antihistamine)
Mr. Sleep (scopolamine and antihistamine)

Proprietary drugs (cold preparations—contain antihistamines)

Coricidin　　　　　Novahistine
Allerest　　　　　Ornex
Contac　　　　　Sinutab
Dristan　　　　　Triaminicin

Toxins

Bittersweet　　　　　Potato leaves and sprouts
Jimson weed　　　　　Deadly nightshade

Despite numerous articles and letters in various journals concerning the value of physostigmine in the treatment of anticholinergic drug toxicity, due to tricyclic antidepressants, antipsychotics, antiparkinson agents, belladonna alkaloids, etc., its use in reversing anticholinergic toxicity is still little appreciated. In 1968, Duvoisin and Katz (8) described the use of physostigmine in the reversal of the central anticholinergic syndrome in 26 patients, and suggested that this drug "deserves a place in therapeutics as an antidote." Seven years later, in 1975, in an article by Granacher and Baldessarini (9), it was revealed in a survey of 20 hospitals in metropolitan Boston that only 6 of these hospitals stocked physostigmine in their pharmacies, indicating a striking lag in the dissemination of knowledge concerning this treatment modality into the general medical community. Indeed, in our own experience, working with interns and residents who have received their training throughout this country and abroad, we find that very few have been instructed in how to use physostigmine in the diagnosis and treatment of either tricyclic antidepressant overdose or other anticholinergic toxicities. It is possible that the potential mortality of anticholinergic intoxication, particularly tricyclic antidepressant overdose, is still not fully appreciated. In 1968, Davis et al. (20) reviewed the literature, finding 203 cases of tricyclic antidepressant poisoning in adults, with 20 fatalities. These cases involved the use of only two drugs. Since that time several additional tricyclic antidepressants have been marketed and the incidence of overdose has increased (4). Additional data concerning tricyclic antidepressants will be presented with the discussion of overdose with this family of drugs.

Specific comments are necessary now concerning the clinical use of physostigmine. In the patient presenting with anticholinergic intoxication, 2 mg. of physostigmine is given, preferably I.V., slowly. Full effect of that dose should appear within 10 minutes. If minimal or no improvement (return of reflexes, improved respiratory exchange, improved state of consciousness, etc.) occurs, the I.V. dose should be repeated. We have not exceeded 8 mgs./hour without seeing some reversal of intoxication regardless of the depth of coma. After the initial reversal of the anticholinergic syndrome, it may be necessary to administer physostigmine, 2 mg. I.M., at 2-hour intervals, depending on the severity of intoxication (and, of course careful monitoring of CNS, respiratory and cardiac functions), for up to 24 hours. In our experience, the I.V. dose takes effect within 10 minutes and lasts 30 to 60 minutes; whereas the I.M. dose takes effect within 20 minutes, and lasts up to 2 to 3 hours. The patient, therefore, requires careful, regular monitoring, both to determine the need for the antagonist, as well as to observe for possible cholinergic overload.

Using physostigmine in the anticholinergic syndrome, we usually have an alert, responsive patient within 24 hours, although careful monitoring should continue for 3 or 4 days. The alternative of using only supportive measures (which we have observed) may result in a prolonged complicated treatment course lasting up to 5 days.

We mentioned briefly that physostigmine can be valuable also diagnostically. It may be used as such when the ingestion of tricyclic antidepressants or other anticholinergics is suspected (10), and also to rule out drug-induced psychosis in patients on combinations of antipsychotic, antidepressant, and antiparkinson drugs (5, 10).

When using physostigmine in either the diagnosis or treatment of anticholinergic toxicity, the clinician must be prepared to deal with any cholinergic problems that might arise. Those of clinical importance would include hypersalivation, increased tracheo-bronchial secretions, emesis and bradycardia. If these cholinergic symptoms should occur, a parenteral quaternary ammonium anticholinergic agent, such as glycopyrrolate (Robinul) 0.4-1.0 mg., or propantheline (Probanthine) 20-30 mg. should be given to counteract them. Remember that a tertiary ammonium anticholinergic agent, such as atropine, *would* cross the blood-brain barrier, resulting in potentiation of the central effects of the original intoxicant (9, 21). It might be wise to intubate the comatose patient prior to diagnostic use of physostigmine to avoid possible emesis, though this is extremely rare with a 1-2 mg. test dose of physostigmine (10).

Although most literature reports encourage the use of physostigmine in anticholinergic toxicity, Newton (4) suggests a doubtful need for this use in routine treatment. He also reports seizures in two patients given physostigmine. However, Snyder (21), in response, emphasizes that the morbidity and mortality in these severely intoxicated patients outweigh the risk of reversible physostigmine side effects. Also, since seizures may occur during severe anticholinergic intoxication, and during the recovery period, it would be difficult to document the seizure as being physostigmine-induced (21). In our experience, one patient had a grand mal seizure ten minutes following a 2 mg. I.V. dose of physostigmine. However, he had had three such seizures prior to physostigmine administration. Also, Granacher (9) cites a report of 1727 successful reversals of central anticholinergic toxicity with no untoward effects.

B. *Naloxone (Narcan)*

Naloxone, perhaps the more widely known and used of the two pharmacologic antagonists in our discussion, is a pure narcotic antagonist. As such, it is capable of reversing the respiratory and circulatory effects of narcotic overdosage. A fact less known and appreciated is that naloxone also reverses respiratory and circulatory depression due to both propoxyphene (Darvon) and pentazocine (Talwin) (22, 23), two narcotic-like analgesics without federal narcotic controls.

Prior to the introduction of naloxone, a partial narcotic antagonist, nalorphine (Nalline) was used to reverse narcotic depression. Nalorphine, however, has some narcotic *agonist* properties, and can potentiate the CNS depressant properties of non-narcotic drugs, such as the sedative-hypnotic agents. Because naloxone is a pure *antagonist*, it can be used diagnostically in the comatose patient in whom the drug ingested is unknown. It should be given in a dose of 0.4 mg. I.V. preferably, or I.M. or S.C. This dose may be repeated at 2-3 minute intervals if necessary for 3 doses. If a narcotic was ingested one would expect to see some reversal of symptoms at this time. If the patient does not respond, one may assume that the drug ingested was an agent other than a narcotic. Naloxone has a duration of action of approximately 3-4 hours. As in the earlier discussion of the use of physostigmine in anti-cholinergic toxicity, it must be emphasized that the patient requires careful monitoring over time. The possibility exists that the duration of action of the narcotic will outlast the duration of action of naloxone resulting in a need for a repeat dose of the antagonist. Failure to recognize this may result in relapse into coma, respiratory and circulatory depression and death. This risk is particularly true in methadone overdose because of its unusually long duration of action.

It is appropriate here to mention that propoxyphene (Darvon) is little appreciated as a highly toxic agent when taken in overdose. As few as 16 capsules of 65 mg. Darvon have resulted in death due to respiratory depression. The immediate treatment, as mentioned above, is naloxone and respiratory support. The danger is that Darvon is still widely prescribed in large quantities, and is viewed by some professionals and laymen as no more than "something a little stronger than aspirin."

III. Specific Drug Families

A. Tricyclic Antidepressants

At present there are six drugs in this class: amitriptyline (Elavil), imipramine (Tofranil, Presamine), nortriptyline (Aventyl), desipramine (Norpramine, Pertofrane), protriptyline (Vivactil), and doxepin (Sinequan, Adapin). Though chemically related to the phenothiazine antipsychotics, these drugs are considerably more toxic following overdosage. They can cause death at 10-30 times the average daily therapeutic dose (1000-3000 mg.) (20). Tricyclic antidepressant overdosage, as mentioned previously, involves peripheral, cardiac and central nervous system symptoms (9, 13, 17, 20, 24-27). Specifically these are: (a) *peripheral:* dry skin and mucous membranes, facial flushing, pupils reacting poorly to light, decreased bowel motility which may progress to ileus, and urinary retention; (b) *cardiac:* tachycardia, widening of the QRS complex, nonspecific S-T changes, atrioventricular and intraventricular conduction disturbances, and serious arrhythmias which may lead to stand still; and (c) *central anticholinergic syndrome:* agitation, choreoathetoid movement, hyper- or hypo-reflexia, confusion, delirium and hallucinations, impaired recent memory, combativeness, aimless picking at bed clothes or imaginary objects, temperature abnormality (hyperthermia or hypothermia), grand mal seizures, coma, shock, respiratory depression and death. The most dangerous of this triad are cardiac arrhythmias and symptoms of the central anticholinergic syndrome (13, 20, 25-28).

Tachycardia is common to all anticholinergic agents. The remaining cardiac effects, however, are thought to be the result of a direct effect of these drugs on the conduction system, since these drugs are apparently deposited in the myocardium (26). Widening of the QRS complex, with marked S-T segment changes, may be of value in the diagnosis of unknown poisoning, suggesting possible tricyclic antidepressant overdose (25). Some late fatalities, after apparent improvement, have occurred, reportedly due to sudden cardiac arrest (28).

Treatment of severe tricyclic antidepressant overdose includes the support of respiration and the cautious use of I.V. fluids (24) (fluids impose an increased workload on the heart and may enhance the cardiac toxicity). One should attempt to remove any unabsorbed drug with repeated gastric lavage with activated charcoal "slurry." Most symptoms, with the exception of some of the serious cardiac effects, of tricyclic intoxication can be reversed by physostigmine salicylate, as described under specific antagonists. In the patient with sufficient respiratory depression to warrant intubation, we must warn against early extubation. Remember, the duration of action of the antagonist is much shorter than that of the tricyclic antidepressants, and respiratory distress may re-occur in one to two hours, requiring possible re-intubation. Seizures may be life threatening and warrant the use of diazepam (Valium) 5 to 10 mg. slow I.V., repeating if necessary. Close monitoring of respiratory function may be critical should the use of anticonvulsants become necessary, due to possible additive respiratory depression. Seizures, like fluids, increase cardiac workload and therefore may enhance the cardiotoxic effects of tricyclic antidepressants. Serious cardiac arrhythmias may require the use of lidocaine 50-100 mg. I.V. bolus, or propranolol (Inderal), 1 mg., slow I.V. Quiet surroundings aid in the control of CNS symptoms. Hyperthermia, in excess of 108°F (42°C) has been reported. Severe hypothermia, below 95°F (35°C), may also occur. These severe temperature changes require immediate treatment with appropriate cooling or heating blankets. In the event of sudden cardiac arrest, institute vigorous resuscitation. Cardiac deaths, as long as 6 days after ingestion of tricyclic antidepressants have occurred (13), suggesting patients be closely monitored for several days. Since tricyclic antidepressants are rapidly deposited in tissue, and only small amounts excreted unchanged, dialysis and forced diuresis are generally ineffective (24, 29).

Whether or not to use physostigmine in the patient experiencing less severe symptoms of the central anticholinergic syndrome such as delirium, hyperactivity, hallucinations, combativeness, etc., depends on clinical judgment. The combative patient may present a danger to himself or others. We have treated these patients with intramuscular physostigmine. The patient often becomes quiet and alert. We will repeat the dose at 2-3 hour intervals until the patient is no longer a management problem. One must also consider that the delirium and agitation may be an early symptom of a more serious overdose. Physostigmine may render the patient alert and responsive at which time he may reveal both the drug ingested and the amount. This information may affect the treatment course. On several occasions, this information correlated well with that given by the family members several hours later. Close observation of the patient, however, must still be continued.

B. *Monoamine Oxidase Inhibitors* (*MAOI's*)

To date, we have not treated an MAOI overdose. Lacking personal experience, we explored the literature for this information in order to make this discussion of overdose treatment more complete. We were surprised to find that recent literature on this subject is sparse, at least in the standard medical reference sources.

The most commonly used monoamine oxidase inhibitors are tranylcypromine (Parnate), phenelzine (Nardil), and iproniazid (Marsilid). Fatalities from tranylcypromine occurred at doses between 170 and 650 mg. Fatalities from phenelzine overdose ranged from 375 to 1500 mg. (20).

We are all aware that, due to a few deaths from the concomitant ingestion of MAOI's and sympathomimetic drugs or tyramine-containing foods and beverages, the routine use of these agents in treatment of depression greatly decreased in this country. It was interesting to learn that Shuckit et al. (30), in their personal communication with the FDA, revealed that this government organization had *no* organized file of case histories to support the warnings imposed on drug companies concerning the cautious use of these products.

Mortalities have occurred with intentional overdose of MAOI's (31), and general guidelines concerning recognition of clinical symptoms and treatment have been proposed.

Symptoms are, for the most part, an extension of pharmacological action. The MAOI's irreversibly inhibit the enzyme monoamine oxidase, resulting in an increased response to endogenous catecholamines. Central nervous system stimulation and increased neuromuscular activity are often present. Severe hypertension with cerebral vascular accidents may occur. Cardiac arrhythmias may also occur. Other symptoms reported are tachycardia, increased respiratory rate, hyperactive deep tendon reflexes, involuntary movements and coma. The most serious, life threatening effect is hyperthermia (20). It is important to remember that because of irreversible inhibition of the oxidase, and subsequent accumulation of catecholamines, there may be a significant "lag time" between drug ingestion and the development of serious toxic symptoms. Therefore, the patient should be observed for several days after suspected drug ingestion.

Treatment of MAOI poisoning is directed primarily toward conservative, supportive care. The manufacturer of tranylcypromine recommends the cautious use of phentolamine (Regitine) 5 mg. I.V. in the event of hypertensive crisis. Increased body temperature should be treated at its onset by external cooling. For excessive neuromuscular activity, the neuromuscular blocker succinylcholine has been used. Ventilation by mechanical means may be required with this treatment. Again, supportive care is of utmost importance in successful treatment.

C. Antipsychotic Agents

Drugs considered in this class are (a) the sedating phenothiazines, chlorpromazine (Thorazine), thioridazine (Mellaril) and promazine (Sparine), (b) the non-sedating phenothiazines such as perphenazine (Trilafon), fluphenazine (Prolixin) and trifluoperazine (Stelazine), and (c) other agents including the thioxanthines, chlorprothixene (Taractan) and thiothixene (Navane), and the butyrophenone haloperidol (Haldol).

A lethal dose for these antipsychotic agents has not been established. The mean dose ingested for what Davis and Termini (32) consider severe intoxication is 6230 mg. for chlorpromazine. Relatively few deaths have been attributed to the overdosage of these drugs. The number of sudden deaths in patients taking large therapeutic doses of phenothiazines such as those described by Hollister and Kosek (33) and others has recently been disputed by Peele and von Loetzen (34), who suggest many of these deaths might be attributed to what was once called "lethal catatonia" occurring in catatonics and manics. They also suggest that some of these deaths are indistinguishable from the autopsy-negative cardiac deaths in the general population.

Symptoms (32, 34, 35) attributed to overdosage of the antipsychotics include agitation, delirium, confusion, twitching, dystonic movement, convulsions, tachycardia, disturbed temperature regulation (usually hypothermia although hyperthermia sometimes occurs), hypotension, cardiovascular collapse and cardiac arrhythmias. Parkinsonism is a common feature. A hyperkinetic state is more apparent with the non-sedating phenothiazines, thioxanthines and butyrophenones than with the sedating phenothiazines.

Treatment of overdosage with these agents includes gastric lavage (most of these agents are water soluble and large amounts may be removed even many hours after ingestion (36)). Hyperthermia, if it occurs, should be treated with a cooling blanket. Hypotension can usually be managed with intravenous fluids, though sometimes may require the cautious use of levarterenol (Levophed), or another alpha adrenergic agent. Epinephrine is *contraindicated* and may potentiate hypotension (most of these drugs are alpha adrenergic blockers, therefore the beta-effects of epinephrine become predominant) (29). Parkinsonism symptoms can be treated with parenteral benztropine (Cogentin) or diphenhydramine (Benadryl) with careful monitoring for arrhythmias. Since antipsychotic drugs are highly bound to protein, and only small amounts are excreted unchanged in the urine, neither hemodialysis, peritoneal dialysis or forced diuresis are beneficial. Some patients seemingly recovering from overdosage have developed sudden late respiratory arrest, cardiac arrest or shock, so management should continue until the patient is well out of CNS depression.

D. *Barbiturates*

The barbiturates have been the drugs most often reported as the cause of poisoning in adults (15,000 hospitalized) and accounted for more than 1,000 deaths per year as reported by Shapiro in 1969 (37). This class of drugs is divided into (a) the short acting barbiturates, secobarbital (Seconal) and pentobarbital (Nembutal), (b) the intermediate acting drug amobarbital (Amytal) and (c) the long acting phenobarbital (Luminal) and mephobarbital (Mebaral). There is a greater incidence of intoxication with the short acting group than with the other two. The lethal dose (3 gm. or 3.5 mg% blood level for short acting and 5 gm. or 8 mg% blood level for long acting) of barbiturates is considered to be about 10 times their *hypnotic* dose.

Symptoms of barbiturate poisoning include drowsiness, mental confusion and ataxia which are rapidly followed by coma with shallow respirations, hypotension, cyanosis, hypothermia or hyperthermia and absent reflexes. The coma continues to deepen and is then associated with pulmonary edema and pneumonia. Death is usually due to pulmonary complications.

Before discussing specific treatment, several factors should be taken into consideration. 1) Gastric lavage is of value only if done within four hours of barbiturate ingestion. 2) Because of differences in pKa values for barbiturates (7.24 for phenobarbital, 7.75 for amobarbital and 7.90-7.96 for secobarbital and pentobarbital, respectively), alkalinization of urine by bicarbonate administration is of value only in the case of phenobarbital (29, 37), as this method will not increase the rate of excretion of the other barbiturates. 3) Since phenobarbital is excreted about 25 percent as the unchanged drug and the other agents are excreted unchanged in only minute amounts, forced diuresis is of significant value only in increasing phenobarbital excretion (29, 37-39). Also, since barbiturates stimulate ADH secretion, it is usually difficult to initiate effective water diuresis (39). 4) The use of analeptic agents is discouraged. Cerebral oxygen requirements are reduced 20 percent in barbiturate coma, therefore, attempts at CNS stimulation increase cerebral oxygen requirements and may cause seizures and greater hypoxic damage to the brain (29, 39). Lastly, while hemodialysis is a most efficient method of removing barbiturates, due to the risks of transferring patients to dialysis units, in addition to the hazards of the dialysis procedures themselves, there has been shown no significant reduction in mortality when compared to treatment employing conservative measures (29, 37-39). This procedure should be reserved for the gravest situations, in which severe cardiovascular depression, renal or liver failure occurs (29, 37-39).

Treatment of barbiturate poisoning with regimens employing conservative measures and good supportive care have proven to be the most successful (29, 37-41). Maintain an adequate airway. Give positive pressure respiratory support with room air or the judicious use of oxygen to patients with respiratory depression. The patient should be positioned with his head 15° lower than his feet. Pulmonary care should include tracheal suction and frequent turning. Delay further drug absorption in the conscious patient using repeated lavage using activated charcoal 50 gm. in 400 ml. of water. Give a cathartic of 60 ml. of either 50 percent magnesium sulfate or Fleets Phosphosoda to facilitate passage of unabsorbed drug through the G.I. tract (remember that lavage is of doubtful value 4 hours following ingestion of drug). Give I.V. fluids, catheterize the patient and maintain an accurate intake and output record. Maintain electrolyte balance. If phenobarbital is ingested, forced diuresis may be helpful: Give dextrose 5% in 0.45% sodium chloride to maintain diuresis of 400 ml./hr. with careful monitoring of central venous pressure and electrolytes; add one amp (50 meq) of sodium bicarbonate to every other bottle to promote pH dependent alkaline diuresis, and monitor blood pH. Sputum and urine cultures should be obtained routinely as pneumonia and urinary tract infections are common complications. Appropriate antibiotics are used depending on culture and sensitivity studies. Record vital signs frequently. Again, good supportive care offers the best survival rate following barbiturate poisoning.

E. Benzodiazepines

The drugs representing this class are chlordiazepoxide (Librium), diazepam (Valium), oxazepam (Serax), chlorazepate (Tranxene), clonazepam (Clonopin), and flurazepam (Dalmane). Benzodiazepines have been available on the commercial market since 1960. These agents are among the most widely used drugs in clinical medicine today. Like all sedative-hypnotic drugs, their abuse potential is high. It is fortunate that the benzodiazepines also have the highest safety index of all CNS depressant drugs. It has been stated often in the literature that there have been no successful suicides when benzodiazepines alone were ingested. As late as 1972, twelve years after the introduction of this drug class into clinical medicine, Greenblatt and Shader (42), in a review of sedative-hypnotic drugs, stated that "fatal doses seldom, if ever, occur." Doses of 2250 mg. of chlordiazepoxide and 1400 mg. of diazepam have been ingested in unsuccessful suicide attempts. In the 1975 edition of Goodman and Gilman (6) it is stated that a few deaths *have* been reported with overdose. Considering their widespread use and abuse, one can only say that this group of drugs has a remarkable margin of safety. When benzodiazepines are combined with other depressant drugs or alcohol, additive effects may occur with possible fatal outcome.

Symptoms of overdose with this class of depressives include drowsiness, weakness, nystagmus, and incoordination. Coma, when it occurs, is usually light and has good prognosis. Conservative treatment with good supportive care is the most effective treatment for pure benzodiazepine ingestion.

F. Glutethimide (Doriden)

Glutethimide must be considered as one of the *most toxic* hypnotic agents available for use today. The mortality rate of patients taking 20 tablets or more has been reported as 45 percent (43). The fatal dose then is considered to be about 10 gm. for the average 70 kg. man.

Symptoms of overdosage are somewhat similar to those of barbiturate poisoning, with emphasis placed on hypotension (29), which is characteristic of glutethimide intoxication. Circulatory shock poses a major therapeutic challenge. Widely dilated pupils, paralytic ileus and urinary retention are also characteristic, all due to the strong anticholinergic effects of the drug (29). Hyperthermia may occur. Central nervous system depression ranges from minimal drowsiness to prolonged coma of up to 100 hours, and there is little correlation between blood level and clinical course of therapy (44).

Several factors must be taken into consideration which are of importance in diagnosis and treatment of glutethimide overdosage. A convulsive phenomenon may develop during the recovery phase of acute toxicity, which is not yet understood. Also, cyclic changes in CNS depression may occur, and sudden apneic episodes with death may occur. Several hypotheses have been offered to explain this cyclic course: 1) low solubility of the drug in the gut (29), 2) the delayed absorption of the drug due to paralytic ileus (29, 44), 3) possible hepatic recycling of deconjugated glutethimide (29), and 4) being lipid soluble, glutethimide is deposited in the fatty tissues, to be re-released when blood levels are lowered. Recently, Hanson et al. reported that a metabolite of glutethimide, referred to as 4-HG (4-hydroxy-2-ethel-2-phenylglutaramide) was discovered and found to be a potent CNS depressant (45). The accumulation of this metabolite, in addition to the already mentioned factors complicating the clinical course, further emphasizes the seriousness of glutethimide intoxication.

Since glutethimide is metabolized by the liver and only insignificant quantities are excreted in the urine (46), forced diuresis is of little value in treatment. Hemodialysis has been used in treatment with questionable results. The conservative approach used in 70 patients treated by Chazan et al. (44) and 31 patients treated by Wright et al. (47) successfully without the use of dialysis, as well as the questionable techniques used in identifying the drug in the dialysate (does not distinguish active drug from metabolites), suggests that the use of hemodialysis is rarely, if ever, indicated in the treatment of glutethimide poisoning.

Treatment involves the initiation of good supportive care as described for barbiturate poisoning. Since glutethimide is lipid soluble, gastric lavage with large volumes of castor oil is of value *at any time* following ingestion of the drug. Lavage is followed by giving 60 ml. of castor oil or Phosphosoda for catharsis. Prior to lavage, intubation with a cuffed endotracheal tube is indicated to avoid lipid aspiration. Severe hypotension should be treated with vasopressors: 1) metaraminol (Aramine) 1 ml. (10 mg.) diluted to 10 ml. with dextrose 5% in water by I.V. push; metaraminol 4 ml. (40 mg.) in 500 ml. dextrose 5% in water dripped at 1-2 ml/min.; or levarterenol 16 mg. in 100 ml. of dextrose 5% in water and titrated to keep systolic pressure above 100 mm Hg. Intravenous fluids should be given with careful monitoring of central venous pressure. Control body temperature by external cooling if necessary to treat hyperthermia. We share with many the opinion that glutethimide should be removed from the commercial market.

G. *Meprobamate*

Meprobamate is marketed as Equanil, Miltown, Meprospan, Kesso-Bamate, etc. It is also marketed generically by several manufacturers. The lethal dose of this drug is difficult to estimate. In their review of meprobamate poisonings, Davis et al. (32, 36) found that while several deaths occurred at doses of 12 to 20 gms., 113 patients survived single doses from 12 to 40 gms. Severe toxicity with possible death must be considered at doses of 10 to 20 times the normal daily dose.

Symptoms of meprobamate overdose are often difficult to distinguish from those of other depressants. Overdose is characterized by coma, hypotensive reactions, slow pulse, low body temperature and occasional atelectasis (29, 32, 36). These effects may in part be due to the muscle relaxing properties of meprobamate (36). Shock and pulmonary edema are the most troublesome complications.

Treatment of meprobamate overdose is similar to that for barbiturates. Intravenous fluids must be administered carefully to avoid pulmonary edema. If severe hypotension occurs, the judicious use of vasopressors, such as metaraminol, may be warranted. Usually a conservative approach, with good surveillance and nursing care, allows complete recovery. Although meprobamate is effectively removed from the body by dialysis (48), this method should be considered only in severe intoxications complicated by hepatic or renal failure. Meprobamate is removed by liver metabolism and urinary excretion at rates much faster than either barbiturates and glutethimide, a fact that should be kept in mind when considering dialysis (29).

H. *Chloral Hydrate*

This drug is marketed as Noctec, Somnos, Felsules, and also generically by several manufacturers. The lethal dose for adults is approximately 10 gms., although death has been reported from as little as 4 gm., and some have survived doses of 30 gms. (49).

Symptoms of chloral hydrate overdose are similar to those of barbiturate poisoning. Pupils may be pinpoint as with morphine overdose. Large doses may cause hemorrhagic gastritis and enteritis (35, 40). Icterus due to hepatic damage and albuminuria from renal irritation may occur (49).

Acute poisoning may occur from the combination of chloral

hydrate and alcohol, the so-called "Mickey Finn." Sellers et al. (50) studied this interaction in man and found that when chloral hydrate and alcohol are taken together, each agent inhibits the metabolic degradation of the other, with increased blood levels of both compounds, resulting in greater CNS depression than when either is taken alone.

The treatment of chloral hydrate poisoning parallels that for barbiturate poisoning.

I. *Miscellaneous Depressants*

This group includes methyprylon (Noludar), methaqualone (Quaalude, Sopor, Parest, Somnafac) and ethchlorvynol (Placidyl). Overdosage with these drugs should be treated by the conservative approach described for barbiturate poisoning.

J. *Lithium Carbonate*

This agent, used to treat the manic-depressive psychotic, is marketed as Eskalith, Lithane and Lithionate. Mortality with this agent is better related to blood levels than dosage. Severe toxicity may occur at blood levels above 2.0 meq/L (51).

Overdosage is manifested primarily by CNS symptoms. Consciousness is severely impaired and coma with total unresponsiveness often develops. Other clinical symptoms are: hypertonic or rigid muscles with hyperactive deep tendon reflexes; muscle tremor or fasciculations, spontaneous attacks of hyperextension of extremities, often combined with wide opening of the eyes, grunting and grasping, and epileptic seizures. Pulmonary complications include atelectasis and/or pneumonia (29, 52). It should be noted that in the presence of sodium and/or water depletion, these toxic effects may appear at "therapeutic" blood levels (53). It is interesting to note that most literature fails to discuss the direct cardiotoxic effects of lithium, described as interstitial myocarditis (54). This mechanism needs further exploration.

In the management of lithium toxicity, the most important principle is care of the comatose patient, with emphasis on prevention of pneumonia. No specific antidote is known. Emphasis is placed on restoring fluid and electrolyte balance. Sodium bicarbonate, acetazolamide (Diamox) and aminophylline are reported to increase lithium excretion, and are probably worth trying when toxicity occurs in patients with normal renal function (29, 55).

REFERENCES

1. POKORNY, A. D.: Myths about suicide. In H. L. P. Resnik (Ed.), Suicidal Behaviors. Diagnosis and Management. Boston: Little Brown, 1968, p. 57.
2. RESNIK, H. L. P. (Ed.): Suicidal Behaviors. Diagnosis and Management. Boston: Little Brown, 1968.
3. RESNIK, H. L. P. and HATHORNE, B. C. (Eds.): Suicide Prevention in the 70's. DHEW Publication No. (HSM) 72-9054. Washington, D. C.: U.S. Government Printing Office, 1973.
4. NEWTON, R. W.: Physostigmine salicylate in the treatment of tricyclic antidepressant overdosage. J.A.M.A., 231:941, 1975.
5. EL-YOUSEF, M. K., JANOWSKY, D. S., DAVIS, J. M. and SEKERKE, H. J.: Reversal of antiparkinsonian drug toxicity by physostigmine: A controlled study. Amer. J. Psychiat., 130:141, 1973.
6. BYCK, R.: Drugs and the treatment of psychiatric disorders. In L. S. Goodman and A. Gilman (Eds.), The Pharmacological Basis of Therapeutics. New York: Macmillan Co., 1975, p. 192.
7. Handbook of Nonprescription Drugs. American Pharmaceutical Association, 1974.
8. DUVOISIN, R. C. and KATZ, R.: Reversal of central anticholinergic syndrome in man by physostigmine. J.A.M.A., 206:1963, 1968.
9. GRANACHER, R. P. and BALDESSARINI, R. J.: Physostigmine—Its use in acute anticholinergic syndrome with antidepressant and antiparkinson drugs. Arch. Gen. Psychiat., 32:375, 1975.
10. SNYDER, B. D.: Physostigmine—Antidote for anticholinergic poisoning. Minnesota Medicine, 58:456, 1975.
11. BERNARDS, W.: Case History Number 74: Reversal of phenothiazine-induced coma with physostigmine. Anesthesia and Analgesia, 52:938, 1973.
12. BURKS, J. S., WALKER, J. E., RUMACK, B. H. and OTT, J. E.: Tricyclic antidepressant poisoning. J.A.M.A., 230:1405, 1974.
13. SLOVIS, T. L., OTT, J. E., TEITELBAUM, D. T. and LIPSCOMB, W.: Physostigmine therapy in acute tricyclic antidepressant poisoning. Clinical Toxicology, 5:451-459, 1971.
14. SNYDER, B. D., BLONDE, L. and MCWHIRTER, W. R.: Reversal of amitriptyline intoxication by physostigmine. J.A.M.A., 230: 1433, 1974.

15. HUSSEY, H. H.: Physostigmine: Value in treatment of central toxic effects of anticholinergic drugs. *J.A.M.A.*, 231:1066, 1975.
16. HEISER, J. F. and WILBERT, D. E.: Reversal of delirium induced by tricyclic antidepressant drugs with physostigmine. *Amer. J. Psychiat.*, 131:1275, 1974.
17. GREENBLATT, D. J. and SHADER, R. I.: Drug therapy—Anticholinergics. *New Engl. J. Med.*, 288:1215, 1973.
18. EL-YOUSEF, M. K., JANOWSKY, D. S., DAVIS, J. M. and SEKERKE, H. J.: Reversal of benztropine toxicity by physostigmine. *J.A.M.A.*, 220:125, 1972.
19. KOELLE, G. B.: Anticholinesterase agents. *In* L. S. Goodman and A. Gilman (Eds.), *The Pharmacological Basis of Therapeutics*. New York: Macmillan Co., 1975, pp. 445-466.
20. DAVIS, J. M., BARTLETT, E. and TERMINI, B. A.: Overdosage of psychotropic drugs: A review, Part II: Antidepressants and other psychotropic agents. *Dis. Nerv. Syst.*, April, 1968, p. 246.
21. SNYDER, B. D.: Physostigmine and anticholinergic poisoning. *J.A.M.A.*, 233:1165, 1975. (Letter to Editor.)
22. EVANS, L. E. J., SWAINSON, C. P., ROSCOE, P. and PRESCOTT, L. F.: Treatment of drug overdosage with naloxone, a specific narcotic antagonist. *Lancet, March*, 1973, p. 452.
23. VLASSES, P. H. and FRAKER, T.: Naloxone for propoxyphene overdosage. *J.A.M.A.*, 229:1167, 1974. (Letter to Editor.)
24. DAVIS, J. M. and TERMINI, B. A.: Attempted suicide with psychotropic drugs: Diagnosis and treatment. (Part two of two parts.) *Medical Counterpoint*, September 1969, p. 59.
25. BARNES, R. J., KONG, S. M. and WU, R. W. Y.: Electrocardiographic changes in amitriptyline poisoning. *Brit. Med. J.*, July, 1968, p. 222.
26. COULL, D. C., CROOKS, J., DINGWALL-FORDYCE, I., SCOTT, A. M. and WEIR, R. D.: Amitriptyline and cardiac disease. *Lancet*, September 1970, p. 590.
27. KANTOR, S. J., BIGGER, J. T., GLASSMAN, A. H., MACKEN, D. L. and PEREL, J. M.: Imipramine-induced heart block. A longitudinal case study. *J.A.M.A.*, 231:1364, 1975.
28. ALEXANDER, C. S. and NINO, A.: Cardiovascular complications in young patients taking psychotropic drugs. *Amer. Heart J.*, 78: 757, 1969.
29. MORRELLI, H. F.: Rational therapy of drug overdose. *In* K. L. Melmon and H. F. Morrelli (Eds.), *Clinical Pharmacology; Basic Principles in Therapeutics*. New York: Macmillan Co., 1972, pp. 605-623.
30. SCHUCKIT, M., ROBINS, E. L. and FEIGHNER, J.: Tricyclic antidepressants and monoamine oxidase inhibitors. Combination therapy in the treatment of depression. *Arch. Gen. Psychiat.*, 24:509, 1971.
31. CIOCATTO, E., FAGIANO, G. and BAVA, G. L.: Clinical features and

treatment of overdosage of monoamine oxidase inhibitors and their interaction with other psychotropic drugs. *Resuscitation*, 1:69, 1972.

32. DAVIS, J. M. and TERMINI, B. A.: Attempted suicide with psychotropic drugs: Diagnosis and treatment (Part one of two parts). *Medical Counterpoint*, July/August, 1969, p. 43.

33. HOLLISTER, L. E. and KOSEK, J. C.: Sudden death during treatment with phenothiazine derivatives. *J.A.M.A.*, 192:93, 1965.

34. PEELE, R. and VON LOETZEN, I. S.: Phenothiazine deaths: A critical review. *Amer. J. Psychiat.*, 130:306, 1973.

35. GLEASON, M. N., GOSSELIN, R. E., HODGE, H. C. and SMITH, R. P. (Eds.): *Clinical Toxicology of Commercial Products*. Williams & Wilkins, 1971, pp. 69-72.

36. DAVIS, J. M., BARTLETT, E. and TERMINI, B. A.: Overdosage of psychotropic drugs: A review. Part I: Major and minor tranquilizers. *Dis. Nerv. Syst.*, March 1968, p. 157.

37. SHAPIRO, F. L. and SMITH, H. T.: The treatment of barbiturate intoxication. *Modern Medicine*, April 1969, p. 104.

38. HADDEN, J., JOHNSON, K., SMITH, S., PRICE, L. and GIARDINA, E.: Acute barbiturate intoxication. Concepts of management. *J.A.M.A.*, 209:893, 1969.

39. SETTER, J. G., MAHER, J. F., and SCHREINER, G. E.: Barbiturate intoxication. Evaluation of therapy including dialysis in a large series selectively referred because of severity. *Arch. Intern. Med.*, 117:224, 1966.

40. ARENA, J. M.: Acute miscellaneous poisoning. *In* H. F. Conn (Ed.), *Current Therapy*. Philadelphia: Saunders, 1973, pp. 874-878.

41. DREISBACH, R. H.: *Handbook of Poisoning: Diagnosis and Treatment*. Lange Medical Publication, 1974, pp. 278-284.

42. GREENBLATT, D. J. and SHADER, R. I.: The clinical choice of sedative-hypnotics. *Annals of Int. Med.*, 77:91-100, 1972.

43. SHARPLESS, S. K.: Hypnotics and sedatives. *In* L. S. Goodman and A. Gilman (Eds.), *The Pharmacological Basis of Therapeutics*. New York: Macmillan Co., 1970, pp. 121-134.

44. CHAZAN,, J. A. and GARELLA, S.: Glutethimide intoxication. A prospective study of 70 patients treated conservatively without hemodialysis. *Arch. Intern. Med.*, 128:215, 1971.

45. HANSEN, A. R., KENNEDY, K. A., AMBRE, J. J. and FISCHER, L. J.: Glutethimide poisoning. A metabolite contributes to morbidity and mortality. *New Engl. J. Med.*, 292:250, 1975.

46. CURRY, S. H., RIDDALL, D., GORDON, J. S., SIMPSON, P., BINNS, T. B., RONDEL, R. K. and MCMARTIN, C.: Disposition of glutetimide in man. *Clin. Pharmacol. Ther.*, 12:849, 1971.

47. WRIGHT, N. and ROSCOE, P.: Acute glutethimide poisoning. Conservative management of 31 patients. *J.A.M.A.*, 214:1704, 1970.

48. MADDOCK, R. K. and BLOOMER, H. A.: Meprobamate overdosage. Evaluation of its severity and methods of treatment. *J.A.M.A.*, 201:123, 1967.
49. HARVEY, S. C.: Hypnotics and sedatives. *In* L. S. Goodman and A. Gilman (Eds.), *The Pharmacological Basis of Therapeutics*. New York: Macmillan, 1975, p. 124-136.
50. SELLERS, C. M., LANG, M., KOCK-WESER, J., LeBLANC, E. and KALANT, H.: Interaction of choral hydrate and ethanol in man, Parts I and II. *Clin. Pharmacol. Ther.*, Jan/Feb. 1972.
51. FRY, D. E. and MARKS, V.: Value of plasma-lithium monitoring. *Lancet*, May 1971, p. 886.
52. AOKE, F. Y. and RUEDY, J.: Severe lithium intoxication: Management without dialysis and report of a possible teratogenic effect of lithium. *Can. Med. Assoc. J.*, 105:847, 1971.
53. LAPIERRE, Y. D.: Lithium intoxication. *Can. Med. Assoc. J.*, 106: 112, 1972. (Letter to Editor.)
54. TSENG, H. L.: Interstitial myocarditis probably related to lithium carbonate intoxication. *Arch. Pathology*, 92:444, 1971.
55. Lithium Carbonate: Package insert. Smith, Kline and French, Roerig and Rowell.

12

Notes on the Psychodynamic Treatment of Childhood Depressions

Carl P. Malmquist, M.D.

Several similarities and differences are present in depressions when they occur in children as contrasted with adults. These points need clarification and they will be elucidated to the extent needed to understand treatment approaches with this age group. It contributes to conceptual confusion and therapeutic mistakes when the differences are not made clear. Rather than simply pose a suggestive list of symptoms and signs of childhood depression, which are still a matter of ongoing work and debate, the emphasis is on a contrast between adults and children who become depressed, and points on psychodynamic treatment. Obviously until we get to a point where sophisticated and experienced clinicians can agree on what childhood depressions are, let alone if they exist, therapies of all sorts remain tentative. Elsewhere I have dealt in great detail with some of the diverse manifestations of depression in children (1).

GENERAL POINTS

1. Foremost, there is a need to keep in mind a developmental framework in work with children. In recent years the term "develop-

mental" has been bandied about a good deal but without clarification of its diverse meanings. While some writers use the term to refer to landmarks of development as correlated with chronological age, others use it for prominent historical events of an individual's life history. Most meaningful with a potentially or already depressed child, is to use a model of the developmental stage of ego functioning for a particular child at a particular time. Using this type of framework, a clinician can evaluate which symptoms, signs and alterations are relevant to evaluation of childhood depressions.

2. Another question of great importance in the treatment of childhood depressions is: Do children really get depressed? The therapeutic implications from the answer to this question need hardly be mentioned. Nor is the question simply rhetorical. Those unsophisticated with theoretical issues in the context of the psychological development of children too readily dismiss this type of question as naive, pointing to the sad affect children manifest as prima facie evidence that children do in fact get depressed. However, this misses the crucial theoretical point in the debate: The experience of depressive affect is not equivalent to the presence of a clinical depression in a child anymore than in an adult. If that is so, what should be prescribed as treatment will obviously differ.

Since we would not want to treat all children who experience sad affect for depression, just who should we treat? As a common example, consider the pre-Oedipal or preschool child who has sustained some type of loss experience. Since this is not an uncommon phenomenon among children by way of divorce, separation, desertion or abandonment in their environment, it allows us to study some rather typical behavioral responses. In the quite young child, a collection of somatopsychic responses get reported, such as sad facies, lethargy, withdrawal, and failure to thrive (2). A variety of direct physical expressions is possible particularly involving the gastrointestinal system or skin disturbances. As the child ages a bit more, he is able physically to move away from whatever seems to be experienced as pain. Hence, a child might find that being with a depressed parent is a painful experience, so that withdrawal from the parent is practiced in turn from their lack of responsiveness to him. The model is then laid down for actively withdrawing as a relief mechanism from pain in general, but more specifically from the emotional pain of sadness with respect to experiencing depressive affect. The picture of a child relying on activity, or hyperactivity, as defensive maneuvers to cope with pain are then witnessed on many levels. Nor is this dissimilar from depressed adults who seek endless engagements in causes and activities as a way of running from their depressions.

What changes over time in such a child? Unquestionably, an increasing degree of complexity in ego functions occurs. Such functions as how events are perceived, their context in different life events, the ability to contain affect, to withhold direct motor discharges from as ready a release, all evolve. These functions all have relevance to coping with depressive affect. However, while some theorists say that such ego functioning is needed before a true clinical depression can occur, this seems to be more of a relative matter rather than an all-or-nothing phenomenon. Hence, while maturation in cognitive ego functioning, including memory, is needed to recall the formal aspects of past events, it is not necessary to the production of a depressive core in a child. A key question is: At what point do we diagnose a child, who continues to experience depressive affect, as having a clinical depression?

A similar type of argument is present involving children at the Oedipal (and post-Oedipal) levels. Again, some argue that clinical depressions in childhood do not really begin until the sadness associated with Oedipal disappointments can be experienced. This position ties in the propensity to react with depression to the disruption of a romanticized closeness in Oedipal attachments. The resultant loss is experienced as a sense of defeat and disappointment. This means that for this group of theorists on the nature of childhood depression, when these developments have occurred, the child is ready to elaborate with depressive responses to other kinds of disappointments. There is also the emergence of overidealized images of parental figures with whom the child identifies. These events parallel the structuralization of a more delineated type of superego structure. An enhanced self-punitiveness may result as well as an ego-ideal which will be difficult to reach. However, some even want to wait until the adolescent period before committing themselves to the possibility that such a clinical state is possible. This is presumably based on the degree of helplessness and hopelessness which is not seen as attaining sufficient clinical intensity until then (3). Of course, which viewpoint one embraces on the nature of childhood depression has some direct correlates with what one believes is needed therapeutically.

3. Some writers differentiate sharply the types of defenses used in adults who get depressed compared to the defenses used by children. Conceding many differences in adult mental functioning from children, one can still remain impressed with how similar many of the defenses used by adults and children are despite different levels of concealment and sophistication. Consider one of the most common examples used by those who argue against the validity of diagnosing clinical depressions until the adolescent age period is reached. They cite the frequent case of children struggling with painful affects relating to a loss. such as helplessness and despair. These critics of childhood depressions point to the increased activity level as the type of defensive effort employed by children to cope with the pain, as though this is not present in adult depressions. However, this appears to be a similar manifestation of dealing with depressive affect as witnessed in an untold number of adults who become depressed as well. In fact, this may be a description of one of the largest categories of adolescent and college age youth who become depressed. The popular resort to drugs or alcohol, the need to be bombarded by many external stimuli, and the rather aimless and tenuous attachment to different groups seem to comprise a large number of depressed young people. Nor do these kinds of activity defenses for dealing with depression disappear once past the period of youth. The flight from painful affect by way of resorting to devices to give reassurance that happiness can be restored often persists. This is one of the reasons why the goal of continuing treatment, once the acute aspects of a depression have been lifted,

becomes more difficult. It is not only that the pain is lifted, but that the psychotherapeutic process raises the spector of bringing the pain back. While children resort to denial and avoidance mechanisms more readily than adults, the prevalence of such mechanisms in an adult population of depressives is equally striking.

Substitute gratifications are another measure to avoid resolving depressive conflicts. These are not as readily satisfying to a child as was once thought; nor are substitute objects as readily available as might be thought. In fact, once object constancy is obtained (at approximately 18 to 36 months), the ability to "plug in" replacements is severely compromised (4). Those who treat children know that a complacent and quiet child is not necessarily one freed from aspects of depression. Nor is it infrequent to see latency-age children with compulsive personality organization dealing with their depressive affect in such a manner analogous to their adult counterparts (5).

4. Confusion abounds when talking about the processes attendant upon childhood mourning versus those in a childhood depression. Mourning is a necessary reaction in the human being once a level of object constancy has been obtained. Thereafter a child must struggle with loss and separation in the external world with accompanying changes in the internal psychological world, depending upon the child's stage of psychological development beyond object constancy.

So many discussions of childhood mourning seem to focus on the reactions of the child to death. Even including reactions to divorce and separation does not do justice to the diverse types of experiences to which children must repeatedly react with the psychological processes of mourning. Some varieties of loss are environmental; some are consequent to developmental changes in the child and adolescent. Difficulties in mourning can often show up as developmental distortions, somatic manifestations (headaches, abdominal complaints, and overeating), learning problems, as well as degrees of experiencing sadness. Mourning can be facilitated by taking a perspective on these symptomatic manifestations which permits mourning to be initiated and then proceed. Again, the question arises, should chronic states of mourning be diagnosed as depression, as they are in adults, when they are not handled with the degree of reparation, restitution, and resolution which mourning requires within a given time period?

5. If depression is viewed as a state experienced by the ego, a variety of responses is called into play. What is the state that the ego is experiencing? As noted, in the young child of preschool age, we can observe a variety of somatic and motor activities which are used to help dispel the pain associated with loss and deprivation. But, once self-observing and self-critical functions develop in the personality, there is the mixed blessing of reacting to oneself with lowered self-esteem accompanied by self-criticism. What appears as accompaniments in the child are expressions of inferiority and guilt (the "I can't do" and "I'm no good" variations of verbalizations).

Bibring, in an attempt to shift the understanding of depression from a focus on oral fixation, libido, and even the role of aggression, elaborated upon the affective state experienced by the ego in terms of its helplessness and the quasi-paralysis of its functioning (6). It is as though the anxiety aroused to meet a threat has itself been subsumed under either defensive measures of withdrawal which can ultimately become a type of "giving up" complex. This type of response has enormous consequences for the physical and emotional integrity of the child. But the key element is the self-esteem component which regulates how far a regression will progress or, for a child, how defective the self-concept was to begin with. Although external events such as loss of a parent, or a depressed parent in the environment, contribute to vulnerabilities in the regulation of self-esteem, there are many subtle phenomena which the ego of the child becomes sensitized to in terms of rejections and rebuffs. Perhaps one of the important variables is not only an unhappy and depressed parent to whom the child is exposed beyond a transient period of time, but the child's sensing the unhappiness or unmet needs of an important adult in his life. Even more is this so if the child begins to feel responsible for the unhappy predicament in those on whom he is dependent for nurturance and, in addition, his well-being.

In the young child, when the personality has differentiated sufficiently so that mourning and giving up the painful object can occur, the damage is done in terms of leaving a high residue of ambivalence. A lack of "fit" or resonance between parental figures and children contributes to diminished self-esteem and such ambivalence (7). Further, there has often been some type of narcissistic impairment such that the child is left seeking repair by way of seeking over-idealized and over-evaluated replacements in others throughout his life. Some children are left struggling with problems of narcissistic slight based on an overinflated but hurt self (8). Other children have problems in differentiating the self from other objects, which can occur at quite an early age. These supersensitive and fragile children are prone to later severe depressions including psychotic depressions. This group is not to be confused with schizophrenic or autistic children even though there may be withdrawal and depersonalization. In the older child of latency age, the damage is done in terms of problems of guilt and their proneness to guilt-based depressions. The child who can experience genuine guilt over transgressions, and can then reintegrate his self-concept by subsequent expiatory efforts, gives us an example of a more integrated superego system in the process of development.

TREATMENT POINTS

1. Children with depression, and with conscious guilt associated with specific behavior, offer a very good prognosis with respect to cathartic therapy with clarification. This is not yet on the level of internalized neurotic conflict although it may become so. When the behavior reflects unconscious guilt, the child may respond by alleviation of certain discomfort via catharsis, but the pattern of guilt-ridden behavior continues. This usually means a call for more intensive treatment and the need for working through.

2. Children in whom shame is prominently associated with the depression have usually been subjected to a good deal of ridicule,

scorn, and intimations that they and their efforts at achievement are intrinsically unacceptable. They believe in the minimal value of themselves and everything associated with them. Consequently, their depression is often concealed behind defenses of guarding themselves from others so that no one will see how defective they are. These children require more extensive treatment because of the defects in their ego ideal formation and self-concept systems.

3. Various types of affect are experienced by the depressed child, and these, coupled with the difficulties in recognizing this condition, create a puzzling phenomenon. I have dealt elsewhere in great detail with some of the diverse expressions of depression in children with the problems these raise for treatment. It is important to know these diverse manifestations so that detection of the situation is not ignored or missed. The component of lowered self-esteem is crucial. While some emphasize object loss as noted above, my own impression is that this type of loss takes its toll in terms of children's not being able to deal with the disappointment and disillusionment that losses entail. Furthermore, the effect of the loss seems mediated by a lowering of self-esteem. It is specious to debate childhood depression in terms of lowered self-esteem versus object loss, since they are both present and ultimately mediated by ego mechanisms. Further, there are many varieties of destructive mechanisms against the self, such as putting oneself down or unwittingly "losing out" on opportunities that present themselves for self-enhancement. Faced with such an ego state, the child calls into play various devices (adaptive or maladaptive) to cope with his predicament. In terms of treatment, these maneuvers may not be seen in perspective, and worked on as responses to depression. One common example is the *aggressive child* whose overtly provocative behavior is seen solely in terms of hyperactivity or hyperaggressiveness, while the defensive nature of such behavior as a protection against painful feelings about himself is missed.

Similarly, the *passive aggressive child* who is manifesting a variety of procrastination techniques in refusing to learn, is to be seen as attempting to repair a damaged self-concept and not let anyone be aware of his private hurts. Conversely, the *overachieving youngster* who has a pressing need to be number one in most activities might be dealing with attempts to ward off depressive affect. A 13-year-old girl had been a class leader and highly praised for all her academic accomplishments during elementary school years. In junior high school she was one among many similarly talented and ambitious adolescent girls. Finding all her tasks now more difficult, and "for the first time since I started school" not being a standout, she became despondent and withdrawn. When she began to overeat, a consultation was requested. In the course of treatment she was able to recall similar feelings at the time she began school when multiple new events had displaced her, such as a sibling's birth, and the realization that she was not really the center of her parent's life as she had then believed. Perhaps one of the most commonly missed situations of depression in the young adolescent is seen in the utilization of drugs and alcohol to handle a depressed state. This therapeutic error is often compounded by many community groups which focus on chemical dependency problems, in some sort of unarticulated framework in which drug usage is seen as the problem and psychological conflict is ignored. A follow-up on these mistreated adolescents into their adulthood would be well worth our while.

SPECIFIC TREATMENT QUESTIONS

The treatment implications from these different ego states can be summarized as follows:

1. The young child who is reacting to depressed adults in his environment, as a major contributing factor to his own depressed state, needs assessment of the level of intensity and appropriate treatment based on this knowledge. It seems obvious that treatment of one or more of the adults, and perhaps the family unit, is needed.

2. The child who appears integrated with a neurotic personality organization, with guilt prominent on a conscious and unconscious level, needs psychotherapy (as any neurotic child) to forestall the consequences of this burden on his development. In all of these situations the need to keep "superego pathology" in mind is important with respect to treatment.

3. A child who appears severely depressed in terms of self-concept deficiencies and guilt-proneness needs intensive treatment to deal with these aspects of himself. In the absence of treatment, there will be an impairment in his development and later functioning as an adult. Not only will he remain depressive-prone, but characterological traits, related to rigidly compulsive defensives or masochistic aspects, are likely. In the presence of shameful aspects of the self, the potential for chronically defective self-esteem regulation is present. Persistent quests for idealized figures go on with the usual disillusionments when the experience is that a loved object has again failed.

4. There is another implication in treating depressed children which needs emphasis: the importance of the family and general environment. Many of these comments apply to treatment of children for any condition, but they have special meaning for depressed children no matter which treatment approach is used. This is not only because of epidemiological and clinical data about the significance of loss of parents as correlated with later depressive reactions in people. It is also from the identification and symbiosis between parental moods, attitudes, and disappointments and what the child experiences in himself. There are also transference and countertransference aspects occurring in the course of treatment which deal with how the psychiatrist perceives and reacts to situations of hopelessness and helplessness in others. This means that somewhere in the course of treatment, the child will express directly (as well as indirectly through defenses) states of depletion, impairment and feelings of emptiness. What does this mean? It means that some of these depressed children have a deep need and hope for an experience of trust and symbiosis with an idealized adult in treatment. When these do not materialize to the idealized degree, a situation of disillusionment gets repeated within the context of the treatment situation itself. This makes difficulties for the adult treater as well as the child treated, especially from the threat and actuality of acting out behavior in the transference but more likely in his environment.

The adult therapist mobilizes his own defenses against letting a child experience suffering again even under therapeutic conditions. It also requires therapeutic acumen in constantly assessing how much depressive affect and reenactment the child should be allowed without the need for unnecessary suffering. However, there is also the need for sufficient experiencing of these painful affects so that working through of old and unresolved conflicts will proceed. Of course, a realistic factor with children is that everything is not in the past. Factors promoting depressive lines of development may be ongoing influences at the present time. While this may be handled by treatment of the parents individually or in family sessions, the ongoing destructive pattern may yet continue. Explicitly, a depressed parent may stay depressed; a divorced parent stays divorced and relatively absent; a parent reenacting parental hate based on his or her own origins continues this with one of his own children. Yet, the child still remains dependent on this adult in a very realistic manner. It is not just a historical working through that is going on in treatment.

5. Among the many types of treatment modalities currently used, are there any that should receive exclusive emphasis for depressed children? Again, a need for consideration of many extraneous factors is needed, such as the availability of a skilled treater, financial means, degree of acute distress, a need for intervention beyond the primary child-patient, etc. Beyond this there is now such a repertoire of treatments in practice, it would take a textbook just to describe them, let alone evaluate the conflicting evidence for their efficacy (9). The comments made in this paper are obviously directed toward some of the psychotherapeutic aspects of treating depressed children. This is not to deny that certain psychopharmacological treatments may not be helpful as adjuncts. In some depressed children who are experiencing a good deal of anxiety, phenothiazine medications may alleviate anxiety and promote the opportunity to deal with the types of defenses which are warding off depressive affect. Although the reports on the use of antidepressant medications with children are meager, at this time they do not appear to be well-validated but rather exist more on a research

level. This is understandable in view of the criteria for the diagnosis
of childhood depressions remaining vague in themselves and needing
clarification.

6. A final point in dealing with depressed children is not to underestimate the value of environmental experiences which can raise the
self-esteem of children. While I believe I have emphasized the ultimate desirability of working through therapy when indicated, and
resolving the symptoms present, which are geared toward avoiding
the pain of depressive effect, the value of improving by way of
a sense of increased competence or mastery should not be ignored.
Some therapies are geared for this goal almost exclusively, but the
ability to deal with the painful affect without denial and self-
destructive behavior can enhance self-esteem in its own right. In
this context the therapist can also gain increased insight and information about the sources of a child's behavior. As with any treatment
modality, simply giving an intellectual recitation appears meaning-
less. But, dealing with defenses, making cognitive connections, rais-
ing questions about alternative choices for behavior that are available, and gaining environmental reinforcements aimed toward resolution are all valuable. In these cases, the child moves forward in
terms of being able to confront and master the narcissistic hurt
from which he has been running in innumerable ways.

CONCLUSION

It is unfortunate that so many adults with depressive problems
have never received treatment when younger. This is partly the
problem of not recognizing the myriad manifestations of childhood
depression, and then proceeding to do something to remedy or alleviate the problem. For those with severe impairments in their self-
concept, later manifestations appear as a mixture of depressive
affect and character psychopathology which is repetitively acted out
as a solution. Another group of adult depressions is composed of
those who had compulsive personality traits as children. These
traits emerge in the course of development as seen in hard work
and achievement as a means of gaining acceptance by others and

of themselves. As long as opportunity exists to keep performing according to high principles, or to strive for success, the emergence of a clinical depression does not occur. Therefore, for many, the day of reckoning does not occur until childhood has passed as well as several years into adulthood. To work, to succeed, and to avoid reflection on the meaning of such diligence are the triad. When these later fail to conceal the narcissistic hurt, to the surprise of many, the honest, good and dedicated person begins to show manifestations of an overt depression. If we would raise more questions, earlier, about the meaning of duty, compulsivity and ideals, we would be well on our way towards lowering the incidence of depression in human beings.

REFERENCES

1. MALMQUIST, C. P.: Depressions in childhood and adolescence, parts I and II. *New Engl. J. Med.*, 284:887-893, 991-996, 1971.
2. SOLNIT, A. J.: Depression and mourning. *In* S. Arieti (Ed.), *American Handbook of Psychiatry*, 2nd Edition. New York: Basic Books, 1975, pp. 107-115.
3. SANDLER, J. and JOFFE, W. G.: Notes on childhood depression. *Int. J. Psycho-Anal.*, 46:88-96, 1965.
4. MAHLER, M., PINE, F. and BERGMAN, A.: *The Psychological Birth of the Human Infant.* New York: Basic Books, 1975.
5. SALZMAN, L.: *The Obsessive Personality.* New York: Science House, 1968.
6. BIBRING, E.: The mechanism of depression. *In* P. Greenacre (Ed.), *Affective Disorders.* New York: International Universities Press, 1953.
7. MAHLER, M.: On sadness and grief in infancy and childhood: Loss and restoration of the symbiotic love object. *Psychoanal. Stud. Child.*, 16:332-351, 1961.
8. KOHUT, H.: *The Analysis of the Self.* New York: International Universities Press, 1971.
9. BERGIN, A. E. and SUINN, R. M.: Individual psychotherapy and behavior therapy. *Ann. Rev. Psychol.*, 26:509-556, 1975.

13

Psychodynamics of Depression: Implications for Treatment

Robert B. White, M.D.,
Harry K. Davis, M.D., and
William A. Cantrell, M.D

> *"Just as the physician might say that there lives
> perhaps not one single man who is in perfect
> health, so one might say perhaps that there lives
> not one single man who after all is not to some
> extent in despair. . . ."*
>
> KIERKEGAARD

Morbid depression is a psychopathologic condition to which
humans are subject from infancy onward. Spitz (1, 2, 3) was
among the first investigators to describe depression in early infancy, and noted that it is a response to physical or emotional
separation from the mother, who at that point is the only meaningful object of the baby's emotional needs. The child's sense of
security and well-being depends almost entirely on her physical
presence and on her emotional capacity to relate to her baby with
what Erikson (4) has called "mutuality." Erikson has also found
that the quality of the mother-infant relationship will largely de-

termine the baby's future emotional health or vulnerability to depressive and other emotional disorders.

Depressive states remarkably similar to those seen in human infants can be produced experimentally in primates by the separation of the infant monkey from its mother or other monkeys to which it has become emotionally attached. There is also abundant data from experiments on monkeys to show that separation early in life from the mother (or other emotionally important monkeys) for one or two periods as short as six days each will produce a later increased vulnerability to react with severe depression when the monkey is separated in adulthood from familiar surroundings and familiar fellow monkeys. A similar increase in vulnerability to emotional loss in adulthood has been demonstrated in people who suffered loss of one or both parents early in life.

There is considerable support (5-16) for the proposition that stressful experiences, especially experiences of loss, are significant factors in the etiology of depressive disorders of either neurotic or psychotic degree. The basic premise of this paper is that loss (real, symbolic, or fantasied) is a necessary condition for the occurrences of most depressive illnesses.

As Gaylin (17, pp. 390, 391) has noted, "What is important to realize is that depression can be precipitated by the loss or removal of anything that the individual over-values in terms of his security. To the extent that one's sense of well-being, safety, or security is dependent on love, money, social position, power, drugs or obsessional defenses—to that extent one will be threatened by its loss." He goes on to note that when a person loses his crucially important sources of security, he will develop a depressed condition characterized by a sense of helplessness and hopelessness. It is this affective state which typifies depressive illness. The importance of the state of helplessness and hopelessness in the etiology of depressions was first emphasized by Bibring (18) and has been elaborated on by Engel (19), Beck (11), Schmale (20), Schmale and Engel (21) and others.

Gaylin comments further: "When the adult gives up hope in his ability to cope and sees himself incapable of either fleeing or

fighting, he is 'reduced' to a state of depression. This very reduction, with its parallel to the helplessness of infancy, becomes, ironi-
cally, one last unconscious cry for help, a plea for a solution to
the problem of survival via dependency. The very stripping of one's
defenses becomes a form of defensive maneuver." Safirstein and
Kaufman (12) have made this same point in another way. They
state: "It is not so important to ask *who* was lost as *what* was lost.
The answer to the question is: tell me what the (depressed) patient
idealizes in himself and others and I will tell you what he has
lost."

The combination of the effect of early childhood loss, primal
parathymia, as Abraham (22) termed it, and recent loss in adulthood is of special importance in the etiology of severe depressive
illnesses, as has been illustrated by numerous studies beginning in
1917 with Freud's seminal paper (23), "Mourning and Melancholia." This has been demonstrated with special clarity by Levi
et al. (24) and by the systematic study by Leff, Roatch, and
Bunney (25). On the other hand Fieve (26), Mendelson (27),
Munro (28, 29), Woodruff, Goodwin, and Guze (30), Winokur
and Pitts (31), and others have presented data which suggest that
depressive disorders often occur without any significant relationship to stressful life events, including events involving loss. How
can these seemingly contradictory findings be explained?

Why Experiences of Loss Are Frequently Overlooked in the History of Depressed Patients

Leff, Roatch, and Bunney (25) help us to understand some of the
reasons for these contradictory findings. They conducted an intensive
study of 40 hospitalized severely depressed patients, including
13 who initially seemed to fulfill completely the usual criteria
for the diagnosis of endogenous depression. In the early phase of
hospitalization, historical data were gathered from these patients and
their families in the manner characteristic of any first-rate psychiatric hospital. Data obtained from both the patient and the members
of his family in this early phase of hospitalization failed to reveal

any stressful life events which could reasonably be considered as causative, or even as precipitating events in the onset of these "endogenous" depressions. In short, a good "routine" history such as any conscientious psychiatrist would obtain in the first few days or weeks of contact with his patient did not uncover significant events of loss in childhood or in the period just prior to the onset of these "endogenous" depressions.

In most studies on the treatment of depressed patients, especially studies of drug or somatic therapy, systematic efforts to gather history would ordinarily stop at this point, that is, after several initial interviews with the patient and members of his family. From the data gathered in this manner, the obvious conclusion would be that the illnesses suffered by patients such as the 13 studied by Leff et al. are truly endogenous in origin, and stressful life events played no significant role in their etiology. However Leff et al. did not stop their search for stressful life events at the end of the first week or so of contact with their patients. Their patients received an average of 60 semi-weekly hour-long psychotherapeutic interviews. The members of the patient's family were also interviewed weekly.

After some weeks or months of continued investigation, additional information was elicited from these "endogenously" depressed patients. This additional information showed that all had suffered severe and clear-cut stressful life events in the year prior to the onset of depressive symptoms. These stressful events tended to cluster in the month immediately preceding the first symptoms. Furthermore, these events involved significant loss of some type. Although the authors do not emphasize that loss characterized the stressful life events in these patients, the descriptions they give make clear that they were events involving loss. For example, one female patient found that her boyfriend was going to marry someone else within a few weeks; a male patient who very much wanted children learned that his marriage was barren because of his low sperm count; another suffered the loss of a close family member by death.

The following case described by Leff et al. (which they indicate was typical of all 13 of their patients with "endogenous" depression) illustrates another issue which we wish to emphasize and about which we will make additional comments later in this paper, namely, the frequency with which the depressed patient and his family collude to withhold crucially significant historical data.

A 23-year-old housewife and mother of a one-year-old child was admitted in a delusional, psychotic state of depression which had culminated in a near-successful suicide attempt with barbiturates. After three interviews the patient continued to insist that she had no idea what might have caused her illness. In initial interviews the husband also denied knowledge of any event that might have depressed his wife, as did the patient's mother. Over a period of three months the patient was seen in psychotherapy three times weekly and the husband was seen weekly. The information obtained in the course of these interviews put a whole new face on the patient's difficulty, and revealed that she had suffered numerous stressful events during her life, events which would probably have depressed anyone under similar circumstances.

The patient was an illegitimate child, and throughout the patient's childhood and adolescence her mother had been sexually promiscuous. Early in life the patient vowed she would never be like her mother. In college the patient fell in love, and during a period when her fiancé was expressing uncertainty about their plans for marriage, she engaged for the first time in intercourse and became pregnant. She experienced great shame at this event because it made her feel that she was like her promiscuous mother. She dropped out of college and married her fiancé. Leaving college and giving up her plan to become a social worker left her angry at the pregnancy which resulted in a child who died soon after birth. The patient considered this to be punishment for her misdeeds. She became withdrawn and irritable as tensions grew in the marriage, and divorce was discussed. However, she soon became pregnant again. After the birth of the second child, the patient's mother became very friendly. Finally the mother came to live with the patient, but they immediately began to quarrel. During one of these fights the patient called her mother a prostitute, and said she never wanted to see her again, dead or alive. Furthermore, she forbade her mother to see the grandchild. Following this fight, the patient became unable to sleep because of worry about

her outburst toward her mother; the mother and other relatives became distant and unfriendly toward the patient.
Tensions grew in the marriage, and quarrels increased between the patient and her husband. Finally a violent quarrel
occurred which lasted past midnight. In the course of this late
night quarrel the husband slapped the patient and said, "You're
a whore, just like your mother." When he awoke the next
morning, his wife was gone. Later that day she was found in
her mother's house in a near fatal coma from an overdose of
barbiturates.

Our own clinical experience (32, 33, 34) strongly supports the
conclusions reached by Leff et al. which were based on data-gathering
techniques similar to those used in our own clinical practices. However this type of clinical data is difficult to quantify, and may be
regarded by many as being insufficiently objective.

From our experience, and from the literature, we have extracted
six factors which help to explain why a number of studies have
failed to note the relationship of life events involving loss to the
onset of depressive disorders, especially depressions which have
symptoms characteristic of the so-called "endogenous" depressive
illnesses.

1. Only an experienced and skilled clinician who repeatedly interviews the depressed patient in depth and over a period of several
days or, in some instances, over a period of weeks or months is
likely to learn of the occurrence of painful losses. To learn of the
losses, the physician must provide the support and emotional
climate in which the patient can resolve his conflicts over the
losses and lessen his defenses against grief to a degree which allows
him to become consciously aware of the loss (and/or the painful
emotional impact of the loss). Only then can the patient gain the
courage to face the reality of his losses.

2. Many psychiatrists underestimate the significance of symbolic
and fantasied losses, and attach importance only to those losses
which are both real and serious, such as the death of a loved one.
The confusion which Kraepelin (35, pp. 179-181) displayed on this

score exemplifies the point. In order to demonstrate the relative unimportance of psychogenic factors in the etiology of depressive psychoses, Kraepelin cited the instance of a woman who had three attacks of depressive illness: the first began after the death of her husband; the second after the death of her pet dog; the third after the death of her pet dove.

3. The patient and the members of his family usually have a strong tendency to avoid volunteering information about the losses that have occurred. They often actively collude to deny that such losses have happened, and resist in various ways the efforts of the psychiatrist to elicit information about them. The patient resists acknowledging the losses because they are exquisitely painful to him, or because his own immature behavior has helped to bring them about. People who develop depressive disorders often have an inordinate need for support and approval from others, and tend to deny or repress characteristics in themselves which put them in an unfavorable light; at least they do so until they decompensate into depressive self-accusations. The family members of depressed patients often resist revealing stressful events which put them in a bad light, as exemplified by the husband cited earlier who slapped his wife and called her a whore, thereby precipitating her near-fatal suicide attempt. Consequently, if the physician does not search actively and skillfully for the presence of loss, the patient and his family may avoid the topic altogether.

4. Those therapists who are dedicated to the proposition that "endogenous" depressive disorders are biochemical disorders which are unrelated to life events may not be attuned to the significance of stressful life events, and consequently may not make active inquiries about them.

5. The severely depressed patient suffers a major degree of ego disorganization. He regresses and uses primitive defenses such as denial, projection, turning against the self, and identification. His depressed mood makes it hard for him to mobilize his energy to talk about anything. Both his depressed mood and his disorganized

ego functions make it difficult for him to communicate and until his depression begins to improve he may be unable to provide important historical data, as Davis et al. (32, 33), Leff et al. (25), Paykel (15), and others have noted.

6. The psychiatrist may unconsciously avoid discussing the patient's losses because this topic is too painful to him. If the psychiatrist has been unduly sensitized by traumatic losses in his own formative years, he may regularly avoid exploring in depth the topic of losses when he gathers historical data from his patient. Any psychiatrist is prone to avoid this topic when he is in a period of stress in his own life, especially stress involving loss which induces a depressive mood.

On the Importance of Distinguishing Various Types of Loss

As indicated earlier, it is our basic proposition that events of loss are a necessary, usually major cause of the vast majority of clinically apparent depressive illnesses, whether neurotic or psychotic in degree. The experience of loss may be an obvious recent loss, as in the instance of grief (36-39). Or it may be a past loss suffered in infancy or childhood (5, 8, 9, 40, 41). Usually it is a combination of past childhood losses and recent losses in adulthood, as Levi et al. (24) have found. Furthermore, to make the matter more complex, the loss in adulthood may be *real, symbolic, fantasied,* or any combination of these, as White and Gilliland (34) have described.

The types of loss in adulthood which are of greatest clinical importance as etiologic factors in depressive illnesses include the following:

1. Loss of a relationship with an emotionally important person because of death, divorce, the waning of affection, geographical separation, and the like.

2. Loss of health, important body functions, physical attractiveness, or physical or mental capacities due to disease, injury, or

aging—in short, some loss of an acceptable self-image or body image.

3. Loss of status or prestige (that is, loss of esteem in the eyes of others).

4. Loss of self-esteem (that is, loss of esteem in one's own eyes).

5. Loss of self-confidence, that is, loss of an adequate sense of competence, as White (42) has termed it.

6. Loss of security such as occupational, financial, social, or cultural.

7. Loss of a fantasy or, more precisely, the loss of hope of fulfilling an important fantasy, especially a fantasy which idealizes one's self or some important person in one's life.

8. Loss of something or someone of great symbolic value, usually referred to as a symbolic loss.

The first six of these categories of loss are easily understood and involve losses that are obvious and real. Category 7, loss of hope of fulfillment of an important fantasy, usually accompanies a real loss but may be more devastating than the real loss itself. The case of a ski instructor who sustained a fracture of his leg which was so severe as to prevent him from jumping in Olympic competition illustrates a devastating loss of a fantasy which accompanies a moderate real loss. Although his fracture would not prevent him from being a ski instructor in the future, it did end his hope of realizing the fantasy of winning a gold medal in the Olympics. This secret fantasy had been an important sustaining factor in the young man's psychological integration for some years. Although his injury was not serious by ordinary standards, and did not impose any major real loss, it produced a serious depressive illness because it destroyed the hope of attaining an important fantasy.

Category 8, symbolic loss, is exemplified by the case of a 49-year-old sports car enthusiast. This man had for years been a successful competitor in sports car rallies, and regularly won many events. He largely attributed his success to the outstanding performance of his crimson Ferrari. Despite the fact that his Ferrari was fully insured, he became significantly depressed when it was destroyed by fire. He felt there could never be another Ferrari such as the one he had lost. Obviously the Ferrari was an important symbol of some things he valued highly and was desperately afraid of losing—youth, agility, physical attractiveness, and sexual potency, to name a few.

Some people who have suffered severe loss in early childhood are sensitized to loss, and become especially prone in later life to react to seemingly trivial symbolic losses with extreme depression. When such an apparently insignificant loss in adulthood is a suitable symbolic representation for a repressed and long forgotten childhood loss, it then may revive all of the despair and depression associated with the earlier trauma. As a consequence, a severe depressive illness may occur which seems out of all proportion to the recent loss. However, as Zetzel (43) has noted, failure to master childhood loss rather than the occurrence of childhood loss may be the major factor in the etiology of later depressions. She notes, and we agree, experiencing and mastering loss are essential for adequate personality development. In other words, loss promotes development under certain circumstances and must not be considered to be an invariably noxious experience.

In summary, losses which evoke depression may be *real, symbolic,* or *fantasied*. Most commonly losses which are sufficiently traumatic to produce a discernible degree of depression involve all or some combination of these three types of loss. As Marris (44) has recently noted, any change in one's life situation produces a loss of the status quo and a grief-like longing for the way things used to be. Holmes and Rahe (45) were the first investigators who systematically studied the stress which life events impose on people. They have consistently found that the most stressful life events are those which involve loss.

THE AFFECT OF DEPRESSION AS A RESPONSE TO LOSS

In this section we shall discuss some studies of human and primate infants which suggest that the affect of depression (and its behavioral and physiological concomitants) is an innate response in the very young to loss of contact with the mother. The adaptive and survival value of such an innate response is obvious, as Zetzel (43), Bowlby (8, 9) and Klerman (13) have noted. Bowlby (5, 6, 8, 9) and Robertson (46) describe three phases in the response of the small child (between the ages of approximately six and 36 months) to physical separation from the mother.

1. *The phase of protest.* This phase involves weeping, wailing, and anxious, agitated, angry searching or calling for the mother. Anger is prominent, and the child may turn this upon himself in such activities as head banging, or he may turn it toward others in temper outbursts. He looks eagerly toward any sight or sound which suggests that his mother might be returning. This phase may last hours or days, rarely longer than a week. This is, of course, very reminiscent of the first phase of grief in the adult, as described by Parkes (38) and others. After some hours or days of this painful, agitated stage of protest, the child enters the second stage, that of despair.

2. *The stage of despair.* This stage may last days or weeks and is characterized by symptoms which are very similar to those exhibited by adults in the second stage of grief, as Heinicke and Westheimer (47) have noted. The child ceases his agitated protesting behavior and becomes quieter and withdrawn. He now looks and acts dejected, depressed, and despairing. He eats poorly, often loses weight, and has little interest in toys or people. When his mother returns, this disturbance subsides. If she does not, this depressed state often changes into the third stage of detachment.

3. *The stage of detachment.* The severity and length of this stage depend on a variety of factors, most important of which is the length of time the mother is absent, although other factors are also of significance. However, beyond a certain time, return of the mother often fails to reverse the child's detachment. Spitz (3) suggests that approximately three months is the critical period of separation, and that beyond that period the child may become in-

creasingly impaired in his ability to form an emotionally close or meaningful, lasting relationship with his mother or anyone else. However, in a given instance, how long is too long for the mother to be absent is variable, and depends on a number of factors such as the child's inborn temperament, the adequacy of the relationship to the mother prior to the separation, the preceding emotional climate in the family, the child's age at the time the separation occurs, the availability of an adequate substitute mothering person, and so on. Once he has entered this phase of detachment, the child shows no joy when reunited with his mother, and for hours, days, or longer he will act as if she were no more important than anyone else. Once the stage of detachment has begun, the child no longer appears sad or depressed. On the surface he may seem to have become adjusted to the separation from the mother. But such a child has not lost his basic need for his mother. Out of necessity he has only apparently relinquished not only his intense emotional investment of his mother, but of people generally. His seemingly improved behavior is not evidence of a healthier mental state; on the contrary, it is a symptom of his despair and loss of hope of ever being able to form a sustaining emotional attachment with anyone. Bowlby's description of the infant's response to loss constitutes what we have earlier referred to as the sensitizing experiences of childhood which create vulnerability to later depressive illness.

EXPERIMENTAL AND CLINICAL STUDIES OF LOSS IN CHILDREN

Numerous studies of the effect of separation in early childhood make clear the extreme importance of loss in the first few years of life (47-51). Ainsworth's unpublished study cited by Bowlby (9, p. 52) is especially instructive. Normal infants were subjected at the age of 12 months to experimental separation from the mother for six minutes—two periods of three minutes each. The experiment was conducted in a bland, non-threatening atmosphere. All of the infants exhibited various degrees of distress which quickly abated after reunion with the mother. However, when the experiment was repeated two weeks later, the infants were significantly more distressed by the mother's brief absences on this second occasion than they had been on the first occasion. Obviously, the six minutes of separation from the mother two weeks earlier had made the children more vulnerable to loss of contact with her than they had originally been. They had developed a minor but detectable sensitization to loss.

If six minutes of separation from the mother affects a 12-month-old infant so profoundly that it can produce symptoms of distress two weeks later, it is not difficult to imagine the greater degree of vulnerability to loss which may be produced by repeated or more prolonged separation from the mother. Winnicott (40) has described one such instance in the case of a little boy separated from his mother for six weeks when he was 18 months old. The separation was due to an illness in the mother. At age 11 years he witnessed his father's accidental death from drowning. This previously normal youngster developed a near psychotic depressive reaction some months after the father's death. Psychoanalytically oriented treatment demonstrated that the boy's extreme response to the father's death was a result of his special sensitivity to loss. This special sensitivity to loss was in large measure a consequence of the separation from his mother when he was 18 months old. This type of gross disruption of the relation between child and parent produces obvious disturbances in the development of the child. But chronic, more subtle disturbances in what Erikson has termed mutuality in the parent-child interaction may be of equal or greater clinical significance than these more circumscribed, dramatic events of loss. Ainsworth, Bell, and Stayton (52) have provided persuasive studies which demonstrate the importance of the subtle and more common aspects of the mother-infant interactions, a study worthy of attention of all psychiatrists.

Loss in the Etiology of Experimentally Induced Depressions in Primates

The profound long-term impact on various non-human primates of loss of contact with the mother or other important sources of security has been experimentally demonstrated by Harlow (53), and Harlow and Suomi (54), as well as by Kaufman (55), Spencer-Booth and Hinde (56), and others. For our purposes, the most instructive of these various experiments is the one performed by Spencer-Booth and Hinde on rhesus monkeys at the age of approximately eight months. The monkeys were separated from their mothers for either one or two periods of six days each. During the separation the babies demonstrated the phases of protest and despair similar to that shown by human infants from the age of about six to 36 months under similar circumstances. All of the baby monkeys tended to cling more or to stay closer to their mothers for up to three months after reunion, as compared to controls. Even more interesting was the long-range effect of such brief separations. At the age of 12 months and at the age of 30 months, two years after the brief separation, the experimental monkeys continued to show a markedly greater degree of needful attachment to their mothers than did controls. In addition, they still showed some of the behavioral manifestations of the depression which were grossly obvious during the period of experimental separation. The twice-separated monkeys showed more marked effects than the monkeys separated only once. Similar results were noted by McKinney, Suomi, and Harlow (57) in a series of somewhat different experiments. They showed that repeated short-term separations of infant rhesus monkeys from either the mother or age mates to whom the babies had become attached produced "a striking arrest of social development. . . ." They comment: "By the techniques of repetitive short-term separations, we have produced monkeys 9 months old that behaved like monkeys 3 months old or younger. . . ."

SUMMARY OF CONCLUSIONS

We wish now to review some of the clinical conclusions that we have reached from the data presented thus far:

1. The affect of depression derives from the biologically innate responses of the human infant to the loss of the physical and/or emotional contact with the mother in the age period of approximately

six months to 36 months, a period during which the mother is the child's primary, perhaps sole, source of security. It seems probable that such childhood experiences of loss are significant in the etiology of depressive illnesses.

2. Loss of contact with the mother in infancy and early childhood may result from either the physical absence of the mother or her emotional absence (that is, her lack of adequate affective responsiveness to the infant). Either type of loss disrupts the normal development of the child and creates a greater than ordinary vulnerability later in life to loss of people, capacities, possessions, or circumstances which provide security. This vulnerability stemming from loss during infancy sensitizes the individual to later loss in childhood, adolescence, or adulthood.

3. Numerous studies (24, 58, 59, 60) demonstrate the relationship between loss of a parent in childhood and the increased incidence and severity of depressive illness in adulthood. Early parental loss sensitizes the person to separation from whatever his security depends upon. Separation from sources of security are inevitable in adulthood. Such separations may lead to severe affective illness in people who are sensitized by early loss or who are constitutionally predisposed.

4. Depression is a response to the loss (or the threat of loss) of someone, something, or some physical or psychological function which is an important source of security and satisfaction.

5. The loss which evokes the affect of depression may be *real, fantasied,* or *symbolic.*

THE CONTINUUM OF THE DEPRESSIVE DISEASES

Kraepelin and the descriptive psychiatrists of the nineteenth and early twentieth century attempted to separate the various categories of mental disorders into discrete entities—in particular, the psychoses were considered qualitatively different from the neuroses and other non-psychotic syndromes. The heritage of Kraepelin is clearly visible in the recent efforts to separate the various types of depressive illnesses into separate categories such as endogenous or exogenous; primary or secondary; neurotic or psychotic; bipolar or unipolar; major or minor, and so on. In the first part of this century Freud and Adolph Meyer were, of course, among the early opponents of this division of psychological disorders into neatly compartmentalized entities. In the last quarter of this century we wish to join them in this opposition.

With regard to the various types of depressive illnesses, we question the validity of making a sharp dichotomy between neurotic disturbances and psychotic disturbances. We concur with investigators such as Beck, Bibring, and others who question whether depressive illnesses of various types and degrees of severity are fundamentally different disorders or whether they differ primarily only in degree. We must note, however, that so distinguished a psychoanalytic investigator of depressive illnesses as Edith Jacobson (61) feels that there are qualitative differences, not just quantitative differences, between the neurotic and psychotic depressive illnesses, the latter being in her view largely the consequence of constitutional factors.

It is our view that the various depressive states can be arranged along a continuum from a normal period of self-limiting low mood at one end to psychotic suicidal hopelessness at the other. This is not to say that we disclaim the significance of possible genetic predispositions or of neurophysiologic factors in the etiology of depressive illnesses. Rather it indicates that we consider emotional loss as a necessary and major factor in causing most depressive illnesses.

Recently, there has been a remarkable swing back toward Kraepelin-like efforts to place the various types of depressive syndromes which differ from one another in some aspect of their phenomenology or family history into different diagnostic pigeonholes. This return to a penchant for classes, subclasses, and sub-subclasses of depressive illnesses very probably reflects the upsurge in interest in the biological-biochemical-genetic aspects of the affective disorders—an upsurge that is partly a consequence of the dramatic breakthrough in the chemotherapy of the affective disorders and partly a result of the tremendous advances in knowledge and technology in the fields of neurophysiology, neuropharmacology, neurochemistry, and genetics. In addition, the remarkable capacity of the computer to analyze large amounts of statistical data has also contributed to this renewed preoccupation with nosology—a preoccupation which has helped to clarify our thinking about mental illness, as the research of Overall (62), Overall, Hollister, Johnson et al. (63) and others has shown.

Nonetheless, it seems to us that the trend toward making mathematical precision the only badge of scientific respectability has led to an unfortunate side effect—a tendency to lose sight of the psychiatric patient as a person with human feelings, relationships, and needs which are not basically different from our own. Karl Menninger (64) has warned of the dangers of undue emphasis on nosology in a manner with which we are very much in agreement.

The patient-physician relationship is a crucial variable in the treatment of depressive conditions or of any other illnesses. It may completely override the pharmacological effect of drugs. For example, Stewart Wolf (65, pp. 156-159) has shown that the influence of the physician on his patient may totally reverse the effect of a large dose of ipecac, causing it to alleviate rather than produce nausea and vomiting. The subtleties of the influence of the doctor on his patient cannot as yet be captured on a rating scale, measured by the computer analysis of data from a double blind study, or certified as being significant by the chi square test.

Controversies Regarding the Treatment of the Depressive Disorders

The lack of unanimity regarding the most effective modes of treatment for depressive illnesses is dramatically exemplified in the seemingly irreconcilable differences among various investigators. For example, Folsom (66) has reported that his psychotherapeutic approach is more effective than either drugs or electroshock therapy in the treatment of depressions, regardless of the type or severity of the depression. Beck (67) has reported that his psychotherapeutic method is as effective as amitriptyline, and in some respects superior. On the other hand, Fieve (26), Paykel et al. (68), Lipton et al. (69) and others present data which suggest that drug or shock therapy is the most effective treatment modality. Fieve as well as Lipton et al. note that a significant number of psychiatrists consider the psychotherapeutic treatment of depressive conditions to be ineffectual or even harmful.

There are ample data to show that electroshock therapy or antidepressant medications alone result in remission of the severe depressive syndromes in about eighty percent of the cases. There is also evidence that depressed patients tend to relapse frequently when they are treated by drug or shock therapy unaccompanied by competent psychotherapy. John Davis (70) reviewed six studies on the effectiveness of electroshock therapy, studies which he considered to be the best available. From this review he concluded that about 10 percent of patients treated with electroshock therapy relapse each month following the use of EST, that 45 percent of the patients in these six studies had relapsed in six months, and 70 percent within one year after treatment was concluded. He states that this relapse rate is essentially identical to that seen when antidepressant drugs or lithium carbonate are discontinued. Lehmann (71) has noted that inadequate response to drug treatment is often related to psychological stress, including stress from disturbing childhood experiences. In cases which are resistant to drug therapy, as well as those which initially respond to drugs but then relapse, Lehmann feels that psychotherapy improves the prognosis. In some reactive depressions he feels that psychotherapy is an essential component of effective treatment.

Having laid forth the confusing and contradictory views in the literature regarding the treatment of depressive illnesses, we wish now to set forth some therapeutic principles which, in our experience, have been helpful, and which we feel offer a rational guide to treatment.

THERAPEUTIC PRINCIPLES FOR THE MANAGEMENT
OF DEPRESSIVE ILLNESSES

1. An understanding of the concept that all depressive states are on a continuum is crucial to the effective treatment of the depressed patient. In addition to the degree of severity, the patient's place on the continuum is determined by other factors. One of these factors which we wish to single out for special emphasis is the nature and severity of early childhood trauma, especially childhood experiences of loss. All individuals suffer greater or lesser experiences of loss in childhood. These experiences largely determine how vulnerable he will be to experiences of loss in adulthood and consequently whether or not he will react to adult losses with depression which may be out of keeping with the severity of those losses.

There are predisposing, sensitizing, and precipitating determinants of depressive disorders. Predisposing determinants may include inborn biochemical errors, physiologic idiosyncracies, or other as yet undiscovered constitutional impairments or vulnerabilities of the organism. Nevertheless, the role of sensitizing and precipitating experiential factors is not lessened by the possible presence of innate biological predispositions. In fact, it can be argued that it is all the more important to be especially attentive to these experiential variables in those who are at greater risk because of biologic vulnerability, as Stainbrook (72) has noted.

2. We wish furthermore to emphasize that early childhood loss is very likely the cause of another factor in the etiology of depression, namely the patient's ambivalence in his relationship with people who are emotionally important to him. When the child loses a parent whom he loves and desperately needs, he invariably reacts with both sadness and anger, as Bowlby (5, 8, 9) has so clearly demonstrated. That is, the very nature of childhood loss is such as to create intense ambivalence. When adult relations retain intense ambivalence because of traumatic childhood losses, loss in adulthood of an emotionally important person will inevitably evoke both longing for and anger at the person who is lost. White and Gilliland

(34, p. 142) have described in detail a case which emphasizes this point.

3. A third principle is that the type of psychotherapy utilized in a given case depends on where that particular patient lies on the continuum of affective illness.

4. A fourth important principle in the management of the depressed patient is the necessity to help him experience and come to terms with his loss and his ambivalent feelings about this loss—that is, to complete his grief. Even though the technique of psychotherapy must be individualized according to the particular needs of each patient, the basic goal of treatment is the same in all depressed patients. *That basic goal is to rediscover and resolve the core of grief, which in our experience inevitably underlies the symptom of depression.* Just as anxiety evoked by a seemingly innocuous external stimulus becomes readily understandable when its *meaning* to the phobic patient is uncovered, so can the depressed person's hopelessness and despair be shown to have meaning, although the meaning may be obscure because the despair is overdetermined and also disguised by the use of various mechanisms of defense such as repression, denial, displacement, and turning against the self.

With these principles in mind, let us now turn to a discussion of therapeutic procedures.

THERAPEUTIC PROCEDURES

As indicated previously, the appropriate treatment for a given patient must be determined by his position on the continuum. On one end of the continuum we find the mild, self-limiting depressive mood which occurs in response to some obvious and significant life stress. At the other end we find the delusional, suicidal, psychotic depression which may initially appear to have no precipitating life event at all. Psychotherapy is an important aspect of treatment, no matter where along the continuum a given patient lies. In addition to individual psychotherapy, group psychotherapy, family therapy, and milieu therapy have been helpful in our experience.

The person with a mild period of reactive depression usually does not see a psychiatrist. Having weathered similar unpleasant and depressing situations in the past, he can rely on his sense of competence derived from coping effectively with adversity to maintain a sense of hope that he will successfully master his current depressive mood.

The next point on the continuum is the reactive depression which causes significant subjective distress and mild to moderate impairment of the patient's capacity to engage in productive activities and to relate satisfactorily with other people. When such a state endures for some weeks or months and does not show promise of spontaneous resolution, the afflicted person usually seeks help. By then he begins to have doubts as to whether or not he will ever recover. In short, he begins to lose hope for the future. In these cases a careful history is essential. One must assess in detail the factors in the patient's past, especially events involving loss, which may have made him unduly prone to overreact to current stresses with depressive symptoms. A searching assessment must be made of the patient's current life circumstances and relationships with other people who are significant to him: spouse, colleagues, parents, siblings, and children. Often such a patient is entangled with friends or family members in pathologic relationships which interfere with treatment and perpetuate his depression; on the other hand, healthy and sustaining relationships can be valuable allies in the treatment.

Individual psychotherapy which has as its aim the gradual clarification of the losses and stresses which the patient has sustained, especially the symbolic and fantasied losses, is the major therapeutic modality indicated in this degree of depressive illness. Conjoint therapy with the spouse or family therapy is often useful and may be a crucial treatment modality for the depressed patient who has become entangled in a network of pathologic family relationships. When pathologic relationships perpetuate the patient's depression, drug or somatic treatment will often remain ineffectual except as an adjunct to the skillful use of individual or family psychotherapy which helps the patient disentangle himself from the pathologic family relations, confront his losses, complete his grief over them, and come to terms with the realities of his life.

The next point on the continuum is exemplified by the patient who has a depressive reaction which seriously impairs his sense of hope for the future. This degree of depression is characterized by suicidal inclinations, serious subjective suffering, and obvious impairment of the capacity to enjoy any activity or to participate effectively in work or personal relationships. Whenever the therapist concludes that there is a significant possibility that the patient might abruptly decompensate into suicidal despair, he is obligated to convey his concern to the patient and to make clear that the patient may contact him at any hour of the day or night if despair becomes unbearable. Regarding a further specification of psychotherapeutic techniques, time allows us only to note that in general we subscribe to the procedures outlined by Beck (11), Weigert (73), Jacobson (74) and Mintz (75). Part of the problem of the psychotherapy of such patients is described by Weigert who states, "The psychotherapist cannot passively wait for the development of a transference neurosis and he cannot hide in an unreachable neutrality. He has to be there with his personality fully present." This degree of activity on the part of the psychotherapist poses problems. If he is unduly active in a seductive way, he will of course promote excessive dependency on the part of his patient. On the other hand, if he is unduly distant, aloof, and analytically impersonal, he will be unable to provide his patient with that degree of emotional support which may be crucial in moments of suicidal despair. In short, the therapist must convey to the patient the firm conviction that he is there, is dependable, and intends to do all that he possibly can to help, but that he cannot solve the patient's problems for him. Patients with this degree of illness are on the borderline between those who need to be hospitalized and those who may be handled on an outpatient basis. Treatment with antidepressant drugs (and in some instances, sedatives or tranquilizers) is usually indicated in such patients as an adjunct to psychotherapy. Conjoint marital therapy or family therapy is also frequently indicated. At the very least, detailed information from family members and reasonable willingness on the part of the therapist to maintain contact with them are important.

The final point on the continuum of depressive illnesses is represented by the patient whose capacity to function in life is so impaired that hospitalization is mandatory. The presence of significant suicidal inclinations constitutes an emergency, and immediate hospitalization is necessary. The seriously depressed patient, whether inert and apathetic or agitated and restless, has suffered a serious regression and impairment of the controlling, organizing, directing, and defensive functions of his ego. Because of this profound regression, the extremely depressed person has a severe derangement in his time sense and his time perspective. Like the very small child, he knows only the now, and has no sustaining capacity to recall the past when things were better for him. Furthermore, he has no capacity to envision the future as being different from the intolerable present. Hence, as Sarwer-Foner (76) has noted, severely depressed patients have a particular delusion regarding time. He states that this delusion ". . . consists of the conviction that their depressed state will . . . never end (and) . . . it will last their entire lifetime. . . ."

Because of his loss of ego integration and his incapacity to believe that he can ever feel better, the depressed person cannot be cheered by the reassurance that his illness has a good prognosis. It is crucial for the psychiatrist to provide those controls and functions which the patient's disorganized ego is incapable of performing. As Lesse (77) has termed it, the psychiatrist must provide an "ego transfusion," or what Robert Knight (78) termed an emotional "rescue force," to help the patient's shattered ego to reintegrate.

Although verbal reassurances sound empty and totally implausible to the seriously depressed patient, the psychiatrist can provide the hopeless patient with some sense of security by decisively taking charge and explaining briefly and simply what he is going to do and why he is going to do it. By thus providing an "emotional rescue force," the psychiatrist supplies even a delusionally hopeless patient with a sense that the depth of his despair has been understood. For a time the doctor relieves the patient of the responsibility for exercising control over his own behavior (especially his suicidal urges), planning his own time, or organizing the basic aspects of day to day living.

Such patients should be told something such as, "I realize you can't possibly believe me when I tell you that your despair is the symptom of an illness, and that I feel confident you can recover from that illness and feel hope again. Because everything seems futile and pointless, I am concerned that you might kill yourself in a moment of despair. Consequently, I am going to put you in a hospital where you will have a nurse with you at all times until you begin to feel some hope for the future. The nurse will never be more than a foot or so away from you. This will intrude on your privacy, and you will not like it. But I am going to do all I can to prevent you from harming yourself until you recover from your illness and can decide rationally whether you want to live or die." Of course, an explanation should also be given at an appropriate time as to what drugs will be used, how frequently psychotherapy sessions will be held, what other programs, such as occupational therapy, the patient will participate in, and the like.

In the most extreme cases of depression which show no improvement after hospitalization, psychotherapy, and appropriate drug therapy have been given an adequate trial, electroshock therapy is indicated. The violent and total opposition to electroshock therapy which has been recently voiced by Friedberg (79) and others is as destructive as the too-ready use of electroshock treatment which unfortunately still occurs in some treatment centers. D'Agostino (80) has recently published a moving personal experience which highlights the irrationality in some of the current opposition to electroshock therapy. The rare but at times serious complications of electroshock treatment have been recently described by Roueché (81).

Some Suggestions for the Further Study of Depressive Illnesses

In closing, we wish to emphasize that depressive illnesses are probably true psychosomatic disturbances which result from the interplay of such factors as inborn temperamental-biochemical disorders, birth trauma, traumatic childhood experiences, and stress later in life, especially experiences of loss. This point of view has recently been summarized in great detail by Akiskal and McKinney (82). The combination of biologic predisposition and sensitizing traumatic experiences early in life make some people more vulnerable than others to the effect of emotional loss in adulthood. It seems probable that the emotional stress created by experiences of loss produce significant alterations in brain chemistry, especially in those individuals predisposed by constitution, birth trauma, early sensitizing experiences, or some combination of these factors. Such a combination of factors seems the most likely explanation for severe depressive illnesses, as the effectiveness of lithium carbonate, antidepressant medications, electroshock therapy, and psychotherapy would suggest. To what degree biochemical factors in depressive illnesses represent a physiological concomitant of the psychological state of depressed affect rather than a cause of the depressed mental state remains open to debate.

The study of infants who suffered anoxia at birth has shed some light on one set of biological factors which produce a predisposition to react to life stresses with depression. As Ucko (83) has shown, infants who suffer significant degrees of anoxia at birth, but who have no obvious intellectual or neurological defects, are more sensitive to changes in their environment when they reach age two or three years than are children who were not anoxic at birth. These anoxic children are unduly sensitive to separation from their mother, as compared to normal children. The genetic influences that may be involved in depressive disorders have recently been summarized by Winokur (84, 85), Cadoret (86), and others.

In addition to the long-range effect of perinatal anoxia or other birth injuries and of genetic predisposition, we now know of a variety of psychological stresses in the early years of life which can profoundly disturb both biological and psychological development. For example, we know that certain types of experiences in a disturbed parent-child relationship can alter such basic biologic functions in the child as the excretion of growth-stimulating hormone from the pituitary, as documented in the syndrome of emotional dwarfism. Stoller (87, 88) and others have defined a particular type of disturbed mother-infant relationship in early childhood which produces irreversible disturbances of gender identity and creates the syndrome of transsexualism. These various studies conclusively demonstrate that infants deprived of adequate care in the first few years of life can be permanently and seriously impaired in their psychological and physical development, as Spitz (1) first demonstrated.

These experiences in the first year or two of life which create irreversible reaction patterns and personality traits seem similar to imprinting in lower species. Furthermore, it seems feasible that experiences in early infancy can permanently skew or distort neuro-physiological-hormonal-enzyme systems and produce a physiologic as well as a psychologic vulnerability to stress in later life, a point of view supported by the work of Harlow and Suomi (54), Mc-Kinney et al. (57), Reite, Kaufman, Pauley, et al. (89), and others who have studied experimental depression in monkeys. These studies offer a promising but as yet incompletely explored method for studying the relationship between the psychological and the neurochemical factors in the etiology of depression.

Although moral, legal, and ethical considerations bar similar laboratory experiments on humans, systematic study of the naturally occurring experiment of grief offers a way to evaluate the interplay of biochemical and psychological factors in depressive states in humans. Grief-stricken people usually show many of the psychologic, behavioral, and vegetative disturbances which are characteristic of severely depressed patients. Serial studies of bereaved people from the moment that they learn that a loved one has a fatal illness until the loved one dies and the symptoms of grief have abated might help settle the question of whether the various biochemical alterations reported in depressed patients are the result of depression or its cause. Although such studies raise obvious ethical and humanitarian problems, if properly done they could not only avoid harm to the bereaved subjects but could potentially be of benefit to them. Every person who experiences the harsh pain of grief seeks to find some meaning in that experience. By helping the bereaved put his painful experience to some use which might benefit others, we may not only lessen the pain of his loss but also shed new light on the most frequent of psychiatric syndromes—depression.

REFERENCES

1. SPITZ, R. A.: Hospitalism: An inquiry into the genesis of psychiatric conditions in early childhood. *Psychoanal. Study Child.,* 1:53, 1945.
2. SPITZ, R. A.: Hospitalism: A follow-up report. *Psychoanal. Study Child,* 2:113, 1946a.
3. SPITZ, R. A.: Anaclitic depression. *Psychoanal. Study Child,* 2: 313, 1946b.
4. ERIKSON, E. H.: *Childhood and Society.* New York: Norton, 1950.
5. BOWLBY, J.: Some pathological processes set in train by early mother-child separation. *J. Ment. Sci.,* 99:265, 1953.
6. BOWLBY, J.: Separation anxiety. *Int. J. Psychoanal.,* 41:89, 1960.
7. BOWLBY, J.: Effects on behavior of disruption of an affectional bond. *In* J. M. Thoday and A. S. Parkes (Eds.), *Genetic and Environmental Influences on Behavior.* Edinburgh: Oliver and Boyd, 1968.
8. BOWLBY, J. *Attachment.* (Vol. 1 of *Attachment and Loss.*) New York: Basic Books, 1969.
9. BOWLBY, J. *Separation.* (Vol. 2 of *Attachment and Loss.*) New York: Basic Books, 1973.
10. ARIETI, S.: Affective disorders: Manic-depressive psychosis and psychotic depression. *In* S. Arieti (Ed.), *American Handbook of Psychiatry,* Second Edition. New York: Basic Books, 1974.
11. BECK, A. T.: *Depression: Cause and Treatment.* Philadelphia: University of Pennsylvania Press, 1967.
12. SAFIRSTEIN, S. L. and KAUFMAN, M. R.: The higher they climb the lower they fall. *Can. Psychiat. Assoc. J.* (Special Suppl.), 11:S229, 1966.
13. KLERMAN, G. L.: Overview of depression. In A. M. Freedman, H. I. Kaplan and B. J. Sadock (Eds.), *Comprehensive Textbook of Psychiatry, II.* Baltimore: Williams and Wilkins, 1975.
14. NEMIAH, J. C.: Depressive neurosis. *In* A. M. Freedman, H. I. Kaplan and B. J. Sadock (Eds.), *Comprehensive Textbook of Psychiatry, II.* Baltimore: Williams and Wilkins, 1975.
15. PAYKEL, E. S.: Life events and depression: A controlled study. *Arch. Gen. Psychiat.,* 21:753, 1969.
16. PAYKEL, E. S.: Life events and acute depressions. In J. P. Scott and E. C. Senay (Eds.), *Separation and Depression.* Washington, D. C.: American Association for the Advancement of Science, 1973.

17. GAYLIN, W. (Ed.): *The Meaning of Despair*. New York: Science House, 1968.
18. BIBRING, E.: The mechanism of depression. *In* P. Greenacre (Ed.), *Affective Disorders, Psychoanalytic Contributions to Their Study*. New York: International Universities Press, 1953.
19. ENGEL, G. L.: *Psychological Development in Health and Disease*. Philadelphia: Saunders, 1962.
20. SCHMALE, A. H.: Adaptive role of depression in health and disease. *In* J. P. Scott and E. C. Senay (Eds.), *Separation and Depression*. Washington, D. C.: American Association for the Advancement of Science, 1973.
21. SCHMALE, A. H. and ENGEL, G. L. Conservation-withdrawal in depressive reactions. *In* E. J. Anthony and T. Benedek (Eds.), *Depression and Human Existence*. Boston: Little, Brown, 1975.
22. ABRAHAM, K. (1924): A short study of the development of the libido, viewed in the light of mental disorders. *In* D. Bryan and A. Strachey (Trans.), *Selected Papers of Karl Abraham*. New York: Basic Books, 1954.
23. FREUD, S. (1917): Mourning and melancholia. *Standard Edition*, Vol. 14, 1957.
24. LEVI, L. D., FALES, C. H., STEIN, M., et al. Separation and attempted suicide. *Arch. Gen. Psychiat.*, 15:158, 1966.
25. LEFF, M. J., ROATCH, J. F. and BUNNEY, W. E.: Environmental factors preceding the onset of severe depression. *Psychiatry*, 33:293, 1970.
26. FIEVE, R. R.: *Moodswing: The Third Revolution in Psychiatry*. New York: William Morrow, 1975.
27. MENDELSON, M.: *Psychoanalytic Concepts of Depression*. New York: Halsted Press, 1974.
28. MUNRO, A.: Parental deprivation in depressive patients. *Brit. J. Psychiat.*, 112:443, 1966.
29. MUNRO, A.: Parent-child separation: Is it really a cause of psychiatric illness in adult life? *Arch. Gen. Psychiat.*, 20:598, 1969.
30. WOODRUFF, R. A., GOODWIN, D. W. and GUZE, S. B.: *Psychiatric Diagnosis*. New York: Oxford University Press, 1974.
31. WINOKUR, G. and PITTS, F. N.: Affective disorder: I. Is reactive depression an entity? *J. Nerv. Ment. Dis.*, 138:541, 1964.
32. DAVIS, H. K. and FARLEY, A. J.: Psychodynamics of depressive illness. *Dis. Nerv. Syst.*, 28:105, 1967.
33. DAVIS, H. K. and FRANKLIN, R. W.: Continuing grief as a method of psychotherapy following E.S.T. *Dis. Nerv. Syst.*, 31:626, 1970.
34. WHITE, R. B. and GILLILAND, R. M.: *Elements of Psychopathology: The Mechanisms of Defense*. New York: Grune and Stratton, 1975.
35. KRAEPELIN, E.: *Manic-Depressive Insanity and Paranoia*. R. Barclay (trans.). Edinburgh: Livingstone, 1921.

36. LINDEMAN, E.: Symptomatology and management of acute grief. *Am. J. Psych.*, 101:141, 1944.
37. GORER, G.: *Death, Grief, and Mourning.* Garden City, N. Y.: Doubleday, 1965.
38. PARKES, C. M.: *Bereavement: Studies of Grief in Adult Life.* New York: International Universities Press, 1972.
39. SCHOENBERG, B., GERBER, I., WIENER, A., et al. (Eds.): *Bereavement: Its Psychosocial Aspects.* New York: Columbia University Press, 1975.
40. WINNICOTT, D. W.: A child psychiatry case illustrating delayed reaction to loss. *In* M. Schur (Ed.), *Drives, Affects, Behavior.* New York: International Universities Press, 1965.
41. MAHLER, M.: Notes on the development of basic moods—the depressive affect. *In* R. M. Loewenstein, L. M. Newman, M. Schur and A. J. Solnit (Eds.), *Psychoanalysis—A General Psychology.* New York: International Universities Press, 1966.
42. WHITE, R. W.: Ego and reality in psychoanalytic theory. *Psychol. Issues,* 3:1, 1963.
43. ZETZEL, E. R.: The predisposition to depression. *Can. Psychiat. Assoc. J.* (Special Suppl.), 11:S236, 1966.
44. MARRIS, P.: *Loss and Change.* Garden City, N. Y.: Anchor Press, 1975.
45. HOLMES, T. H. and RAHE, R. H.: The social readjustment rating scale. *J. Psychosom. Res.,* 11:213, 1967.
46. ROBERTSON, J.: Some responses of young children to the loss of maternal care. *Nursing Times,* 49:382, 1953.
47. HEINICKE, C. M. and WESTHEIMER, I. J.: *Brief Separations.* New York: International Universities Press, 1965.
48. BERGMANN, T. and FREUD, A.: *Children in the Hospital.* New York: International Universities Press, 1965.
49. PROVENCE, S. and LIPTON, R. C.: *Infants in Institutions.* New York: International Universities Press, 1962.
50. HEINICKE, C. M.: Some effects of separating two-year-old children from their parents: A comparative study. *Hum. Relat.,* 9:105, 1956.
51. HEINICKE, C. M.: Parental deprivation in early childhood: A predisposition to later depression? *In* J. P. Scott and E. C. Senay (Eds.), *Separation and Depression.* Washington, D. C.: American Association for the Advancement of Science, 1973.
52. AINSWORTH, M. D. S., BELL, S. M. and STAYTON, D. J.: Infant-mother attachment and social development. *In* M. P. M. Richards (Ed.), *The Integration of a Child Into a Social World.* New York: Cambridge University Press, 1974.
53. HARLOW, H. F.: *Learning to Love.* New York: Jason Aronson, 1974.
54. HARLOW, H. F. and SUOMI, S. J.: Induced depression in monkeys. *Behav. Biol.,* 12:273, 1974.
55. KAUFMAN, I. C.: Mother-infant separation in monkeys. *In* J. P.

Scott and E. C. Senay (Eds.), *Separation and Depression.* Washington, D. C.: American Association for the Advancement of Science, 1973.

56. SPENCER-BOOTH, Y. and HINDE, R. A.: Effects of brief separation from mothers during infancy on behavior of rhesus monkeys 6-24 months later. *J. Child Psychol. Psychiat.*, 12:157, 1971.

57. McKINNEY, W. T., SUOMI, S. J. and HARLOW, H. F.: New models of separation and depression in rhesus monkeys. *In* J. P. Scott and E. C. Senay (Eds.), *Separation and Depression.* Washington, D. C.: American Association for the Advancement of Science, 1973.

58. BROWN, F.: Depression and childhood bereavement. *J. Ment. Sci.*, 107:754, 1961.

59. BRUHN, J. G.: Broken homes among attempted suicides and psychiatric out-patients: A comparative study. *J. Ment. Sci.*, 108: 772, 1962.

60. BRUHN, J. G. and McCULLOCH, W.: Parental deprivation among attempted suicides. *Brit. J. Psychiat. Soc. Work*, 6:186, 1962.

61. JACOBSON, E.: *Depression.* New York: International Universities Press, 1971.

62. OVERALL, J. E.: The brief psychiatric rating scale in psychopharmacologic research. *In* R. Pichot and R. Olivier-Martin (Eds.), *Psychological Measurements in Psychopharmacology.* Basel: S. Karger, 1974.

63. OVERALL, J. E., HOLLISTER, L. E., JOHNSON, M., et al.: Nosology of depression and differential response to drugs. *J.A.M.A.*, 195:946, 1966.

64. MENNINGER, K., MAYMAN, M. and PRUYSER, P.: *The Vital Balance.* New York: Viking Press, 1963.

65. WOLF, S. G.: *The Stomach.* New York: Oxford University Press, 1965.

66. FOLSOM, J. C.: The antidepressant regimen. *In* W. E. Fann, A. D. Pokorny, I. Karacan, et al. (Eds.), *Phenomenology and Treatment of Depression.* New York: Spectrum, 1976.

67. BECK, A. T.: New rapid forms of psychotherapy for depressed outpatients. Unpublished paper presented at National Conference on Depressive Disorders, sponsored by The National Association of Mental Health, Arlington, Va., Oct. 23, 1975.

68. PAYKEL, E. S., DIMASCIO, A., HASKELL, D., et al.: Effects of maintenance amitriptyline and psychotherapy on symptoms of depression. *Psychol. Med.*, 5:67, 1975.

69. LIPTON, M. A., ELDRED, S. H., GOTTSCHALK, L. A., et al.: Pharmacotherapy and psychotherapy of depression. *In: Pharmacotherapy and Psychotherapy: Paradoxes, Problems and Progress* (Vol. IX, No. 93). New York: Group for the Advancement of Psychiatry, 1975.

70. DAVIS, J. M.: Which patients need ECT. *Medical World News*, Oct. 27, 1975, pp. 19-29.

71. LEHMANN, H. E.: Somatic treatment methods, complications, failures. This volume, 1977.

72. STAINBROOK, E.: Depression: The psychosocial context. This volume, 1977.

73. WEIGERT, E.: The psychotherapy of the psychoses. *In* A. Burton (Ed.), *Psychotherapy of the Psychoses.* New York: Basic Books, 1961.

74. JACOBSON, E.: The psychoanalytic treatment of depressive patients. *In* E. J. Anthony and T. Benedek (Eds.), *Depression and Human Existence.* Boston: Little, Brown, 1975.

75. MINTZ, R. S.: Basic considerations in the psychotherapy of the depressed suicidal patient. *Amer. J. Psychother.*, 25:56, 1971.

76. SARWER-FONER, G. J.: A psychoanalytic note on a specific delusion of time in psychotic depression. *Can. Psychiat. Assoc. J.* (Special Suppl.), 11:S221, 1966.

77. LESSE, S.: Combined drug and psychotherapy of severely depressed ambulatory patients. *Can. Psychiat. Assoc. J.* (Special Suppl.), 11:S123, 1966.

78. KNIGHT, R. P. (1953): Borderline states. *In* S. C. Miller (Ed.), *Clinician and Therapist: Selected Papers of Robert P. Knight.* New York: Basic Books, 1972.

79. FRIEDBERG, J.: Electroshock therapy: Let's stop blasting the brain. *Psychology Today,* 9:18, 1975.

80. D'AGOSTINO, A. M.: Depression: Schism in contemporary psychiatry. *Am. J. Psychiat.*, 132:629, 1975.

81. ROUECHE, B.: As empty as Eve. *New Yorker*, Sept. 9, 1974, pp. 84-100.

82. AKISKAL, H. S. and McKINNEY, W. T.: Overview of recent research in depression. *Arch. Gen. Psychiat.*, 32:285, 1975.

83. UCKO, L. E.: A comparative study of asphyxiated and non-asphyxiated boys from birth to five years. *Dev. Med. Child Neurol.*, 7:643, 1965.

84. WINOKUR, G.: Genetic aspects of depression. *In* J. P. Scott and E. C. Senay (Eds.), *Separation and Depression.* Washington, D. C.: American Association for the Advancement of Science, 1973.

85. WINOKUR, G.: Heredity in the affective disorders. *In* E. J. Anthony and T. Benedek (Eds.), *Depression and Human Existence.* Boston: Little, Brown, 1975.

86. CADORET, R. J.: Genetics of affective disorders. This volume, 1977.

87. STOLLER, R.: *Sex and Gender.* New York: Science House, 1968.

88. STOLLER, R.: Facts and fancies: An examination of Freud's concept of bisexuality. *In* J. Strouse (Ed.), *Women and Analysis.* New York: Viking, 1974.

89. REITE, M., KAUFMAN, I. C., PAULEY, J. D., et al.: Depression in infant monkeys: Physiological correlates. *Psychosom. Med.*, 36:363, 1974.

Index